ATLAS OF HUMAN ANATOMY

Commissioning Editor: Timothy Horne, Richard Furn
Project Development Manager: Janice Urquhart
Project Manager: Frances Affleck
Design direction: Judith Wright, George Ajayi
Page layout: Jim Farley

ATLAS OF HUMAN ANATOMY

S. JACOB MMBS MS (Anatomy)
Senior Lecturer
Department of Biomedical Science
University of Sheffield;
Formerly Member of the Court of Examiners
Royal College of Surgeons of England

Dissections by
David J. Hinchcliffe

Photography by
Mick A. Turton

Illustrated by
Amanda Williams

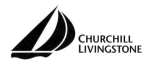
CHURCHILL
LIVINGSTONE

EDINBURGH LONDON NEW YORK PHILADELPHIA ST LOUIS SYDNEY TORONTO 2002

CHURCHILL LIVINGSTONE
An imprint of Harcourt Publishers Limited

Harcourt Publishers Limited 2002

 is a registered trademark of Harcourt Publishers Limited

The right of Sam Jacob to be identified as author of this work has been asserted by him in accordance with the Copyright, Designs and Patents Act 1988

First published 2002

ISBN 0 443 05364 2

British Library Cataloguing in Publication Data
A catalogue record for this book is available from the British Library

Library of Congress Cataloging in Publication Data
A catalog record for this book is available from the Library of Congress

Note
Medical knowledge is constantly changing. As new information becomes available, changes in treatment, procedures, equipment and the use of drugs become necessary. The author and publishers have taken care to ensure that the information given in this text is accurate and up to date. However, readers are strongly advised to confirm that the information, especially with regard to drug usage, complies with the latest legislation and standards of practice.

The
publisher's
policy is to use
paper manufactured
from sustainable forests

Printed in Spain

PREFACE

Human gross anatomy is one of the most important subjects in the study of Medicine and Allied Health Sciences. Dissection of the cadavers is the best means of studying gross anatomy. However, this is often difficult because of limitations of facilities, the short time available in the curriculum and the growing shortage of cadavers for dissection. By using a combination of fully labelled photographs of dissections, radiological anatomy, and drawings, along with a comprehensive descriptive text, this book aims to provide the student with a real understanding of the anatomy of the human body. The *Atlas of Human Anatomy* contains illustrations of surface anatomy, osteology, dissections, radiological, CT and MRI images and line artwork. The background text, concise but comprehensive, describes the most important features of each area with special emphasis on clinical relevance and application. Organised on a regional basis the *Atlas* contains illustrations and descriptions on upper limb, thorax, abdomen and pelvis, vertebral column and spinal cord, lower limb, and head and neck. Each chapter starts with a relevant account of surface anatomy and osteology. Features of anatomy that are of clinical importance are indicated with an 🔦 icon in the margin.

In planning this book I took into account the time constraint affecting most modern anatomy courses as well as the wide variety of teaching methodology used. It is hoped that the book will act as a useful companion for those who learn anatomy by dissection or by using prosections and plastinated specimens. The level of detail contained in it is more than adequate for most undergraduate medical and dental courses. The book is also useful for students of Biological, Biomedical and Allied Health Sciences where human anatomy is part of the curriculum. Surgeons in training can use this for a rapid review of anatomy while preparing for post-graduate examinations.

I would like to express my gratitude to many co-workers and friends who gave me invaluable help and encouragement towards the production of this book. I am greatly indebted to David Hinchcliffe for producing the excellent dissections and to Mick Turton for his exceptional expertise in photography. The *Atlas* would not have been possible without their dedicated efforts and unswerving enthusiasm. Jill Revill, Caroline Couldwell, Andy Fitzgerald and Malcolm Hinchcliffe also deserve credit for facilitating this work. Professor Rachel Koshi and the late Dr Thomas Koshi (Christian Medical College, Vellore) provided many of the radiographs. The MRI and CT scans were obtained from Dr Matthew Bull, Consultant, Northern General Hospital, Sheffield. Emily Evans carried out the dissection of the female pelvis under the supervision of my colleague Geoff Cope. I am grateful to them all. Thanks are also due to Professor Peter Andrews, Chairman of the Department, and Mr Ivan Dart, Laboratory Manager, for the facilities in the department of Biomedical Science, University of Sheffield. Finally my sincere thanks to Janice Urquhart and her production team for the expertise and care with which they made possible the preparation of this *Atlas* and to Timothy Horne and Richard Furn at Harcourt Health Sciences for entrusting me with this project.

Sheffield 2001   S. Jacob

CONTENTS

WHAT IS ANATOMY?

Anatomy is the study of the structure of the body. The word anatomy is derived from the Greek word anat'ome which means to cut up. The Latin equivalent of this is dissecare from which the word dissection is derived. Of all the basic science courses offered to students of medicine, dentistry and allied health sciences there is none more directly related to their professional practice than gross anatomy and its application.

The arrangement of structures in the body is very complex. The first task in the study of anatomy is the visualisation of the different structures, appreciating especially the way they are packaged in the body and their relationship to one another. Study of dissection illustrations along with that of diagnostic images such as plain radiographs, angiograms, CT and MRI scans play a major role in achieving this goal. Surface anatomy is the art of projecting on to the surface the underlying structures. Many definitive elements of the living body can be easily identified on the surface. Ignorance of this part of anatomy will be a serious handicap during the physical examination of a patient.

The main divisions of the body are the head, neck, thorax, abdomen and the upper and lower limbs (Figs 1.1, 1.2). The internal organs are located within the various cavities of the body. The cranial cavity contains the brain and the vertebral canal in the vertebral

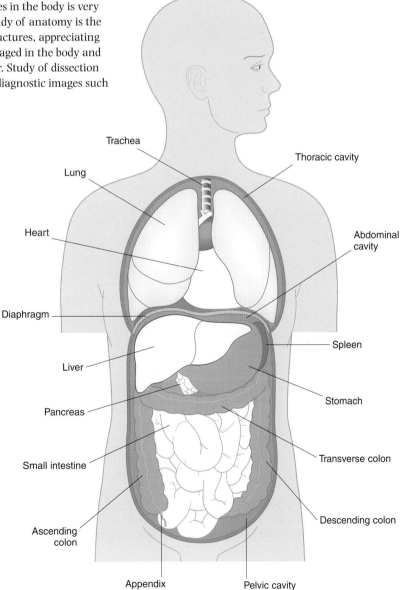

Fig. 1.1 *The internal organs within the various cavities of the body — anterior view*

Trachea

Thoracic cavity

Lung

Heart

Abdominal cavity

Diaphragm

Spleen

Liver

Stomach

Pancreas

Transverse colon

Small intestine

Descending colon

Ascending colon

Appendix

Pelvic cavity

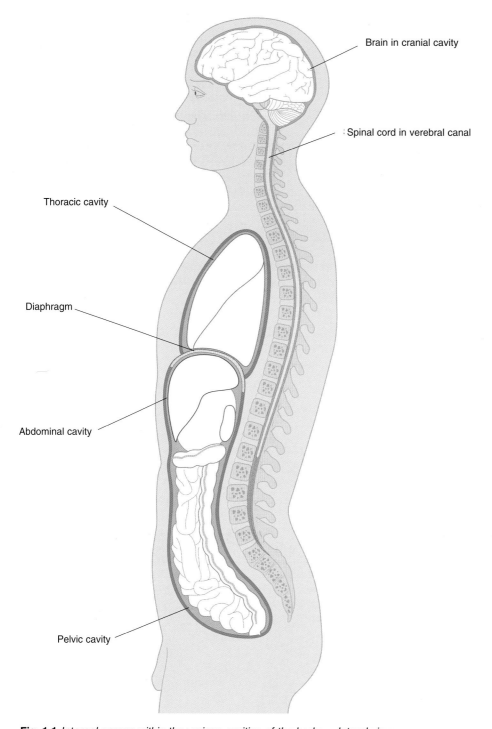

Fig. 1.1 *Internal organs within the various cavities of the body — lateral view*

column contains the spinal cord. The right and left lungs and the heart are in the thoracic cavity. Each lung is surrounded by the pleural cavity and the heart by the pericardial cavity. The thoracic cavity is separated from the abdominal cavity by the dome-shaped diaphragm, which is a sheet of muscle. The abdominal cavity is further divided into the abdominal cavity proper, which contains the liver, stomach, small intestine, parts of the large intestine, pancreas, spleen and kidneys, and the pelvic cavity which has the sigmoid colon, rectum, urinary bladder and parts of the reproductive system.

Anatomy has a highly specialised vocabulary, most of them derived from Greek or Latin. It is the language of medicine. Communications between health professionals can be severely hampered without the accurate use of anatomical nomenclature.

The anatomical position, about which the anatomical relations of structures are described, is that in which the person stands erect, arms by the sides, palms of the hands facing forwards (Fig. 1.3). Structures in front are termed anterior and those behind, posterior. Structures above are superior and those below, inferior. Structures nearer the midline of

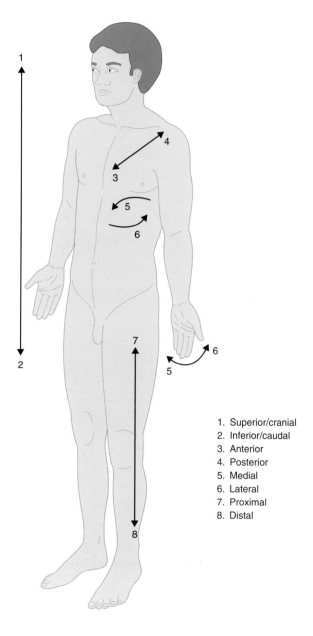

1. Superior/cranial
2. Inferior/caudal
3. Anterior
4. Posterior
5. Medial
6. Lateral
7. Proximal
8. Distal

Fig. 1.3 *Commonly used positional and directional terms when the body is in standard anatomical position.*

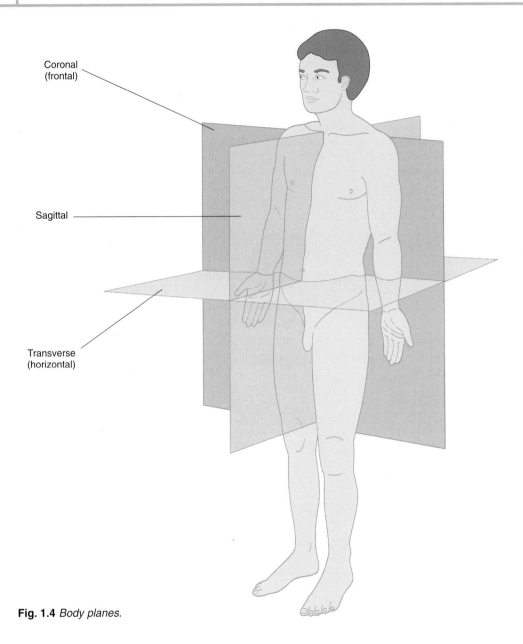

Coronal
(frontal)

Sagittal

Transverse
(horizontal)

Fig. 1.4 *Body planes.*

the body are medial and those away from the midline, lateral. Structures nearer to the surface are superficial and those further from the surface are deep. In the limbs, the term proximal is used to describe structures nearer to the trunk and distal for those away from the trunk. A sagittal plane passes vertically anteroposteriorly through the body and the coronal plane is at right angles to the sagittal plane. A plane that passes at right angles to both the coronal and sagittal plane dividing the body into cross sections is the transverse or horizontal plane (Fig. 1.4).

Movement in the coronal plane away from the midsagittal plane is called abduction, return towards the midsagittal plane is adduction. Bending of any part in the sagittal plane is flexion and straightening is extension. Rotation occurs around a vertical axis. It may be medial rotation, towards the midline, or lateral, away from it.

UPPER LIMB

INTRODUCTION

The human upper limb, which is primarily used for grasping and manipulating objects, consists of the following five regions (Fig. 2.1):

- shoulder
- axilla
- arm
- forearm
- hand.

The shoulder has a wide range of mobility by virtue of the movements of the humerus, the clavicle and the scapula. The axilla or the armpit is the space between the chest wall and the upper part of the arm and contains the principal nerves and vessels. The bone of the arm, the region between the shoulder and the elbow, is the humerus (Fig. 2.2). In the arm the muscles are arranged in two compartments, flexors anteriorly and extensors posteriorly. A similar arrangement is seen in the forearm as well. The forearm is the region between the elbow and the wrist. The radius and the ulna of the forearm articulate with the humerus at the elbow joint and with each other at the superior and inferior radioulnar joints. Pronation and supination to rotate the forearm and hand for grasping and manipulating objects occur at the radioulnar joints; flexion and extension of the forearm take place at the elbow joint.

The wrist containing the carpal bones connects the forearm and hand. The skeleton of the hand is formed by the five metacarpal bones and that of the fingers by the phalanges. The anterior aspect of the hand is the palm of the hand. The hand can act as a tactile organ as the skin of the palm has a rich sensory innervation. The hand is for grasping objects. In the precision grip, as in holding a pen, the thumb is in the opposed position where the pulp of the thumb faces the pulp of the index finger. The thumb is of great functional value in all grips especially in the precision grip. In a power

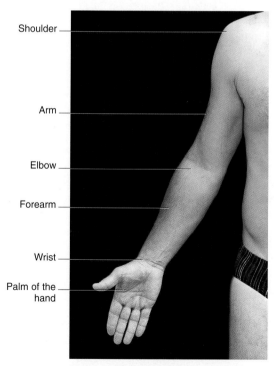

Fig. 2.1 *Regions of the upper limb.*

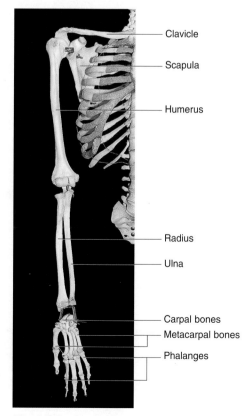

Fig. 2.2 *Bones of the upper limb.*

Flexed fingers

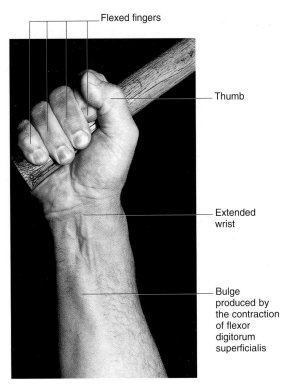

Thumb

Extended wrist

Bulge produced by the contraction of flexor digitorum superficialis

Fig. 2.3 *Power grip.*

grip as in holding a hammer, the wrist is kept extended and the powerful long flexors of the digits contract to make the fingers flex to hold the handle (Fig. 2.3). The thumb reinforces the grip. All grips and manipulations rely on normal mobility of all the fingers. A single immobile finger can make the whole hand clumsy.

SURFACE ANATOMY AND BONES OF THE SHOULDER AND PECTORAL REGIONS

The clavicle which is subcutaneous is palpable throughout and its movements during the movements of the upper limb can be felt by holding it between finger and thumb. The jugular notch (suprasternal notch) is felt between the prominent medial end of the clavicle. The clavicular and sternal heads of the sternocleidomastoid are visible (Fig. 2.4). The pulsation of the subclavian artery is felt on deep palpation against the first rib in the supraclavicular region just lateral to the clavicular head of the muscle. More posteriorly in the root of the neck the upper lateral border of the trapezius is visible. The muscle can be felt contracting by elevating the shoulder against resistance. The pectoralis major, as it bridges across the chest wall and arm, forms the anterior wall of the axilla. Its lower border is the anterior axillary fold. The muscle can be felt contracting when the arm is adducted against resistance. The clavicular and the sternocostal heads of the muscle may be visible in a muscular person. Below and lateral to the pectoralis major the digitations of the serratus anterior may be seen (Fig. 2.4).

The acromion of the scapula (Fig. 2.5) forms the highest bony point of the shoulder region. This point is used to measure the length of the upper limb. The coracoid process of the scapula is felt on deep palpation below the clavicle at its junction between the lateral third and the medial two-thirds. The muscle covering the whole of the shoulder region and giving it its

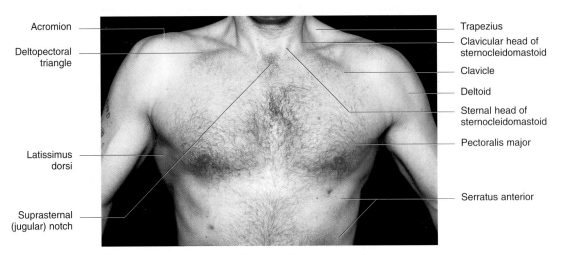

Acromion

Deltopectoral triangle

Latissimus dorsi

Suprasternal (jugular) notch

Trapezius

Clavicular head of sternocleidomastoid

Clavicle

Deltoid

Sternal head of sternocleidomastoid

Pectoralis major

Serratus anterior

Fig. 2.4 *Surface anatomy of the shoulder and pectoral region.*

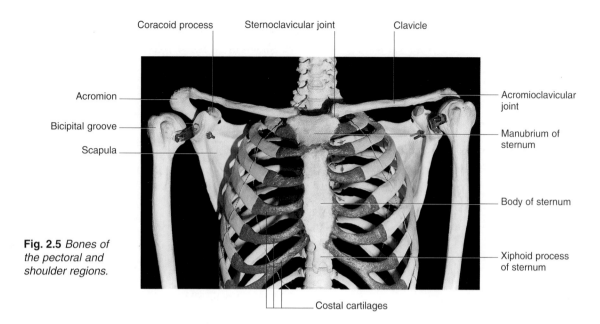

Coracoid process Sternoclavicular joint Clavicle

Acromion

Bicipital groove

Scapula

Acromioclavicular joint

Manubrium of sternum

Body of sternum

Xiphoid process of sternum

Costal cartilages

Fig. 2.5 *Bones of the pectoral and shoulder regions.*

rounded contour is the deltoid. The cephalic vein, a superficial vein of the upper limb, lies subcutaneously in the deltopectoral triangle which is the gap between the deltoid and the pectoralis major.

Pectoralis major (Fig. 2.6)

Origin
Medial third of the clavicle (clavicular head) and the sternum and costal cartilages (sternocostal head).
Insertion
Lateral lip of the bicipital groove on the shaft of the humerus.

Nerve supply
Lateral and medial pectoral nerves.
Action
The sternocostal fibres adduct and medially rotate the humerus at the shoulder joint. The clavicular fibres flex the humerus. If the upper limb is abducted and fixed the muscle can move the ribs and act as an accessory muscle of respiration.
Test
For clavicular head — abduct the arm to 90° and ask the patient to push the arm forward against resistance. For sternocostal head — abduct the arm to 60° and adduct it against resistance. The contracting heads can be seen and felt.

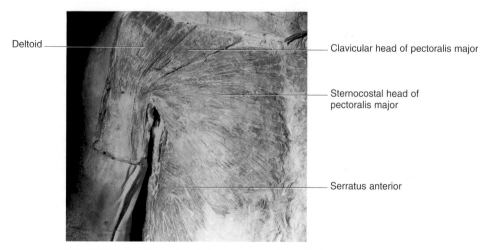

Deltoid

Clavicular head of pectoralis major

Sternocostal head of pectoralis major

Serratus anterior

Fig. 2.6 *Pectoralis major, deltoid and serratus anterior.*

Pectoralis minor (Fig. 2.7)

Origin
Third to fifth (often second to fourth) ribs.
Insertion
The coracoid process of the scapula.
Nerve supply
Medial pectoral nerve.
Action
Draws the scapula (hence the arm) forwards — protraction of shoulder. It can also depress the shoulder.

Serratus anterior

Origin
By a series of digitations from the upper eight ribs.
Insertion
The costal surface of the scapula along its medial border. The muscle forming the medial wall of the axilla lies between the scapula and the chest wall before reaching its insertion.
Nerve supply
Long thoracic nerve from the roots of the brachial plexus (see Fig. 2.32). The nerve lies on the surface of the muscle on the medial wall of the axilla and is vulnerable in surgical procedures such as 'axillary clearance' of lymph nodes for the treatment of carcinoma of the breast. Nerve damage causes winging of the scapula where its medial border is seen more raised and prominent.
Action
Protraction (forward movement) of the scapula as in pushing, punching and fencing.

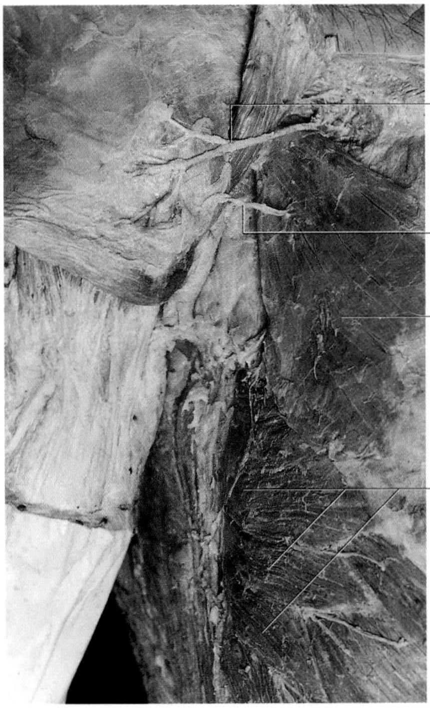

THE SKELETON VIEWED FROM THE BACK (Fig. 2.8)

The most prominent point in the midline on the occipital bone is the external occipital protuberance from which the superior nuchal line, a transverse ridge, extends laterally. The vertebral column consists of seven cervical, twelve thoracic and five lumbar vertebrae, and the sacrum. The upper border of the hip bone, the iliac crest, forms the border between the back of the trunk and the gluteal region of the lower limb. The spinous processes of the vertebrae to which the latissimus dorsi and the trapezius muscles are attached project backwards in the midline. The scapula whose concave costal surface lies against the convex rib cage has a projection backwards, the spine of the scapula. When the arm is by the side of the trunk the medial end of the spine known as the root of the spine of the scapula lies at the level of the third rib.

SURFACE ANATOMY OF THE BACK (Fig. 2.9)

Surface features of the trapezius and the latissimus dorsi can be examined at the back. The superolateral border of the trapezius is seen and felt in the lower part of the neck. This can be made more prominent by raising the point of the shoulder against resistance. The spinous processes of the vertebrae are palpable in the midline. They can be made more prominent by bending the trunk forward. The lateral border of the latissimus dorsi is visible as the posterior axillary fold. The muscle can be palpated here by adducting the abducted arm against resistance. The medial border, the inferior angle and the spine of the scapula and the acromion are also seen. As the scapula contributes to the movement of the shoulder, the mobility of the shoulder joint (glenohumeral joint) is assessed by immobilising the scapula by holding on to it at the back.

Lateral pectoral nerve

Medial pectoral nerve

Pectoralis minor

Digitations of serratus anterior

Fig. 2.7 *Pectoralis minor.*

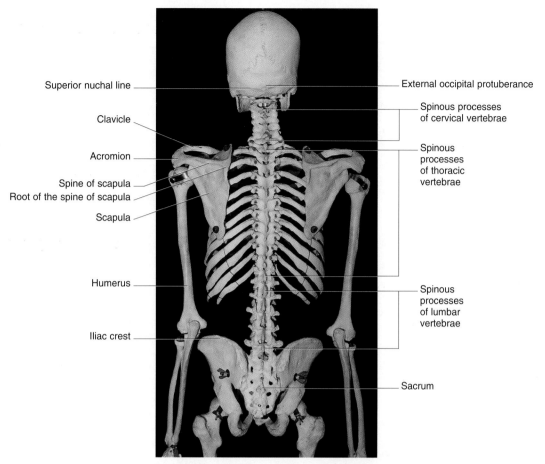

Superior nuchal line

External occipital protuberance

Clavicle

Spinous processes
of cervical vertebrae

Acromion

Spinous
processes
of thoracic
vertebrae

Spine of scapula
Root of the spine of scapula

Scapula

Humerus

Spinous
processes
of lumbar
vertebrae

Iliac crest

Sacrum

Fig. 2.8 *The skeleton viewed from the back.*

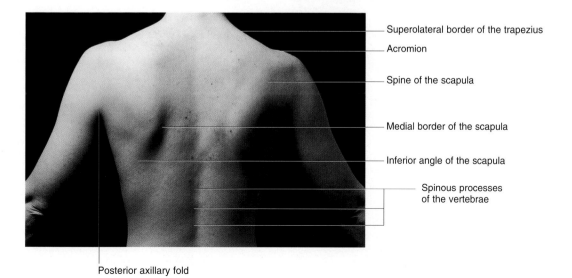

Superolateral border of the trapezius

Acromion

Spine of the scapula

Medial border of the scapula

Inferior angle of the scapula

Spinous processes
of the vertebrae

Posterior axillary fold

Fig. 2.9 *Surface anatomy of the back.*

SUPERFICIAL MUSCLES OF THE BACK
(Fig. 2.10)

Trapezius

Origin
- External occipital protuberance and the superior nuchal line.
- Ligamentum nuchae — fibroelastic tissue connecting the muscle to the spines of the cervical vertebrae.
- Spinous processes of seventh cervical to twelfth thoracic vertebrae.

Insertion
- Upper fibres to the lateral third of the clavicle.
- Middle fibres to the acromion.
- Lower fibres to the spine of the scapula.

Nerve supply
Spinal part of the accessory nerve.

Actions
Assisted by the lower fibres of the serratus anterior the trapezius rotates the scapula so that the glenoid fossa faces upwards. This action is important for raising the arm above the level of the shoulder. The shoulder is elevated by the upper fibres (as in shrugging the shoulder). All fibres of the muscle help to retract the scapula.

Test
Shrug the shoulder against resistance. The upper part of the muscle can be seen and felt as contracting.

Latissimus dorsi

This large superficial muscle is seen in the lower half of the back. It wraps around the chest wall and as it comes to be inserted in the bicipital groove of the humerus, contributes to the posterior axillary fold.

Nerve supply
The thoracodorsal nerve (C6,7,8) from the posterior cord of the brachial plexus. It is vulnerable in operations on the axilla.

Actions
Extension, medial rotation and adduction of the shoulder (as in scratching the opposite scapular region). The muscle is used as a myocutaneous flap in reconstructive breast surgery.

Test
Abduct the arm and adduct it against resistance. The muscle can be felt contracting in the posterior fold of the axilla.

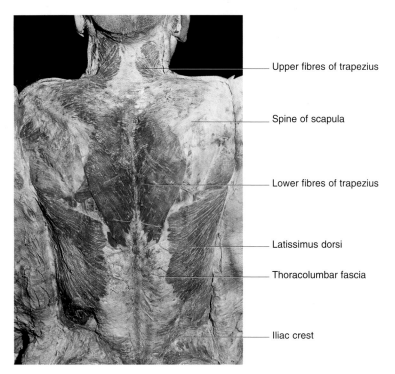

Upper fibres of trapezius

Spine of scapula

Lower fibres of trapezius

Latissimus dorsi

Thoracolumbar fascia

Iliac crest

Fig. 2.10 *Superficial muscles of the back.*

STRUCTURES DEEP TO THE TRAPEZIUS (Fig. 2.11)

The levator scapulae and the two rhomboids lying deep to the trapezius are inserted on the medial border of the scapula.

BONES OF THE SHOULDER GIRDLE

Clavicle (Figs 2.12, 2.13)

The clavicle holds the upper limb away from the trunk and allows it to have a wide range of movements in the shoulder region. It is subcutaneous throughout and is easily palpable. It has two curves, the lateral third being concave forward and the medial two-thirds convex forward. The junction between the two curves is the weakest point and is the commonest site of clavicular fractures. After a fracture the lateral fragment of the clavicle may get displaced downwards due to the weight of the upper limb. The classic injury for fracture is a fall on the outstretched hand when the body weight is transmitted through the clavicle to the sternum. Medially the clavicle articulates with the sternum at the sternoclavicular joint and laterally with the acromion of the scapula at the acromioclavicular joint. The lateral end of the clavicle is held firmly on to the coracoid process by the strong coracoclavicular ligament attached to the conoid tubercle and the trapezoid ridge. Through this ligament the scapula, and hence the upper limb, is held suspended from the clavicle. Four major muscles of the shoulder region are attached to the clavicle, medially the pectoralis major and the clavicular head of the sternocleidomastoid and laterally the deltoid and the trapezius. The small subclavius muscle arising from the first rib is attached to the groove on the under surface.

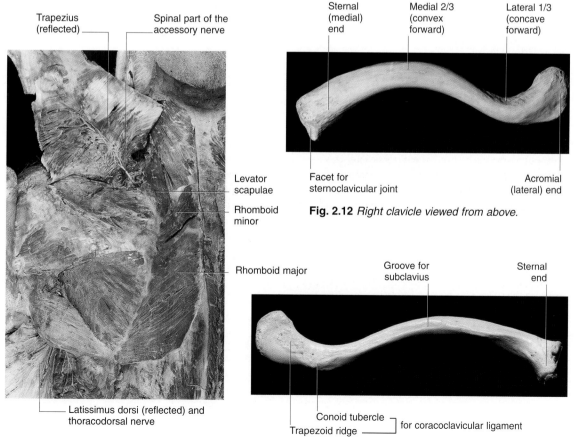

Fig. 2.11 *Structures deep to the trapezius.*

Fig. 2.12 *Right clavicle viewed from above.*

Fig. 2.13 *Right clavicle viewed from below.*

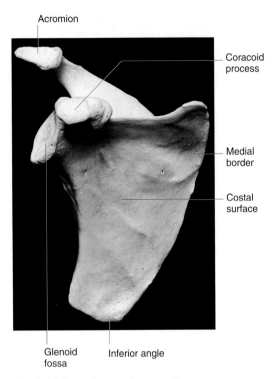

Fig. 2.14 *Scapula anterior aspect.*

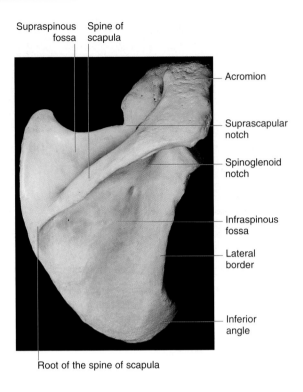

Fig. 2.15 *Scapula posterior aspect.*

Scapula — anterior aspect (Fig. 2.14)

The scapula whose mobility is essential to facilitate the wide range of movements of the shoulder is rarely fractured as the bone is almost completely encased in muscles. From the anterior aspect of the scapula (the costal surface) which covers the thoracic cage the subscapularis muscle originates. The surface is marked by ridges for the attachment of fibrous septae of this multipennate muscle. The serratus anterior muscle which moves the scapula forward (protraction of scapula) is inserted on the medial margin on the costal surface. The glenoid fossa, seen at the lateral aspect in the upper part, faces forward as well as laterally. Above this is the acromion which is the uppermost bony point in the shoulder region. The coracoid process projecting anteriorly receives the attachments of three muscles, i.e. short head of biceps, coracobrachialis and the pectoralis minor. The coracoclavicular and the coracoacromial ligaments are also attached to the coracoid process.

Scapula — posterior aspect (Fig. 2.15)

The lateral end of the spine projects forwards as the acromion. The medial end of the spine, the root of the spine, lies at the level of the spinous process of the third thoracic vertebra. The spine of scapula and the acromion are subcutaneous and are palpable. The trapezius and the deltoid are attached to the spine of the scapula and the acromion. The teres minor arises from the lateral border of the scapula, and the teres major from the inferior angle. The upper border of the scapula has the suprascapular notch near the root of the coracoid process. This lodges the suprascapular nerve. The notch is bridged by the supraspinous ligament which separates the suprascapular artery from the nerve. The nerve and the artery after supplying the supraspinatus enter the infraspinous fossa by passing through the spinoglenoid notch.

Lateral view of the scapula (Fig. 2.16)

This view shows the glenoid fossa, the coracoid process and the acromion more fully. The shallow glenoid fossa or the glenoid cavity articulates with the head of humerus. Its upper end has the supraglenoid tubercle for the long head of the biceps. The infraglenoid tubercle is below its lower border. The glenoid fossa is lined by articular cartilage and is slightly deepened by the fibrocartilagenous glenoid labrum attached to its

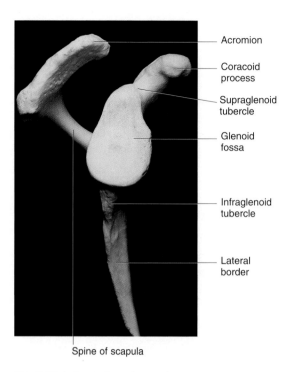

Acromion

Coracoid process

Supraglenoid tubercle

Glenoid fossa

Infraglenoid tubercle

Lateral border

Spine of scapula

Fig. 2.16 *Lateral view of scapula.*

margins. The capsule of the shoulder joint is attached to the labrum and the surrounding bone. The origin of the long head of the biceps from the supraglenoid tubercle is within the capsule of the joint whereas the long head of the triceps arising from the infraglenoid tubercle is extracapsular.

JOINTS OF THE SHOULDER GIRDLE

Sternoclavicular joint (Fig. 2.17)

This is a synovial joint between the medial end of the clavicle, the manubrium sternum and the first costal cartilage. The joint is atypical in that unlike most synovial joints the articular cartilage covering the articular surfaces is fibrocartilage and not hyaline. Besides, the cavity is separated into two by a fibrocartilagenous articular disc. The disc may act as a shock absorber when forces are transmitted to the joint through the clavicle. The joint is surrounded by strong ligaments which stabilise it. The clavicle moves like a 'see-saw'. Elevation of the shoulder end (lateral end) of the clavicle makes the sternal end move downwards. Protraction (forward movement) of the shoulder end makes the sternal end move backwards.

Acromioclavicular joint

This is a synovial joint between the lateral end of the clavicle and the medial border of the acromion. The sloping surfaces of the two bones, as seen in Fig. 2.18, make the articulation weak. The clavicle will override the acromion when the joint is subluxated or dislocated. Like the sternoclavicular joint the articular surfaces are covered by fibrocartilage. There is also an incomplete fibrocartilagenous intraarticular disc. The gap between the two bones as seen in the radiograph (Fig. 2.18) is mostly occupied by the disc.

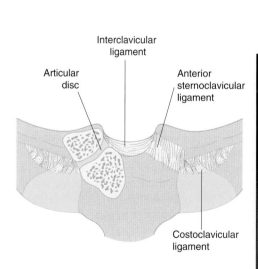

Interclavicular ligament

Articular disc

Anterior sternoclavicular ligament

Costoclavicular ligament

Fig. 2.17 *The sternoclavicular joint. The right-hand side shows the interior.*

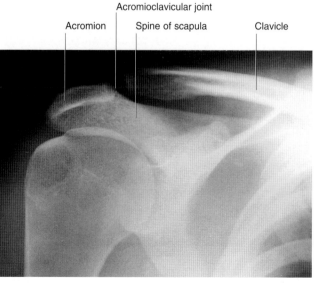

Acromioclavicular joint

Acromion

Spine of scapula

Clavicle

Fig. 2.18 *Radiograph of the acromioclavicular joint.*

MOVEMENTS OF THE PECTORAL GIRDLE (SCAPULA AND CLAVICLE)

Movements of the scapula make the coracoclavicular ligament taut and from then on the clavicle and the scapula move as a single unit at the sternoclavicular joint. Following are the movements of the shoulder girdle (Fig. 2.19).

Movements	Muscles
Protraction — scapula moves forward hugging the chest wall	Serratus anterior Pectoralis minor
Retraction — as in bracing the shoulder backwards	Trapezius Rhomboids
Elevation (shrugging the shoulder)	Trapezius (upper fibres) Levator scapulae
Depression	Serratus anterior Pectoralis minor
Forward rotation of the scapula making the glenoid face upwards — a mechanism to increase the range of abduction of the shoulder	Trapezius Lower fibres of the serratus anterior

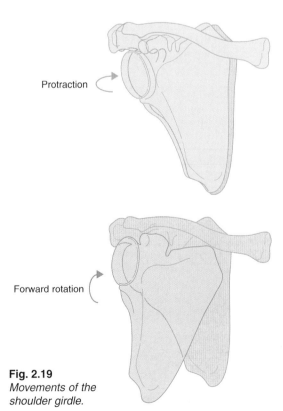

Protraction

Forward rotation

Fig. 2.19
Movements of the shoulder girdle.

THE SHOULDER JOINT

The shoulder joint is completely surrounded by the massive deltoid muscle.

Deep to the deltoid lies the supraspinatus, infraspinatus and teres minor and subscapularis, the four muscles connecting the various aspect of the scapula to the humerus. These reinforce the capsule of the shoulder joint and are collectively known as the rotator cuff muscles or SITS.

Scapula and the upper end of humerus — anterior view (Fig. 2.20)

The upper end of humerus shows the spherical head which articulates with the glenoid fossa and the greater and lesser tubercles which receive muscle attachments. The area of the head of humerus is about four times larger than that of the shallow glenoid fossa making the shoulder joint unstable but very mobile. The capsule of the joint is attached to the anatomical neck of humerus except in the lower part where it extends on to the surgical neck. The upper part of the greater tubercle receives the attachment of the supraspinatus. The subscapularis is inserted to the lesser tubercle. The intertubercular sulcus or the bicipital groove lodges the tendon of the long head of biceps arising from the supraglenoid tubercle. Three muscles are inserted in the region of the intertubercular sulcus; the pectoralis major to its lateral lip, teres major to the medial lip and the latissimus dorsi to its floor.

Subscapularis and the anterior aspect of shoulder joint (Fig. 2.21)

The dissection shows the subscapularis arising from the costal surface of scapula, its insertion to the lesser tubercle of the humerus as well as the anterior aspect of the capsule of the shoulder joint. The short head of biceps and the coracobrachialis, both arising from the coracoid process, are removed to expose the anterior aspect of the shoulder joint. The surgical exposure to the anterior aspect of the shoulder can be done through the deltopectoral groove leading to detachment of the tip of the coracoid process with coracobrachialis and short head of the biceps. This will expose the anterior surface of the capsule covered by the subscapularis. The long head of biceps emerging from the capsule of the shoulder joint and the teres major inserting to the medial lip of the biciptal groove are also seen.

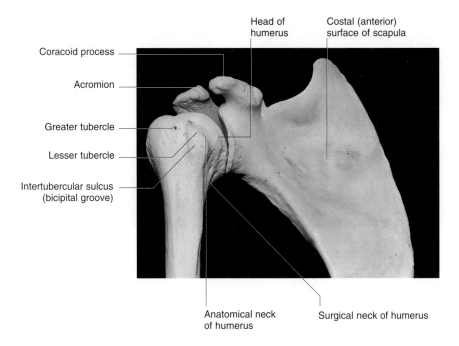

Coracoid process

Acromion

Greater tubercle

Lesser tubercle

Intertubercular sulcus
(bicipital groove)

Head of
humerus

Costal (anterior)
surface of scapula

Anatomical neck
of humerus

Surgical neck of humerus

Fig. 2.20 *Scapula and the upper end of the humerus — anterior view.*

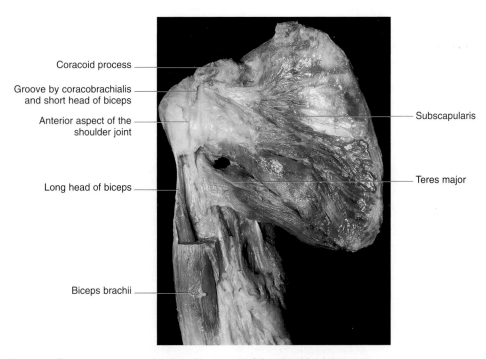

Coracoid process

Groove by coracobrachialis
and short head of biceps

Anterior aspect of the
shoulder joint

Long head of biceps

Biceps brachii

Subscapularis

Teres major

Fig. 2.21 *Subscapularis and the anterior aspect of the shoulder joint.*

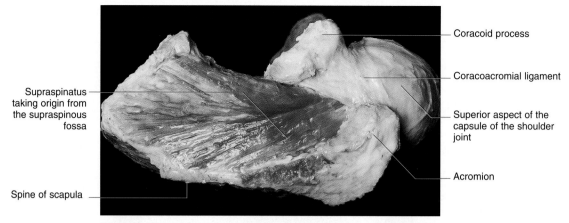

Fig. 2.22 *Supraspinatus and the superior aspect of the shoulder joint.*

Supraspinatus and the superior aspect of shoulder joint (Fig. 2.22)

This view of the superior aspect of shoulder shows the supraspinatus arising from the supraspinous fossa of scapula. The tendon of the muscle passes deep to the coracoacromial ligament to gain insertion to the greater tubercle and the superior aspect of the capsule of the shoulder joint. It is supplied by the suprascapular nerve. Besides stabilising the shoulder joint by reinforcing the capsule it assists the deltoid in abduction. The supraspinatus initiates abduction which is then continued by the deltoid. Together the two muscles abduct the shoulder up to about 120°. The subacromial bursa which is continuous with the subdeltoid bursa separates the tendon of the supraspinatus from the coracoacromial ligament.

Degenerative disorders causing supraspinatus tendinitis can lead on to subacromial bursitis, both conditions producing pain during abduction of the shoulder. Pain is worse as the arm traverses the arc between 60° and 120° (painful arc) when the impingement is maximal.

Scapula and the upper end of the humerus — posterior aspect (Fig. 2.23)

The features of the posterior aspect of the scapula and the upper end of the humerus are shown in Fig. 2.23.

Infraspinatus and the posterior aspect of shoulder joint (Fig. 2.24)

This dissection of the posterior aspect of the shoulder joint and the scapular region shows the infraspinatus

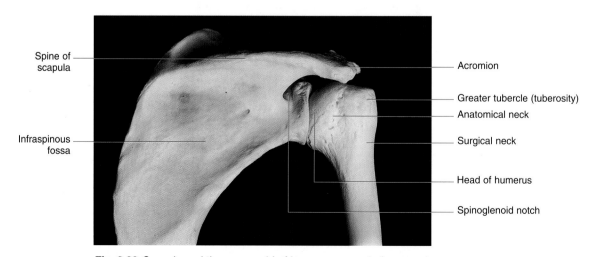

Fig. 2.23 *Scapula and the upper end of humerus — posterior aspect.*

arising from the infraspinous fossa. Its tendon lies across the posterior aspect of the shoulder joint to reach the posterior surface of the greater tubercle for its insertion. The teres minor which is inserted on the greater tubercle below the infraspinatus arises from the lateral border of the scapula. The tendons of these two muscles along with those of the supraspinatus and the subscapularis fuse with the capsule of the shoulder joint. The rotator cuff thus formed by these four muscles is the main factor stabilising the shoulder joint. For surgical exposure via a posterior approach the deltoid is detached to expose the infraspinatus and teres minor. These are cut to expose the capsule. Care is taken not to damage the branches of the axillary nerve and the accompanying posterior circumflex humeral artery which emerges through the quadrangular space to supply the deltoid. The space is bounded by the surgical neck of the humerus laterally, the long head of the triceps medially, teres minor above and teres major below (also see Fig. 2.39).

The interior of the shoulder joint

The shoulder joint is a synovial joint of the ball and socket type where the head of the humerus articulates with the glenoid fossa of the scapula (Fig. 2.25). The area of the rounded head of the humerus is about four times larger than that of the shallow glenoid fossa. The humeral head and glenoid fossa are lined by articular cartilage (hyaline) and additionally the labrum glenoidale (fibrocartilage) forms a ring around the margin of the glenoid fossa (Fig. 2.25).

The fibrous capsule is attached to the scapula beyond the labrum and to the humerus around its anatomical neck, except inferiorly, where its attachment is lower, into the surgical neck. The capsule is thin and loose

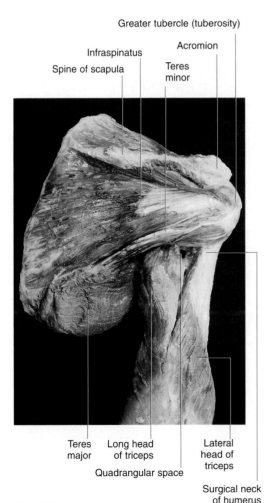

Greater tubercle (tuberosity)

Infraspinatus

Acromion

Spine of scapula

Teres minor

Teres major Long head of triceps Lateral head of triceps

Quadrangular space

Surgical neck of humerus

Fig. 2.24 *Infraspinatus and the posterior aspect of the shoulder joint.*

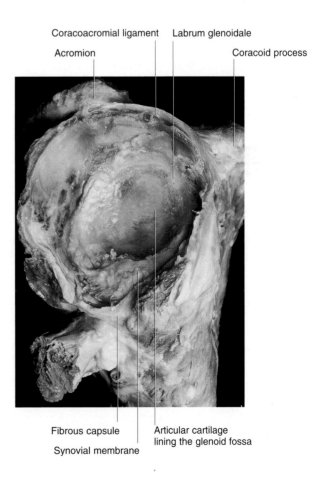

Coracoacromial ligament Labrum glenoidale

Acromion

Coracoid process

Fibrous capsule

Synovial membrane

Articular cartilage lining the glenoid fossa

Fig. 2.25 *Interior of the right shoulder joint — medial aspect.*

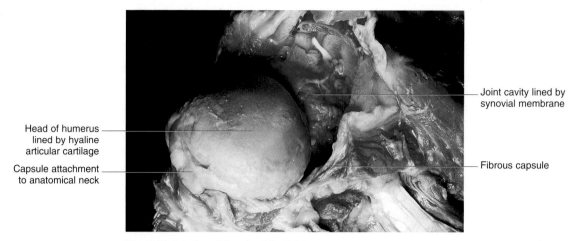

Head of humerus lined by hyaline articular cartilage

Capsule attachment to anatomical neck

Joint cavity lined by synovial membrane

Fibrous capsule

Fig. 2.26 *Interior of the shoulder joint.*

facilitating mobility at the expense of stability (Fig. 2.26).

The inner surface of the fibrous capsule and all intracapsular structures except the articular cartilage are lined by the synovial membrane. It herniates through the hole in the capsule to communicate with the subscapularis bursa. It may also communicate with the infraspinatus bursa. It forms a sleeve around the tendon of the long head of biceps which traverses the joint.

Movements of the shoulder joint
(Fig. 2.27)

Movement	Muscles
Abduction	Supraspinatus Deltoid (lateral part)
Adduction	Pectoralis major (sternocostal head) Teres major Latissimus dorsi
Flexion	Pectoralis major (clavicular head) Deltoid (anterior fibres)
Extension	Teres major Deltoid (posterior fibres) Latissimus dorsi
Medial rotation	Pectoralis major, teres major, subscapularis Deltoid (anterior), latissimus dorsi
Lateral rotation	Infraspinatus, teres minor, deltoid (posterior)

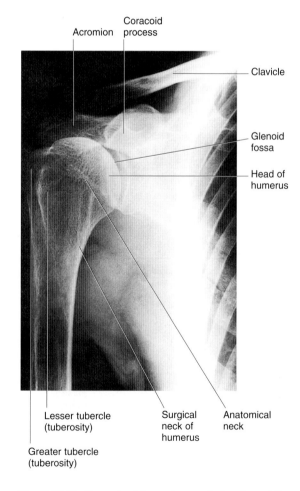

Acromion

Coracoid process

Clavicle

Glenoid fossa

Head of humerus

Lesser tubercle (tuberosity)

Surgical neck of humerus

Anatomical neck

Greater tubercle (tuberosity)

Fig. 2.27 *Radiograph of the anteroposterior view of the shoulder.*

The wide-ranging movements of the shoulder are allowed by complex mechanisms. All the movements of the shoulder joint are accompanied by movements of the shoulder girdle. The first 30° of abduction mostly takes place in the shoulder joint. Subsequently the shoulder joint and the shoulder girdle move simultaneously. For every 15° of abduction 10° takes place in the shoulder joint and 5° in the shoulder girdle. The movement of the shoulder girdle is achieved by the contraction of the trapezius and the lower fibres of the serratus anterior facilitating forward rotation of the scapula to make the glenoid to face upwards. If this is prevented (as in trapezius paralysis) the arm cannot be raised much above the level of the shoulder. The latter part of abduction of the shoulder is also accompanied by a lateral rotation of the humerus.

AXILLA (Fig. 2.28)

The axilla is the space between the trunk and the upper arm. It is pyramidal in shape and its boundaries are:

- Anterior wall — pectoralis major and the pectoralis minor muscles.
- Posterior wall — subscapularis, teres major and the latissimus dorsi muscles.
- Lateral wall — upper end of the humerus with the biceps brachii and the coracobrachialis muscles.
- Medial wall — the serratus anterior muscle covering the ribs and intercostal spaces.
- Apex — formed by the first rib medially with the clavicle in front and the scapula behind. It is the channel of communication between the posterior triangle and the axilla.
- Base — skin and deep fascia extending between the chest wall and the arm.

The axilla contains:

- Fat and lymph nodes.
- Axillary artery and vein.
- Brachial plexus.

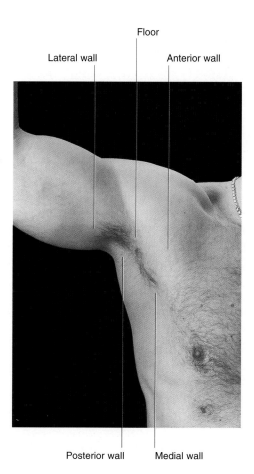

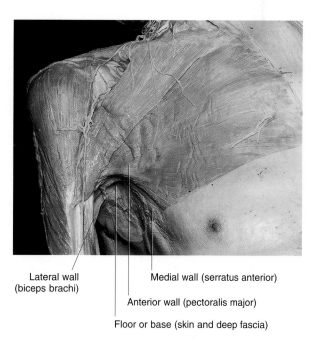

Fig. 2.28a *Walls of the axilla — surface anatomy.*

Fig. 2.28b *Walls of the axilla — viewed from the front.*

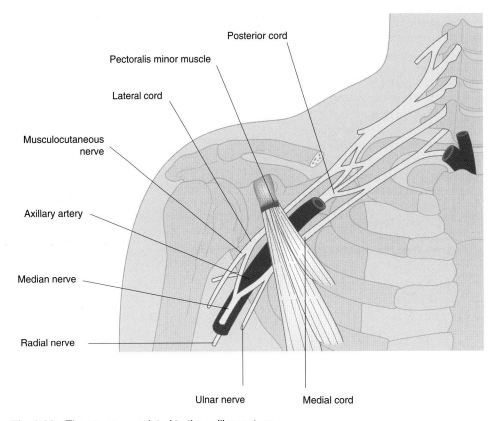

Fig. 2.29a *The structures related to the axillary artery.*

Axillary artery (Fig. 2.29a)

The axillary artery is a continuation of the subclavian artery and it extends from the outer border of the first rib to the lower border of the teres major from where it continues as the brachial artery. For descriptive purposes it can be divided into three parts by the pectoralis minor. The part above the muscle is the first part, the part underneath is the second and the part below being the third part. The three cords of the brachial plexus are arranged around the second part of the artery in the following manner:

- Lateral cord — lateral to the artery.
- Medial cord — medial to the artery.
- Posterior cord — posterior to the artery.

i.e. The three cords are named after their relation to the second part of the artery.

The axillary vein is medial to the artery separated from it for most of its course by the medial cord and its branches. The major branches are:

- acromiothoracic
- lateral thoracic
- posterior circumflex humeral
- subscapular.

Branches of the axillary artery anastomose with those of the subclavian around the scapula (Fig. 2.29b), which may be an important collateral channel in case of obstruction to the distal part of the subclavian artery.

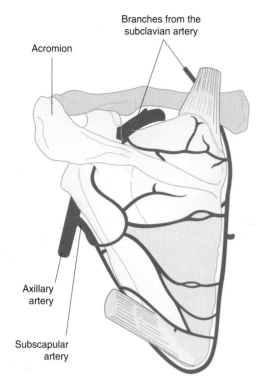

Acromion

Branches from the
subclavian artery

Axillary
artery

Subscapular
artery

Fig. 2.29b *Arterial anastomoses over the scapula.*

Surface marking of the artery

Draw a line from the middle of the clavicle to the groove behind the coracobrachialis. Pulsation of the artery can be felt by deep palpation of the axilla after abducting the arm.

Surgical exposure

The first part of the artery lies deep to the clavicular head of the pectoralis major and can be exposed by splitting the muscle fibre and incising the clavipectoral fascia which connects the upper border of the pectoralis minor to the clavicle.

Axillary vein

This vein commences at the lower border of the teres major as a continuation of the basilic vein and it continues into the neck as the subclavian vein in front of the scalenus anterior muscle. The venae comitantes of the brachial artery join it near its commencement. As seen in Fig. 2.30, the cephalic vein drains into it in its upper part. The lateral thoracic vein which is a tributary of the axillary vein is connected to the tributaries of the great saphenous vein of the lower limb. These connecting veins on the side of the chest wall enlarge in inferior vena caval obstruction.

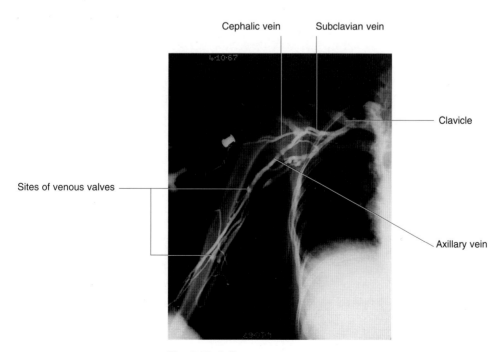

Cephalic vein

Subclavian vein

Clavicle

Sites of venous valves

Axillary vein

Fig. 2.30 *Axillary venogram.*

Brachial plexus (Fig. 2.31)

The brachial plexus is described as having:

Roots

Anterior rami of C5–T1 spinal nerves.

Trunks

The upper trunk formed of roots from C5 and C6, the middle trunk by C7 and the lower trunk by union of roots from C8 and T1.

Cords

The anterior divisions of upper and middle trunks join to form the lateral cord, the anterior division of the lower trunk continues as the medial cord and the posterior divisions of all the three trunks join together to form the posterior cord.

Branches

   Medial cord:

- medial pectoral nerve, ulnar nerve
- medial root of the median nerve
- medial cutaneous nerve of the forearm
- medial cutaneous nerve of the arm.

   Lateral cord:

- lateral pectoral nerve
- lateral root of the median nerve
- musculocutaneous nerve.

Posterior cord:

- subscapular nerves
- axillary nerve
- thoracodorsal nerve
- radial nerve.

Nerves and vessels of the axilla

The dissection of the lower part of the neck and axilla as illustrated in Fig. 2.32 shows the subclavian artery continuing as the axillary artery. The axillary vein which continues into the neck as the subclavian vein lies medial to the axillary artery. The formation of the median nerve by its medial and lateral roots is seen. The musculocutaneous nerve is seen entering the corachobrachialis. Also seen are the long thoracic nerve supplying the serratus anterior and the thoracodorsal nerve supplying the latissimus dorsi.

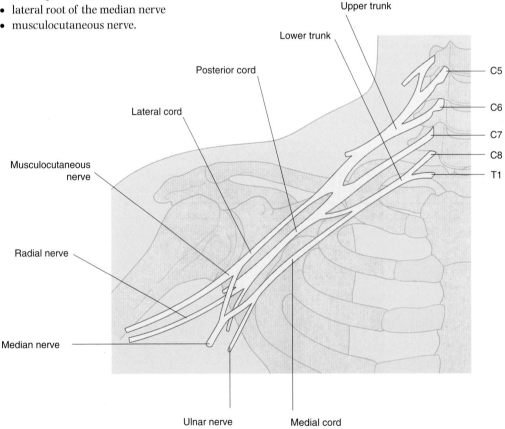

Fig. 2.31 *The brachial plexus.*

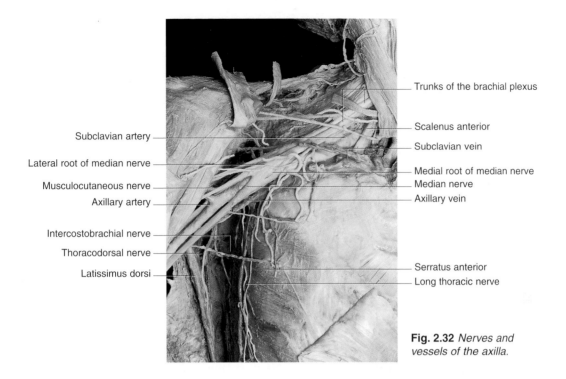

Trunks of the brachial plexus

Scalenus anterior

Subclavian artery

Subclavian vein

Lateral root of median nerve

Medial root of median nerve

Musculocutaneous nerve

Median nerve

Axillary artery

Axillary vein

Intercostobrachial nerve

Thoracodorsal nerve

Latissimus dorsi

Serratus anterior

Long thoracic nerve

Fig. 2.32 *Nerves and vessels of the axilla.*

The intercostobrachial nerve which is a branch of the second intercostal nerve supplies a small area of skin of the medial aspect of the arm. This is the only nerve supplying the upper limb without passing through the brachial plexus. This nerve as well as the long thoracic nerve and the thoracodorsal nerve are vulnerable in 'axillary clearance', a surgical dissection to remove the axillary lymph nodes, in the treatment of carcinoma of the breast.

Posterior cord branches (Fig. 2.33)

The subscapular nerves, axillary nerve, thoracodorsal nerve and the radial nerve are seen.

The axillary nerve leaves the axilla winding round the surgical neck of the humerus, passing below the shoulder joint. It is accompanied by the posterior circumflex humeral branch of the axillary artery (see Fig. 2.39). The nerve may be paralysed in dislocation of the shoulder joint as well as in a fracture of the surgical neck of the humerus. The thoracodorsal nerve lies in the loose areolar tissue in front of the subscapularis muscle and can be traced to the latissimus dorsi

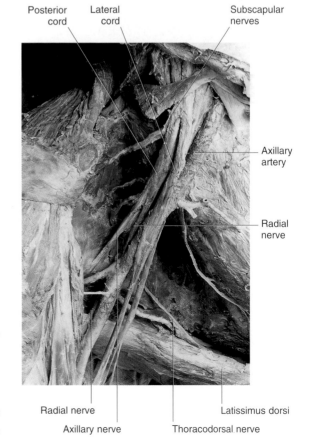

Posterior cord

Lateral cord

Subscapular nerves

Axillary artery

Radial nerve

Radial nerve

Axillary nerve

Thoracodorsal nerve

Latissimus dorsi

Fig. 2.33 *Posterior cord branches (axillary artery and the lateral and medial cords are displaced medially).*

muscle. The muscle on which the posterior cord lies is the subscapularis. Two or three nerves enter the subscapularis from the posterior cord. The radial nerve which is the continuation of the posterior cord will supply the extensor muscles in the arm and forearm.

Segmental innervation of the upper limb

Knowledge of the dermatomes (segmental innervation of the skin) and myotomes (segmental innervation of muscles) are important for testing for nerve root compression and assessing the level of spinal cord injuries (Fig. 2.34). The dermatomes of the upper segments of the brachial plexus (C5,C6) are on the lateral aspect, the lower segments (C8,T1) on the medial aspect and C7 in the middle. There is considerable overlap across adjoining dermatomes. However there is no overlap across the axial line as it separates discontinuous segments.

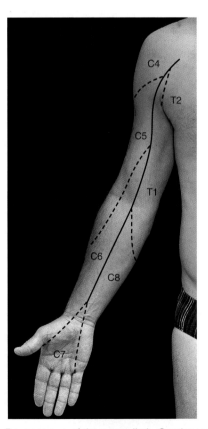

Fig. 2.34 *Dermatomes of the upper limb. Continuous line represents the axial line across which there is no overlap. However there is considerable overlap across the interrupted lines which demarcate adjoining dermatomes.*

The pattern of the myotomes is more complex. There is a proximal to distal gradient as the C5 supplies the shoulder and T1 the intrinsic muscles of the hand. The flexors of the elbow are by C5 and C6, whereas C7 and C8 supply the extensors (triceps). The biceps tendon jerk therefore tests C5,C6 segments and the triceps jerk C7,C8.

Lymph nodes of the axilla (Fig. 2.35)

The lymph nodes in the axilla are of tremendous clinical importance as they drain the mammary gland. There are about 20–30 lymph nodes scattered in the fibro-fatty tissue.

- Anterior or pectoral group: Lies along the lateral thoracic artery at the lower border of the pectoralis minor.
- Posterior or subscapular group: Lies along the posterior wall of the axilla in its posterior part related to the subscapular artery.
- Lateral group: Lies on the lateral wall of the axilla along the axillary vein.
- Central group: Lies in the fat of the axilla and receives afferent vessels from the above groups.

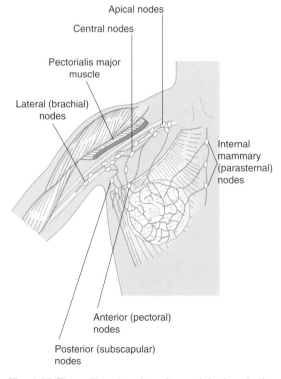

Fig. 2.35 *The axillary lymph nodes and the lymphatic drainage of the breast.*

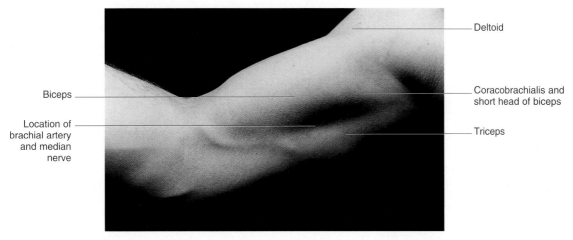

Fig. 2.36 *Surface anatomy of the front of arm.*

- Apical group: Lies in the apex of the axilla. The apical nodes are also connected to the supraclavicular or lower deep cervical lymph nodes (of the neck).

ANTERIOR ASPECT OF THE ARM

Surface anatomy of the front of arm
(Fig. 2.36)

The medial border of the biceps is known as the danger zone of the arm as it is related to the brachial artery and its venae comitantes and the median nerve. Surgical exposure of the humerus is preferably done by incisions along the lateral border of the muscle to avoid cutting the artery and the nerve. Brachial artery pulsation is felt by palpating the artery against the humerus. The upper part of the medial border of the biceps has the coracobrachialis along with its short head. The musculocutaneous nerve enters the coracobrachialis at this level and can be blocked by intramuscular injection of local anaesthetic agents in this area. The median nerve along with the axillary artery lies in the groove behind the coracobrachialis. Laterally the prominent deltoid is easily visible and it can be seen tapering to its insertion on the deltoid tuberosity at the middle of the humerus.

The superficial veins of the arm
(Fig. 2.37)

The upper limb is drained by two sets of veins, superficial and deep. The superficial veins lie superficial to the deep fascia and are clinically important as they are frequently used for cannulation. The deep veins accompany the arteries as venae comitantes until the middle of the arm where the axillary vein is formed. The cephalic and the basilic are the two major superficial veins. Both are formed in the dorsal venous

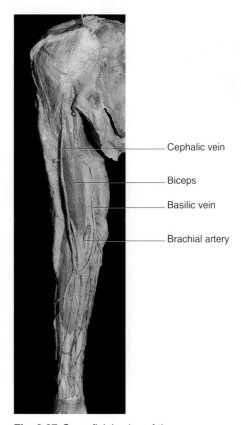

Fig. 2.37 *Superficial veins of the arm.*

arch at the back of the hand. In the arm the cephalic vein lies on the lateral border of the biceps and ascends to the shoulder region to reach the deltopectoral groove where it pierces the deep fascia to join the axillary vein.

The basilic vein lies along the medial border of the biceps up to the middle of the arm where it pierces the deep fascia to join the venae comitantes of the brachial artry to become the axillary vein.

Deltoid (Fig. 2.38)

Origin
Lateral third of the clavicle, acromion and the spine of the scapula.
Insertion
Deltoid tuberosity at the middle of the shaft of the humerus.
Action
Anterior fibres help pectoralis major to flex the shoulder. Lateral fibres combine with the supraspinatus to abduct the shoulder, whereas the posterior fibres along with the latissimus dorsi and teres major extend the joint.
Nerve supply (Fig. 2.39)
Axillary nerve, a branch of the posterior cord of the brachial plexus, passes through the quadrangular space winding round the surgical neck of the humerus to enter the muscle. The nerve can be damaged in dislocation of the shoulder as well as in fracture of the surgical neck of the humerus.
Test
Hold the arm in the abducted position against resistance. Inability to do so suggests paralysis of the muscle. Damage to the axillary nerve will cause atrophy of the muscle and flattening of the contour of the shoulder.

Anterior fibres of deltoid

Lateral (middle) fibres of deltoid

Insertion of deltoid

Biceps

Triceps

Posterior fibres of deltoid

Fig. 2.38 *Deltoid lateral view.*

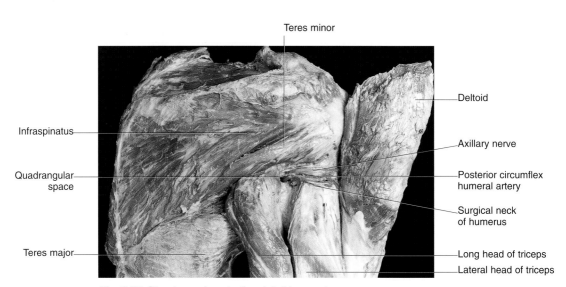

Teres minor

Infraspinatus

Quadrangular space

Teres major

Deltoid

Axillary nerve

Posterior circumflex humeral artery

Surgical neck of humerus

Long head of triceps

Lateral head of triceps

Fig. 2.39 *Structures deep to the deltoid aspect.*

Biceps brachii (Fig. 2.40)

Biceps

Origin

Short head — coracoid process.

Long head — supraglenoid tubercle of the scapula.
The tendon of the long head, lined by synovial sheath,
passes through the shoulder joint to enter the bicipital
groove of the upper part of the humerus.

Insertion

Tendon of biceps — posterior aspect of the radial
tuberosity. In the cubital fossa the tendon gives off a
medial expansion, the biciptal aponeurosis, which
merges with the deep fascia to be inserted to the
subcutaneous border of the upper end of the ulna.

Action

The biceps is a powerful flexor of the elbow and a
supinator of the forearm. The tendon of the long head
may contribute to the stability of the shoulder as it
runs over the head of the humerus. It is a weak flexor
of the shoulder.

Test

Flex the supinated forearm against resistance, the
biceps can be seen and felt as contracting.

Brachialis (Fig. 2.41)

This takes origin from the anterior surface of the lower
half of the humerus. It covers the anterior surface of
the elbow joint before getting inserted to the coronoid
process of the ulna. The muscle is supplied by the
musculocutaneous nerve. The lateral half is also
supplied by the radial nerve. The radial nerve emerges
between its lower part and the brachioradialis. It is a
flexor of the elbow joint.

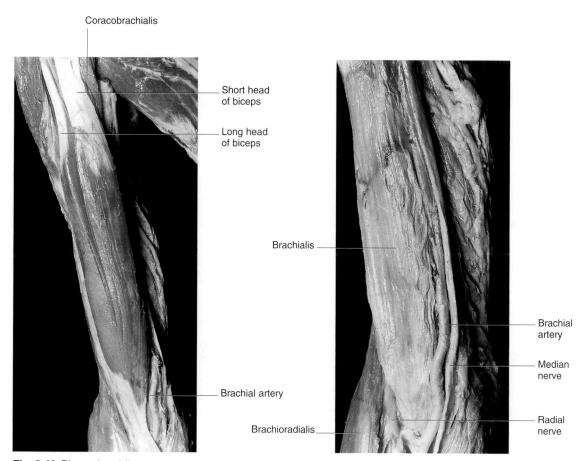

Fig. 2.40 *Biceps brachii.*

Fig. 2.41 *Brachialis (after removal of biceps).*

Nerves and vessels of the front of arm
(Fig. 2.42)

Brachial artery
The brachial artery which is the continuation of the axillary artery terminates in the cubital fossa by dividing into the radial and ulnar. The profunda brachii accompanying the radial nerve is one of its major branches.

The lower part of the brachial artery can be damaged in supracondylar fractures of the humerus especially in children. Intense spasm of the artery may lead to Volkmann's ischaemic contracture (ischaemic damage of the forearm muscles).

The musculocutaneous nerve (C5,6,7)
This is a branch of the lateral cord of the brachial plexus. The nerve, after supplying the coracobrachialis, biceps and brachialis, continues as the lateral cutaneous nerve of the forearm.

Median nerve
This nerve is formed by contributions from the lateral and medial cords. In the upper part the nerve is lateral to the brachial artery but crosses anterior to the artery to its medial side as it descends. It gives off no branch in the arm.

POSTERIOR COMPARTMENT OF THE ARM

The posterior compartment of the arm contains the triceps muscle through which runs the radial nerve accompanied by the profunda brachii artery. The ulnar nerve lies in the lower part closely behind the medial epicondyle.

Triceps (Fig. 2.43)

The origins of the triceps are as follows:

- Long head from the infraglenoid tubercle of the humerus.
- Lateral head from the back of the humerus above the groove for the radial nerve.
- Medial head from the back of the humerus below the groove for the radial nerve.

The muscle has a tendon lower down which is inserted to the upper surface of the olecranon of the ulna.

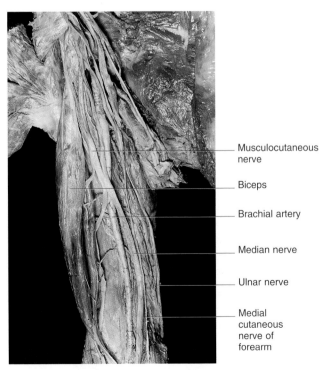

Musculocutaneous nerve

Biceps

Brachial artery

Median nerve

Ulnar nerve

Medial cutaneous nerve of forearm

Fig. 2.42 *Nerves and vessels of the front of arm. (Biceps is displaced laterally.)*

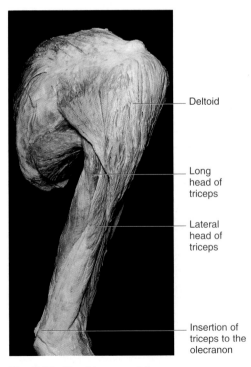

Deltoid

Long head of triceps

Lateral head of triceps

Insertion of triceps to the olecranon

Fig. 2.43a *The triceps and the deltoid viewed from the back.*

Nerve supply (Fig. 2.44)

The long and medial heads of the triceps are supplied by branches from the radial nerve given off in the axilla. A branch to the lateral head and an additional branch to the medial head are given off from the radial nerve in the spiral (radial) groove of the humerus.

Fractures of the middle of the shaft of the humerus damaging the radial nerve will not paralyse the triceps as it is supplied by branches given off in the axilla.

Ulnar nerve

This nerve from the medial cord of the brachial plexus as it descends pierces the medial intermuscular septum to enter the posterior compartment. At the elbow the nerve lies in the groove behind the medial epicondyle where it is palpable. It gives off no branch in the arm.

Radial nerve in the spiral groove

RADIAL NERVE

The nerve which is almost the continuation of the posterior cord passes obliquely down from medial to lateral closely related to the posterior surface of the shaft of the humerus lying in the groove for the radial nerve (spiral groove). The nerve then pierces the lateral intermuscular septum to enter the anterior

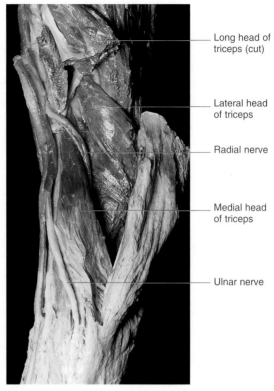

Fig. 2.43b *The triceps viewed from the medial aspect.*

Long head of triceps (cut)

Lateral head of triceps

Radial nerve

Medial head of triceps

Ulnar nerve

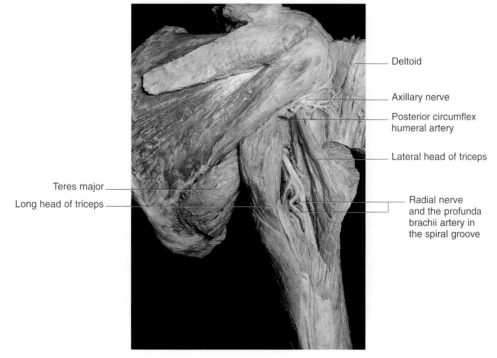

Deltoid

Axillary nerve

Posterior circumflex humeral artery

Lateral head of triceps

Teres major

Long head of triceps

Radial nerve and the profunda brachii artery in the spiral groove

Fig. 2.44 *Nerves and vessels in the posterior aspect of arm.*

compartment where it lies between the brachialis and brachioradialis. Just above the elbow the radial nerve gives off branches to the brachioradialis, extensor carpi radialis longus and lateral half of the brachialis. In front of the lateral epicondyle it divides into its two terminal branches, the superficial radial branch and the posterior interosseous nerve

SURFACE MARKING OF THE RADIAL NERVE
This is seen as a line from the junction of the posterior wall of the axilla and arm obliquely downwards along the back of the arm to the junction of the lower and middle third of its lateral surface and from there to the front of the lateral epicondyle.

ANATOMY OF THE FOREARM

The cubital fossa

The cubital fossa is a triangular area in front of the elbow. Superficial veins here are often used for intravenous injections. Such injections can inadvertently be made into the brachial artery or the median nerve which are closely related to the veins, resulting in disastrous consequences.

Surface anatomy (Fig. 2.45)
Superficial veins are made visible by compressing the arm and occluding the venous return. The tendon of the biceps is easily felt in the middle of the fossa as it reaches its insertion on the radial tuberosity. The bicipital aponeurosis which separates the superficial veins from the brachial artery and the median nerve is palpated by flexing and supinating the forearm against resistance.

Pulsation of the brachial artery is felt medial to the biceps tendon. The median nerve lies medial to the artery. The brachioradialis is visible and can be felt contracting if the forearm is flexed against resistance in the midprone position. Similarly the pronator teres forming the medial boundary of the fossa is made prominent by pronating the forearm against resistance. The lateral and medial epicondyles of the humerus are felt easily at the lower end of the humerus. The radial nerve is located deeply in the cubital fossa in front of the lateral epicondyle, a site often used to induce local anaesthesia.

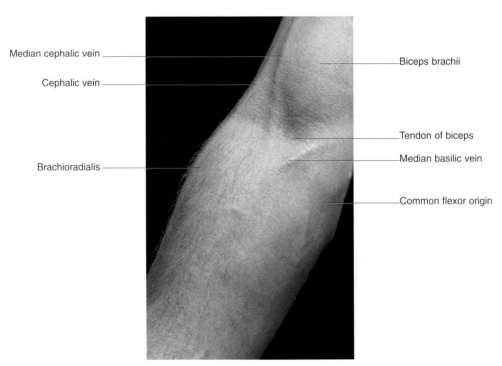

Median cephalic vein

Cephalic vein

Brachioradialis

Biceps brachii

Tendon of biceps

Median basilic vein

Common flexor origin

Fig. 2.45 *Cubital fossa — surface anatomy.*

Superficial dissection of the cubital fossa
(Fig. 2.46)

The arrangement of the superficial veins in the cubital fossa is variable. In the dissection shown a median vein of the forearm gives off the median cephalic and median basilic ('M' arrangement). Alternatively a large median cubital vein may run obliquely upwards from the cephalic vein to join the basilic vein ('H' arrangement). The dissection also shows the brachial artery and the median nerve medial to the tendon of biceps being separated from the vein by the bicipital aponeurosis.

Boundaries and floor of the cubital fossa
(Fig. 2.47)

The dissection where most of the contents except the median and the radial nerves are removed shows the structures forming the boundaries and floor of the cubital fossa:

- Lateral boundary — the brachioradialis.
- Medial boundary — the pronator teres.
- Roof — deep fascia reinforced by the bicipital aponeurosis.
- Floor — mostly brachialis, supinator laterally.

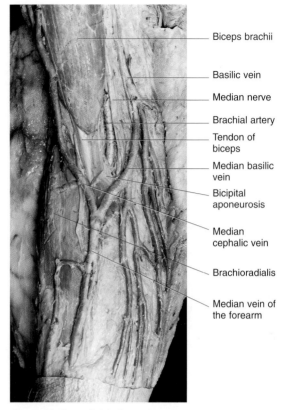

Biceps brachii

Basilic vein

Median nerve

Brachial artery

Tendon of biceps

Median basilic vein

Bicipital aponeurosis

Median cephalic vein

Brachioradialis

Median vein of the forearm

Fig. 2.46 *Superficial dissection of the cubital fossa.*

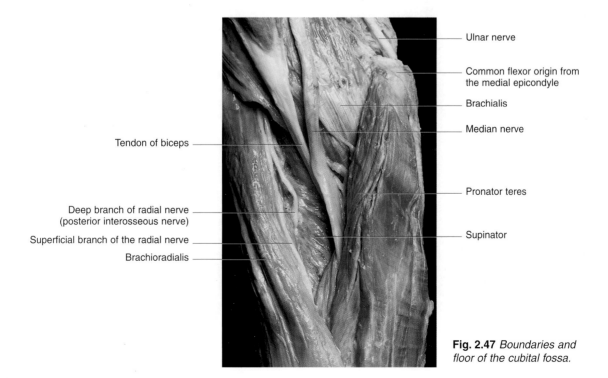

Tendon of biceps

Deep branch of radial nerve (posterior interosseous nerve)

Superficial branch of the radial nerve

Brachioradialis

Ulnar nerve

Common flexor origin from the medial epicondyle

Brachialis

Median nerve

Pronator teres

Supinator

Fig. 2.47 *Boundaries and floor of the cubital fossa.*

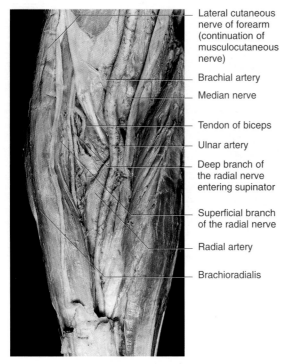

Lateral cutaneous
nerve of forearm
(continuation of
musculocutaneous
nerve)

Brachial artery

Median nerve

Tendon of biceps

Ulnar artery

Deep branch of
the radial nerve
entering supinator

Superficial branch
of the radial nerve

Radial artery

Brachioradialis

Fig. 2.48 *Contents of the cubital fossa.*

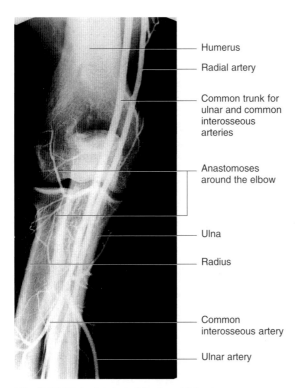

Humerus

Radial artery

Common trunk for
ulnar and common
interosseous
arteries

Anastomoses
around the elbow

Ulna

Radius

Common
interosseous artery

Ulnar artery

Fig. 2.49 *High division of the brachial artery (angiogram).*

Contents of the cubital fossa (Fig. 2.48)

From lateral to medial are the tendon of the biceps, brachial artery and the median nerve. The brachial artery divides into the radial and ulnar arteries in the middle of the cubital fossa. Deep to the brachioradialis in the lateral part of the fossa the radial nerve divides into its superficial (cutaneous) branch and the posterior interosseous nerve, the latter then passes through the supinator which clasps the upper end of the radius.

High division of the brachial artery (angiogram) (Fig. 2.49)

The brachial artery normally divides into its two terminal branches, the radial and ulnar arteries in the cubital fossa. However this division can be at a higher level and in this case one of the branches, often the radial, can be superficial in the cubital fossa and can be mistaken for a vein. The angiogram shows the high origin of the radial artery, the other branch being a common trunk for the ulnar and common interosseous arteries, the latter a major branch of the ulnar in the forearm. Also seen are the rich anastomoses around the elbow between ulnar, radial and common interosseous branches.

Lower end of the humerus and the radius and ulna (Fig. 2.50)

The upper end of the radius has a palpable head which articulates with the capitulum and it can be felt to rotate during pronation and supination of the forearm below the lateral epicondyle of the humerus. The annular ligament runs around the head. The supinator wraps around the neck and the proximal shaft. Within the supinator the posterior interosseous nerve (deep branch of radial nerve) winding around the neck is vulnerable. The radial (bicipital) tuberosity receives the insertion of the tendon of biceps. At the upper end of the ulna the coronoid process projects anteriorly. Between this and the olecranon lies the trochlear notch for articulation with the trochlea of the lower end of humerus. The shaft of the radius which is convex laterally receives the insertion of the pronator teres in its middle. The interosseous membrane connecting the radius and ulna is attached to the medial borders of the two bones and it separates the anterior (flexor) and posterior (extensor) compartments of the forearm. The deep muscles of the flexor and extensor compartments arise from interosseous membrane as well as the shafts of the two forearm bones. The expanded lower end of the radius articulates with the scaphoid and lunate at the wrist joint. The grooves in its posterior aspect hold

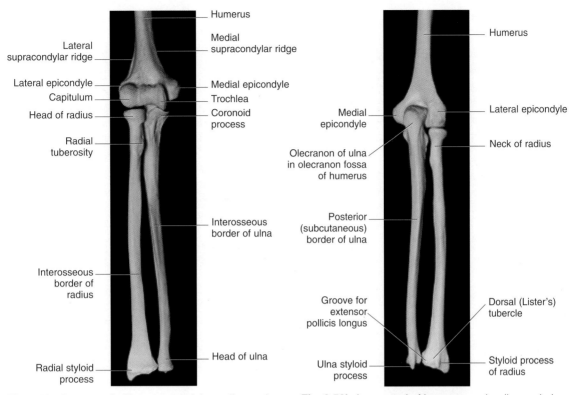

Fig. 2.50a *Lower end of humerus and the radius and ulna — anterior aspect.*

Fig. 2.50b *Lower end of humerus and radius and ulna — posterior aspect.*

the extensor tendons crossing the wrist. The tendon of the extensor pollicis longus lies in the groove medial to the Lister's (dorsal) tubercle of the radius. The ulna does not articulate with any carpal bone. The head of the ulna is covered by a fibrocartilagenous disc connecting the radius and ulna and forming a part of the inferior radioulnar joint. The shaft has a subcutaneous posterior border which gives attachment to an aponeurosis from which the flexor digitorum profundus, flexor carpi ulnaris and the extensor carpi ulnaris take origin. Surgical exposure of the ulna is usually done by incising along this border. Both radius and ulna have styloid processes. The styloid of the former is at a lower level compared to that of the latter.

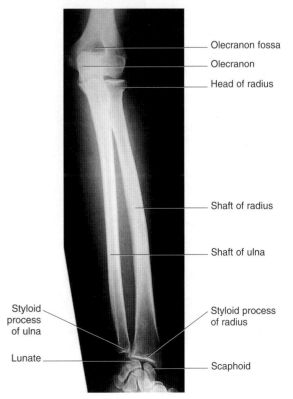

Fig. 2.50c *Radiograph of the lower end of humerus and the radius and ulna.*

Skeleton of the hand (Fig. 2.51)

The skeleton of the hand consists of eight carpal bones, five metacarpal bones and the phalanges of the fingers. The carpal bones are arranged in two rows. The proximal row from lateral to medial contains the scaphoid, lunate and triquetral with the pisiform articulating with the triquetral. The distal row has the trapezium, trapezoid, capitate and hamate. The metacarpal bones have expanded bases proximally and rounded heads at their distal ends. The first metacarpal is shorter and thicker than the others. Proximally it articulates with the trapezium to form the versatile carpometacarpal joint of the thumb. The thumb has only two phalanges, proximal and distal, whereas each of the remaining four fingers has a proximal, middle and distal phalanx.

MUSCLES OF THE FRONT OF THE FOREARM

The flexor compartment of the forearm has the muscles arranged in two groups, the superficial group containing five muscles and the deep three muscles. The bulkier flexor compartment muscles act to make the grip powerful.

The superficial muscles (Figs. 2.52, 2.53)

All the superficial muscles of the front of forearm take origin from the anterior surface of the medial epicondyle — the common flexor origin. There are additional attachments to the forearm bones as well as the deep fascia.

Pronator teres
Origin (Fig. 2.52)
The superficial head from the medial epicondyle, the deep head from the ulna.
Insertion
On the lateral surface of the middle of the shaft of the radius.
Nerve supply
The first muscular branch of the median nerve (C6,C7).
Action
It is a pronator of the forearm and a weak flexor of the elbow.

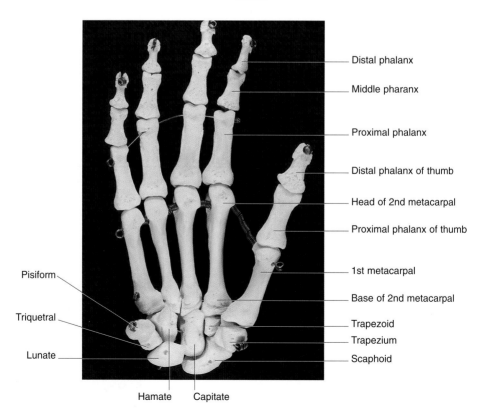

Distal phalanx

Middle pharanx

Proximal phalanx

Distal phalanx of thumb

Head of 2nd metacarpal

Proximal phalanx of thumb

1st metacarpal

Base of 2nd metacarpal

Trapezoid

Trapezium

Scaphoid

Pisiform

Triquetral

Lunate

Hamate   Capitate

Fig. 2.51 *Skeleton of the hand (also see Fig. 2.70).*

Test
Pronate the forearm against resistance and feel the muscle at the medial border of the cubital fossa.

Brachioradialis

The brachioradialis, a muscle of the extensor compartment, lies along the lateral border of the forearm.
Origin
Lateral supracondylar ridge of the humerus.
Insertion
On the base of the styloid process of the radius.
Nerve supply
By a branch of the radial nerve, given off above the elbow.
Action
It is a powerful flexor of the elbow when the forearm is in the midprone position. The muscle can be seen and felt if this action is produced against resistance.

Flexor carpi radialis

The tendon of flexor carpi radialis, enclosed in a synovial sheath, passes through the carpal tunnel to lie in the groove on the trapezium before inserting to the bases of the second and third metacarpals. In the region of the wrist the radial artery lies lateral to the tendon and the median nerve with the overlying palmaris longus medial to it.
Nerve supply
Median nerve (C6,C7).
Action
Flexes the wrist as well as abducts it (radial deviation).
Test
Flex the wrist against resistance. The tendon of the flexor carpi radialis can be seen and felt at the lateral aspect of the front of the wrist (see Fig. 2.58a).

Palmaris longus

The long flat tendon of the muscle passes in front of the flexor retinaculum to merge with the palmar aponeurosis. Just above the wrist the tendon covers the median nerve. This muscle supplied by the median nerve may be absent in about 13% of arms.

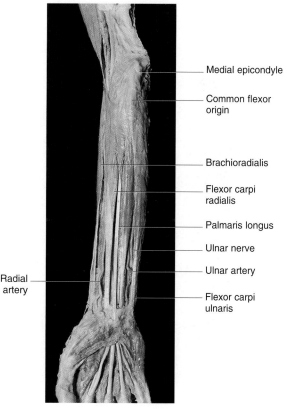

Fig. 2.52 *Common flexor origin, pronator teres.*

Common flexor origin

Pronator teres

Radial artery

Insertion of pronator teres

Brachioradialis

Fig. 2.53 *Superficial muscles of the front of forearm — flexor carpi, radialis, palmaris longus.*

Medial epicondyle

Common flexor origin

Brachioradialis

Flexor carpi radialis

Palmaris longus

Ulnar nerve

Ulnar artery

Radial artery

Flexor carpi ulnaris

Flexor digitorum superficialis (Fig. 2.54)

This muscle has four tendons which traverse the palm to be inserted to the middle phalanx of the digits. In the forearm the muscle has the median nerve adherent to its deep surface where it can be easily mistaken for a tendon during exploration.

Nerve supply
Median nerve (C7,C8).

Action
It is a flexor of the proximal interphalangeal joints and its continued action may flex the metacarpophalangeal joints and the wrist joint. It contracts to make a power grip.

Test
Flex the fingers at the proximal interphalangeal joints against resistance while the distal interphalangeal joints are held extended (to prevent the action of flexor digitorum profundus).

Flexor carpi ulnaris

At the wrist the tendon of the flexor carpi ulnaris lies medial to the ulnar artery and nerve and can be palpated. It is inserted to the pisiform, hamate and fifth metacarpal bone.

Nerve supply
Ulnar nerve.

Action
It flexes as well as adducts (ulnar deviation) the wrist.

Test
It can be tested by adducting the little finger or by flexing the wrist against resistance.

Deep muscles

Flexor digitorum profundus (Fig. 2.55)

Taking origin mostly from the anterior surface of the ulna and the interosseous membrane, this has four tendons which pass through the carpal tunnel enclosed in the same synovial sheath as the tendons of the superficialis — the ulnar bursa. In the palm the tendons proceed towards their insertion on the base of the terminal phalanx.

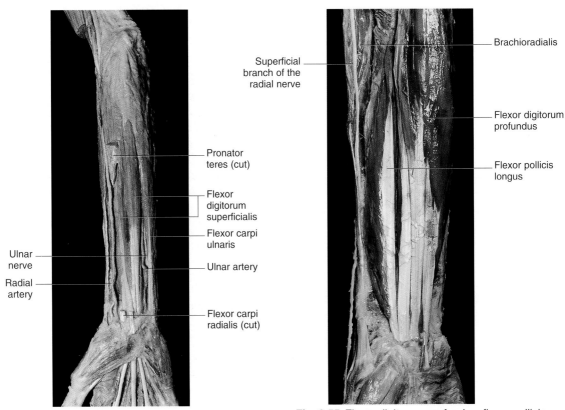

Pronator teres (cut)

Flexor digitorum superficialis

Flexor carpi ulnaris

Ulnar artery

Ulnar nerve

Radial artery

Flexor carpi radialis (cut)

Superficial branch of the radial nerve

Brachioradialis

Flexor digitorum profundus

Flexor pollicis longus

Fig. 2.54 *Flexor digitorum superficialis, flexor carpi ulnaris.*

Fig. 2.55 *Flexor digitorum profundus, flexor pollicis longus after removal of superficial muscles.*

Nerve supply

The muscle is supplied by the anterior interosseous branch of the median nerve as well as the ulnar nerve (through C8,T1 fibres).

Action

It is the only flexor of the distal interphalangeal joints and its continued action will flex the proximal interphalangeal, metacarpophalangeal and wrist joints. The power of digital flexion is maximum when the wrist is extended. Along with the superficialis this muscle makes the power grip.

Test

Flex the distal phalanx against resistance with the middle and proximal phalanges held extended.

Flexor pollicis longus

This, the long flexor of the thumb (pollex), is the only flexor of its interphalangeal joint. It takes origin from the anterior surface of the radius and the interosseous membrane and its tendon passes through the carpal tunnel ensheathed by the radial bursa (synovial sheath). It is inserted to the base of the distal phalanx of the thumb.

Nerve supply

By the anterior interosseous branch of the median nerve (C8,T1).

Action

This muscle primarily is a flexor of the interphalangeal joint of the thumb but it can also flex the metacarpophalangeal joint and the carpometacarpal joint of the thumb as well as the wrist joint.

Test

Hold the proximal phalanx of the thumb steady and flex the distal phalanx.

Pronator quadratus (Fig. 2.56)

This quadrangular muscle arises from the distal end of the shaft of the ulna and is inserted to the anterior surface of the lower fourth of the radius. It is supplied by the anterior interosseous nerve (C7,C8). It is a pronator of the forearm and it also helps to hold the radius and ulna together when the hand is weight bearing.

Space of Parona

This is a fascial space of surgical importance. It is anterior to the pronator quadratus and extends upwards up to the oblique line of attachment of the flexor digitorum superficialis to the radius. Into the space of Parona protrude the synovial sheaths of the flexor tendons and infection can extend into it when the sheaths are affected. Drainage is facilitated by incisions on either side of the flexor tendons.

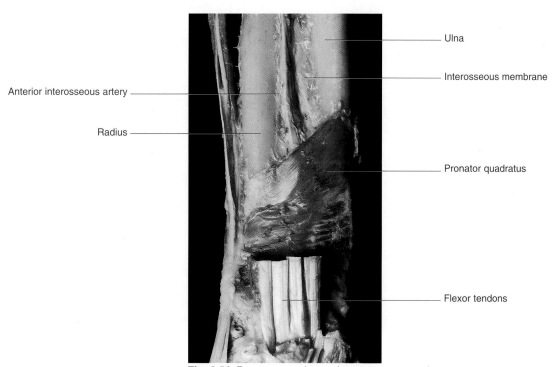

Fig. 2.56 *Pronator quadratus, interosseous membrane.*

Median nerve

Brachial artery

Ulnar artery

Pronator teres (cut)

Radial artery

Median nerve

Flexor carpi ulnaris

Ulnar nerve

Ulnar artery

Flexor carpi radialis (cut)

Median nerve

Fig. 2.57a *Arteries and nerves in the front of the forearm.*

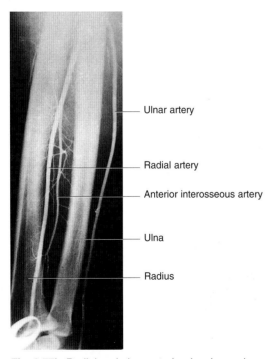

Ulnar artery

Radial artery

Anterior interosseous artery

Ulna

Radius

Fig. 2.57b *Radial and ulnar arteries (angiogram).*

ARTERIES AND NERVES OF THE FOREARM (Fig. 2.57)

The division of brachial artery into radial and ulnar arteries is seen in the cubital fossa, and the latter is seen going deep to the pronator teres. As it descends the ulnar artery lies on the flexor digitorum profundus and is accompanied by the ulnar nerve on its medial side. The artery and the nerve are under cover of the flexor carpi ulnaris, except at the lower end where they lie lateral to the tendon of the muscle. The nerve and the artery enter the palm passing superficial to the flexor retinaculum. In the forearm the ulnar artery gives off the common interosseous artery which in turn divides into anterior and posterior interosseous branches. The radial artery as it descends lies on the supinator, the insertion of the pronator teres, radial origin of the flexor digitorum superficialis, flexor pollicis longus and the pronator quadratus. Distally it winds round the radius deep to the tendons of the abductor pollicis longus and extensor pollicis brevis to reach the anatomical snuff box. In the upper part the artery is covered by the brachioradialis. In the lower part of the forearm it is more superficial and its pulsation can easily be felt lateral to the tendon of the flexor carpi radialis.

The median nerve leaves the cubital fossa by passing between the two heads of the pronator teres. At the distal aspect of the forearm the nerve lies medial to the tendon of the flexor carpi radialis almost covered by the tendon of the palmaris longus. It then passes through the carpal tunnel to enter the palm. The median nerve and its anterior interosseous branch given off in the forearm together supply all the muscles in the front of the forearm except flexor carpi ulnaris and the medial half of the profundus which are supplied by the ulnar nerve.

PALM OF THE HAND

Surface anatomy of the wrist and hand (Fig. 2.58)

The proximal wrist crease is at the level of the wrist joint. On flexing the wrist the flexor carpi radialis, the palmaris longus, the flexor digitorum superficialis as well as the flexor carpi ulnaris can be seen and felt. The radial artery pulsation is felt lateral to the flexor carpi radialis. This is the usual site for arterial cannulation. The surface marking of the radial artery is along a line connecting a point medial to the tendon of the biceps to the point where its pulsation is felt.

The pulsation of the ulnar artery can be felt at the distal end of the forearm lateral to the tendon of the flexor carpi ulnaris. It can be exposed in the lower part of the forearm by displacing the flexor carpi ulnaris and by safeguarding the ulnar nerve.

The median nerve is located between the flexor carpi radialis and the palmaris longus and the ulnar nerve and artery lateral to the flexor carpi ulnaris.

The skin of the palm is adherent to the underlying connective tissue. The fixity will prevent the skin from slipping over objects whilst gripping. The flexure creases (lines of the palm) and papillary ridges also improve the grip. There is an abundance of sweat glands on the palm. The cutaneous innervation of the palm and digits are through the median and ulnar nerves. The palm is supplied by the palmar branches of the nerves. The digital branches of the median nerve supply the skin of the lateral three and a half fingers and that of the ulnar nerve the medial one and a half fingers.

The proximal limit of the flexor retinaculum is in level with the distal skin wrist crease. The tubercle of the scaphoid and the pisiform are palpable at this level. The trapezium and the hook of the hamate are felt deep to the overlying thenar and hypothenar muscles. Tenderness can be elicited by pressing the ulnar nerve against the hook of the hamate.

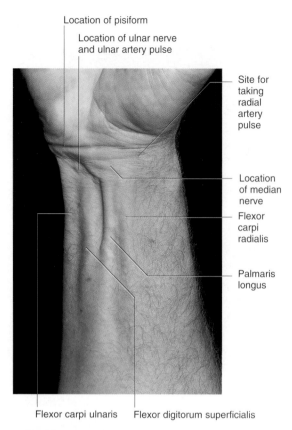

Fig. 2.58a *Surface anatomy of the wrist.*

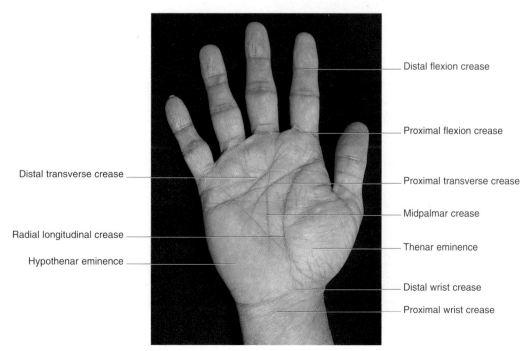

Fig. 2.58b *Surface anatomy of the hand.*

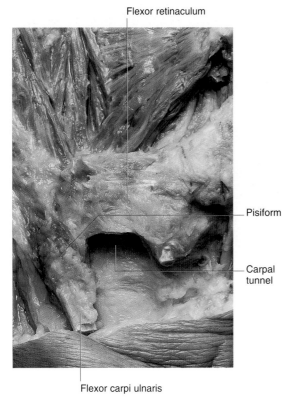

Flexor retinaculum

Pisiform

Carpal tunnel

Flexor carpi ulnaris

Fig. 2.59a *Flexor retinaculum and the carpal tunnel (after removal of most of the related structures).*

Flexor retinaculum and the carpal tunnel (Fig. 2.59)

The flexor retinaculum is a thickening of the deep fascia bridging the concavity across the anterior surfaces of the carpal bones to prevent 'bow stringing' of the flexor tendons passing deep to it. It is attached to the scaphoid and trapezium laterally and to the pisiform and hook of the hamate medially. The carpal tunnel is the space between the flexor retinaculum and the anterior concavity of the carpal bones.

The carpal tunnel is packed with the flexor tendons entering the hand. The median nerve goes through the tunnel. The nerve can be compressed by swelling of the tendons or by arthritis affecting the joints of the carpal bones increasing pressure in the tunnel. The condition is known as carpal tunnel syndrome, which manifests as pain and diminished sensation on the skin along the distribution of the median nerve to the digits as well as weakness of the thenar muscles. The thenar and hypothenar muscles take origin from the flexor retinaculum. The ulnar nerve as well as the palmar cutaneous branch of the median nerve (supplying skin over the thenar eminence) lie superficial to the retinaculum. The ulnar nerve along with the artery is covered by a band of fibrous tissue forming the Guyon's canal (also see Fig. 2.61a) as it passes over the flexor retinaculum. The ulnar nerve may become compressed

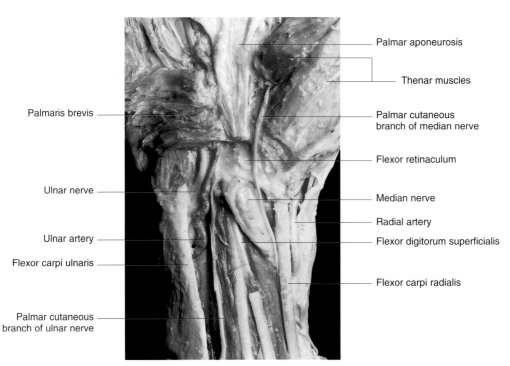

Palmar aponeurosis

Thenar muscles

Palmar cutaneous branch of median nerve

Flexor retinaculum

Median nerve

Radial artery

Flexor digitorum superficialis

Flexor carpi radialis

Palmaris brevis

Ulnar nerve

Ulnar artery

Flexor carpi ulnaris

Palmar cutaneous branch of ulnar nerve

Fig. 2.59b *Flexor retinaculum and carpal tunnel with related structures.*

as it lies in the Guyon's canal and it is not that easily blocked by local anaesthetic agents at the flexor retinaculum because of its fibrous covering.

The palmar aponeurosis (Fig. 2.60)

This lies immediately deep to the subcutaneous tissue of the palm. It extends distally from the flexor retinaculum and divides into four slips, one to each finger, to be attached to the fibrous flexor sheath. The palmar aponeurosis is clinically important as it can be affected by Dupuytren's contracture in its medial part. In this condition the aponeurosis undergoes fibrosis to produce flexion deformity of the medial two fingers.

The subcutaneous palmaris brevis muscle which stretches across the hypothenar muscles is supplied by the superficial branch of the ulnar nerve. Its contraction may steady the grip on the ulnar side of the palm.

Superficial and deep palmar arches (Fig. 2.61)

Deep to the palmar aponeurosis lies the superficial palmar arch, the arterial arcade formed by the ulnar artery with a small contribution from the radial artery. This contribution may be missing and hence the arch incomplete (Fig. 2.61a).

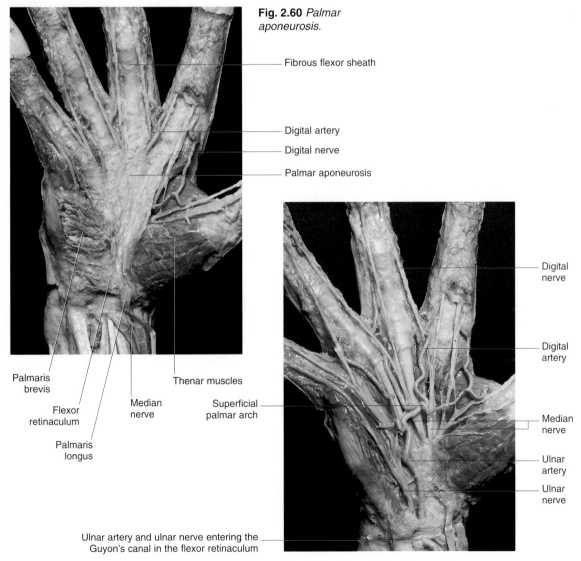

Fig. 2.60 *Palmar aponeurosis.*

Fibrous flexor sheath

Digital artery

Digital nerve

Palmar aponeurosis

Palmaris brevis

Flexor retinaculum

Palmaris longus

Median nerve

Thenar muscles

Superficial palmar arch

Digital nerve

Digital artery

Median nerve

Ulnar artery

Ulnar nerve

Ulnar artery and ulnar nerve entering the Guyon's canal in the flexor retinaculum

Fig. 2.61a *Superficial palmar arch.*

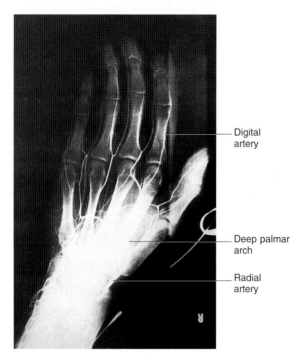

Fig. 2.61b *Angiogram of radial artery and the deep palmar arch. (The deep palmar arch is partly obscured by the opacity of the metacarpal bones.)*

The arch gives off four digital branches; the first three run distally to the webs of the fingers where they divide to supply the adjacent fingers. The fourth digital branch supplies the medial surface of the little finger. The digital arteries are accompanied by the digital branches of the ulnar and the median nerves.

The deep palmar arch lies deep to the flexor tendons and is usually complete. It runs across the palm about 1 cm proximal to the superficial arch.

The radial artery is usually selected for arterial cannulation (Fig. 2.61b). Checking for the integrity of the palmar arches is carried out before cannulation as there is a small risk of thrombosis of the artery. This is done by the Allen's test in which the arterial flow to the hand is stopped by occluding the arteries by firm finger pressure. The hand is then exsanguinated by clenching the fist a few times. The pressure on the radial artery is maintained while that on the ulnar is removed. If the hand flushes rapidly the ulnar inflow is satisfactory. The test is repeated keeping the ulnar artery occluded and releasing the radial artery to test the radial inflow.

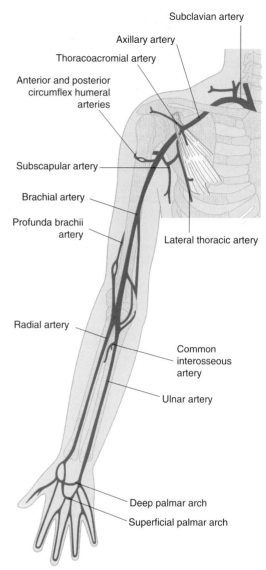

Fig. 2.61c *Summary diagram showing the arteries of the upper limb.*

The median and the ulnar nerves
(Fig. 2.62)

The ulnar nerve divides into a superficial and a deep branch as it leaves the flexor retinaculum. The superficial branch, which can be palpated as it lies on the hook of the hamate, gives off two digital branches that supply the ulnar one and a half fingers. The deep branch passes deeply between the hypothenar muscles and supplies all the interossei, both heads of the adductor pollicis, the medial two lumbricals and the three hypothenar muscles.

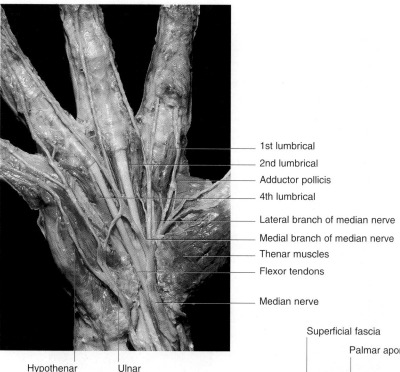

1st lumbrical
2nd lumbrical
Adductor pollicis
4th lumbrical
Lateral branch of median nerve
Medial branch of median nerve
Thenar muscles
Flexor tendons
Median nerve

Hypothenar muscles   Ulnar nerve

Fig. 2.62 *Median and ulnar nerves in the hand (flexor retinaculum is partially removed).*

The median nerve divides into a medial and a lateral branch, the former dividing again to supply the ring, middle and the index fingers as well as the second lumbrical muscle. The lateral branch divides further to supply the radial side of the index finger and the whole of the thumb. The branch to the index finger supplies the first lumbrical.

The palmar digital branches at the distal aspect wind around the fingers to supply the skin on the dorsum of the terminal phalanges as well.

The thenar muscles (Fig. 2.63)

There are three muscles in this group — the abductor pollicis brevis, flexor pollicis brevis and the opponens. They take origin from the flexor retinaculum and the adjoining carpal bones. The abductor and the flexor are inserted to the lateral aspect of the first phalanx of the thumb. The opponens lies deep to these two muscles and is inserted to the first metacarpal bone. Distal to the flexor retinaculum the median nerve gives a recurrent branch which curls backwards over the retinaculum to supply the three thenar muscles. The

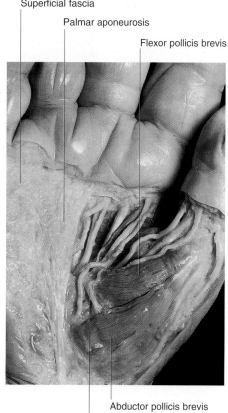

Superficial fascia
Palmar aponeurosis
Flexor pollicis brevis
Abductor pollicis brevis
Recurrent branch of median nerve supplying thenar muscles

Fig. 2.63 *Thenar muscles and the recurrent branch of median nerve.*

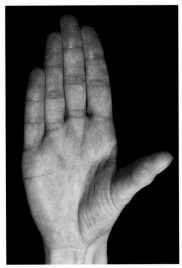

Fig. 2.64a *Palmar abduction of thumb.*

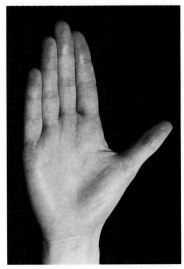

Fig. 2.64b *Radial abduction of thumb.*

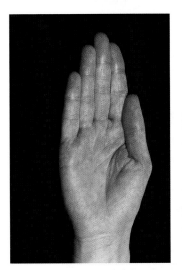

Fig. 2.64c *Adduction of thumb.*

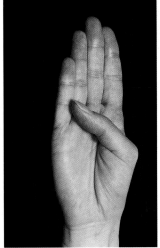

Fig. 2.64d *Transpalmar adduction of thumb.*

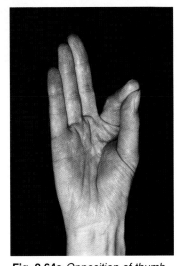

Fig. 2.64e *Opposition of thumb.*

 recurrent branch is relatively superficial and can easily be damaged by superficial cuts and incisions in this area. Such an injury will impair the grip by affecting the movements of thumb.

Test

The abductor pollicis brevis being superficial can easily be tested. Bring the thumb forward at right angles to the plane of the palm against resistance and feel the muscle contracting.

Movements of the thumb (Fig. 2.64)

The following are the movements of the thumb redefined by the International Federation of Societies for Surgery of the Hand:

- Palmar abduction — In this movement, produced by abductor pollicis brevis, the thumb moves away from the index finger at right angles to the plane of the palm keeping the thumbnail in a plane at right angles to that of the four fingernails.

- Radial abduction — The thumb is moved away from the index finger in the plane of the palm by abductor pollicis longus and extensor pollicis brevis. The

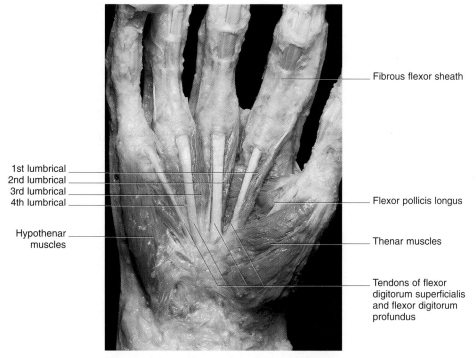

1st lumbrical
2nd lumbrical
3rd lumbrical
4th lumbrical

Hypothenar muscles

Fibrous flexor sheath

Flexor pollicis longus

Thenar muscles

Tendons of flexor digitorum superficialis and flexor digitorum profundus

Fig. 2.65a *Long flexor tendons, lumbricals and hypothenar muscles.*

opposite movement of adduction is produced by adductor pollicis and can be continued across the palm by flexor pollicis brevis.

- Opposition — In this the pulp of the thumb is made to face the pulp of another finger (as in holding a pin between thumb and index finger) by medially rotating and adducting the first metacarpal bone at its joint with the trapezium. This is done mostly by the opponens pollicis.

The flexor tendons (Fig. 2.65)

The tendons of the flexor digitorum superficialis and profundus lie deep to the superficial palmar arch. The tendons of the profundus lie deep to those of the superficialis. They pass in pairs into the fibrous flexor sheaths of fingers. At the proximal part of each finger the superficialis is tunnelled through by the profundus tendon. The superficialis is inserted to the base of the middle phalanx and the profundus to the terminal phalanx. The tendon of the flexor pollicis longus is inserted to the base of the terminal phalanx of the thumb.

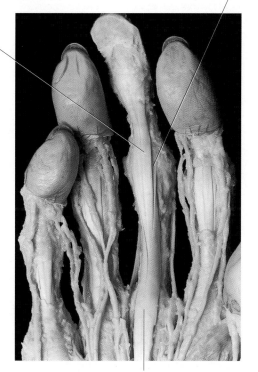

Flexor digitorum superficialis

Flexor digitorum profundus

Flexor digitorum superficialis

Fig. 2.65b *Insertion of flexor digitorum superficialis and flexor digitorum profundus.*

The lumbrical muscles

There are four lumbrical muscles in the hand, one for each finger. Each muscle takes origin from the flexor digitorum profundus tendon, crosses the root of the finger laterally and is inserted to the dorsal digital expansion at the back of the finger. How the lumbrical muscles of the hand function is not clearly understood. Many anatomists are of the view that the muscles are used to simultaneously flex the metacarpophalangeal and extend the interphalangeal joints. The lateral two lumbricals are usually supplied by the median nerve and the medial two lumbricals by the ulnar nerve.

The attachments of the hypothenar muscles — abductor, flexor and opponens digiti minimi — are mirror images of those of the thenar muscles and they act on the little finger.

Synovial sheath

The flexor tendons are enclosed by synovial sheaths. In the fibrous flexor sheath both tendons are invested by a common synovial sheath. The tendons receive their blood supply through synovial folds known as vincula, each tendon having two, vincula longa and vincula brevia. The sheath of the little finger is continuous with the ulnar bursa covering the flexor tendons in the palm. The flexor pollicis longus is covered by a single sheath throughout, the radial bursa. The arrangement of the synovial sheaths for these tendons is illustrated in Fig. 2.66. Synovial sheaths can be infected producing tenosynovitis. Infection can spread throughout the sheath. Infection of the sheath of the little finger can thus spread up the distal aspect of the forearm into the space of Parona.

Fibrous flexor sheath (Fig. 2.67)

The flexor tendons are held on to the front of the finger by the fibrous flexor sheath. The tendons move inside the sheath during flexion and extension. However narrowing of the space in the sheath can occur by thickening of the sheath or nodular thickening of the tendon. The finger may then click painfully when

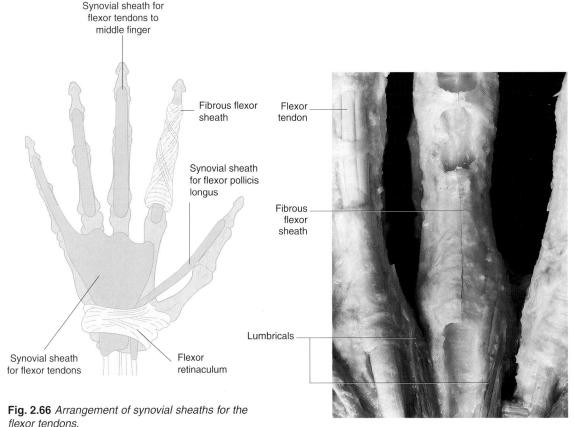

Fig. 2.66 *Arrangement of synovial sheaths for the flexor tendons.*

Synovial sheath for flexor tendons to middle finger

Fibrous flexor sheath

Synovial sheath for flexor pollicis longus

Synovial sheath for flexor tendons

Flexor retinaculum

Flexor tendon

Fibrous flexor sheath

Lumbricals

Fig. 2.67 *Fibrous flexor sheath.*

attempting to bend it, or when the hand is unclenched the affected finger can remain bent and may suddenly straighten with a snap — a 'trigger finger'.

Adductor pollicis (Fig. 2.68)

This muscle located deep in the palm has two heads of origin, the transverse head arising from the third metacarpal bone and the oblique head from the bases of the second and third metacarpal bones and the capitate. The two heads converge to its insertion to the medial aspect of the first phalanx of the thumb. It is supplied by the deep branch of the ulnar nerve.

Interosseous muscles (Fig. 2.69)

The interosseous muscles lie in the interosseus spaces between the metacarpal bones. They are in two groups, palmar and dorsal. The palmar interossei are arranged in such a way that they produce adduction of the fingers by moving them towards the middle finger. The dorsal interossei are abductors of the fingers, i.e. moving the fingers away from the axis of the movement going through the middle of the middle finger. It is easier to work out the arrangement of the

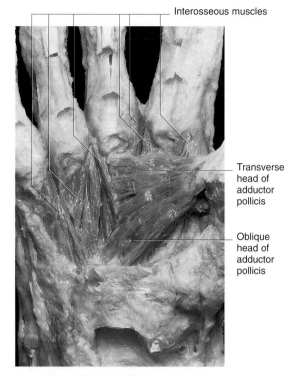

Interosseous muscles

Transverse head of adductor pollicis

Oblique head of adductor pollicis

Fig. 2.68 *Adductor pollicis.*

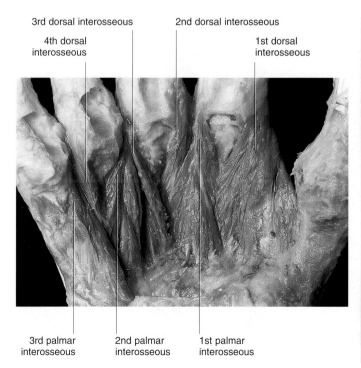

3rd dorsal interosseous

4th dorsal interosseous

2nd dorsal interosseous

1st dorsal interosseous

3rd palmar interosseous

2nd palmar interosseous

1st palmar interosseous

Fig. 2.69a *Palmar and dorsal interosseous muscles.*

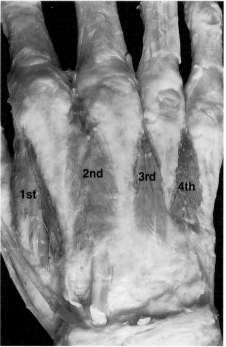

Fig. 2.69b *Dorsal interossei seen from the posterior aspect of hand (dorsum of hand).*

interosseous muscles by remembering the words PAD (palmar interossei adducts) and DAB (dorsal interossei abduct). When the palmar and the dorsal interossei act together they, like the lumbricals, can flex the metacarpophalangeal joints and extend the interphalangeal joints. All the interossei are supplied by the deep branch of the ulnar nerve.

Injuries to the carpal bones

Fracture of the scaphoid and dislocation of the lunate are common injuries sustained by the carpal bones. The scaphoid fractures through its waist (middle portion). The artery to the bone usually enters its distal half and hence when it fractures the proximal half will be without blood supply and may undergo avascular necrosis. A fall on the hand may dislocate the lunate bone or may dislocate the whole carpus backwards with the lunate remaining stationary (perilunar dislocation). These injuries tear the soft tissue and produce avascular necrosis of the bone and may also damage the median nerve.

BACK OF THE FOREARM AND HAND

The superficial extensor muscles at the back of the forearm (Fig. 2.71)

The extensor carpi radialis longus takes origin from the lateral supracondylar ridge just below the origin of the brachioradialis. The extensor carpi radialis brevis, the extensor digitorum, the extensor carpi ulnaris and the extensor digiti minimi have a common origin from the front of the lateral epicondyle (common extensor origin). The extensors of the carpus are inserted into the metacarpal bones. Four tendons arise from the extensor digitorum which pass deep to the extensor retinaculum to enter the dorsum of the hand where they spread out to reach their insertions on the dorsal aspect of the digits. All these muscles are supplied by the posterior interosseous branch of the radial nerve, except the extensor carpi radialis longus, which like the brachioradialis is supplied by the radial nerve just above the elbow (see wrist drop, p. 59).

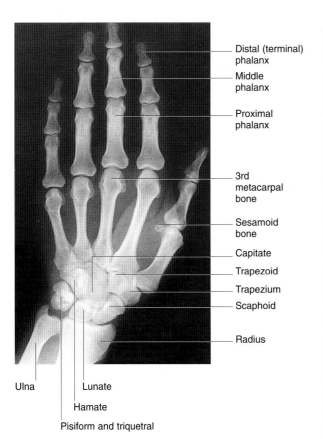

Distal (terminal) phalanx
Middle phalanx
Proximal phalanx
3rd metacarpal bone
Sesamoid bone
Capitate
Trapezoid
Trapezium
Scaphoid
Radius
Ulna
Lunate
Hamate
Pisiform and triquetral

Fig. 2.70 *Radiograph of the hand.*

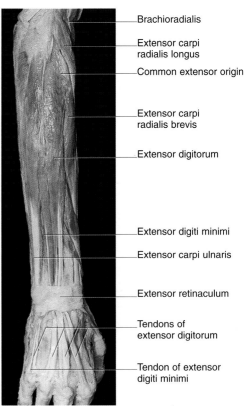

Brachioradialis
Extensor carpi radialis longus
Common extensor origin
Extensor carpi radialis brevis
Extensor digitorum
Extensor digiti minimi
Extensor carpi ulnaris
Extensor retinaculum
Tendons of extensor digitorum
Tendon of extensor digiti minimi

Fig. 2.71 *Superficial extensor muscles at the back of forearm.*

Extensor retinaculum (Fig. 2.72)

The extensor retinaculum is a thick band of deep fascia attached proximally to the anterolateral border of the radius above the styloid process and distally and medially to the pisiform and triquetral bones. It has no attachment to the ulna. The retinaculum which is comparable to the flexor retinaculum prevents bowstringing of the extensor tendons when the hand is hyperextended. The extensor tendons lie in six separate compartments deep to the retinaculum. The tendons are enclosed in synovial sheaths. The abductor pollicis longus and the extensor pollicis brevis can be seen superficially in the distal part of the forearm winding round the radius before passing deep to the retinaculum.

The deep extensors (Fig. 2.73)

This group contains the long abductor and the extensors of the thumb as well as the extensor indicis. They are attached to both the ulna and radius and the interosseous membrane. The extensor pollicis longus tendon winding round the dorsal tubercle (Lister's tubercle) of the radius on its way to its insertion to the distal phalanx of thumb can rupture spontaneously or as a consequence of fracture of the lower end of the radius (Colles' fracture). The flexor pollicis longus will then overact producing a flexion deformity of the distal phalanx of the thumb (hammer thumb). The extensor indicis is an additional extensor for the index finger. Its tendon joins the ulnar side of the extensor digitorum tendon on the index finger. This muscle can be connected on to the tendon of the extensor pollicis longus to repair a hammer thumb.

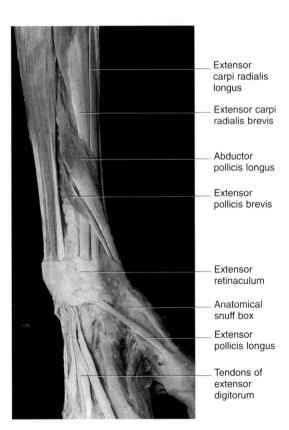

Extensor carpi radialis longus

Extensor carpi radialis brevis

Abductor pollicis longus

Extensor pollicis brevis

Extensor retinaculum

Anatomical snuff box

Extensor pollicis longus

Tendons of extensor digitorum

Fig. 2.72 *Extensor retinaculum and the extensor tendons on the lateral aspect of wrist and hand.*

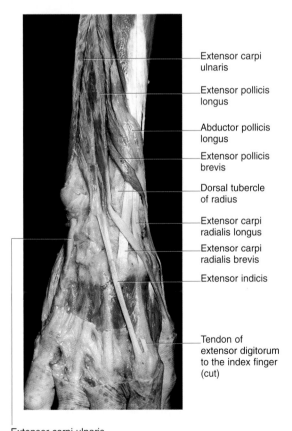

Extensor carpi ulnaris

Extensor pollicis longus

Abductor pollicis longus

Extensor pollicis brevis

Dorsal tubercle of radius

Extensor carpi radialis longus

Extensor carpi radialis brevis

Extensor indicis

Tendon of extensor digitorum to the index finger (cut)

Extensor carpi ulnaris

Fig. 2.73 *Deep extensors at the back of the forearm. (All the superficial extensors except extensor carpi radialis longus and brevis and extensor carpi ulnaris have been removed.)*

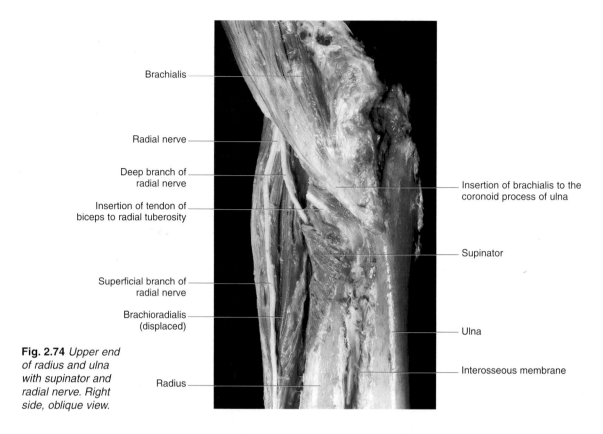

Brachialis

Radial nerve

Deep branch of radial nerve

Insertion of tendon of biceps to radial tuberosity

Superficial branch of radial nerve

Brachioradialis (displaced)

Radius

Insertion of brachialis to the coronoid process of ulna

Supinator

Ulna

Interosseous membrane

Fig. 2.74 *Upper end of radius and ulna with supinator and radial nerve. Right side, oblique view.*

Supinator (Fig. 2.74)

This muscle covering the upper part of the back of the radius lies deep to the brachioradialis and the superficial extensors. The muscle is closely related to the radial nerve. The posterior interosseous branch of the radial nerve (deep branch of the radial) passes through the supinator before giving its branches to the extensor muscles in the forearm. The supinator which is inserted into the posterolateral aspect of the upper part of the radius supinates the forearm in the extended position.

Dorsum of the hand, anatomical snuff box — surface anatomy (Fig. 2.75)

The space proximal to the thumb bounded medially by the extensor pollicis longus and laterally by the tendons of the abductor pollicis longus and the extensor pollicis brevis is the anatomical snuff box. The scaphoid bone forms its floor. The radial artery lies in it and the cephalic vein and the superficial branch of the radial nerve cross it superficially. After a fall on the outstretched hand, tenderness in the anatomical snuff box is suggestive of a fracture of the scaphoid bone. The

tendons of the extensor digitorum are also visible as the wrist is extended against resistance. The metacarpal bones are easily palpable on the dorsum of the hand.

Superficial structures at the dorsum of the hand (Fig. 2.76)

The veins in the digits drain into a dorsal venous arch from which the cephalic and basilic veins are formed. The former crosses the anatomical snuff box and courses upwards along the lateral aspect in the front of the forearm. The basilic vein arising from the medial aspect of the venous arch runs upwards along the posteromedial aspect of the forearm. The superficial branch of the radial nerve and the dorsal branch of ulnar nerves innervate the skin of the dorsum of the hand and digits. The radial nerve supplies the lateral two and a half or even three and a half fingers (variable) and the corresponding region of the dorsum of the hand. The remaining medial aspect is supplied by the ulnar nerve. The dorsal aspect of the terminal phalanges are supplied by the palmar digital branches (median and ulnar nerves) winding round the borders of the digits to reach the dorsal aspect. The radial artery reaches the anatomical snuff box by winding

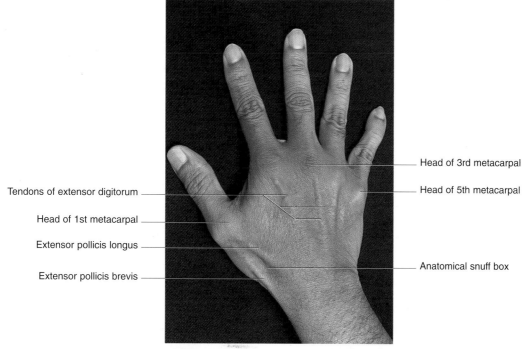

Tendons of extensor digitorum

Head of 1st metacarpal

Extensor pollicis longus

Extensor pollicis brevis

Head of 3rd metacarpal

Head of 5th metacarpal

Anatomical snuff box

Fig. 2.75 *Dorsum of the hand — surface anatomy.*

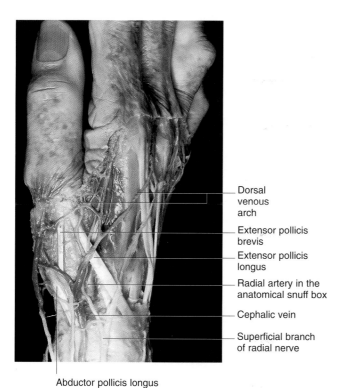

Dorsal venous arch

Extensor pollicis brevis

Extensor pollicis longus

Radial artery in the anatomical snuff box

Cephalic vein

Superficial branch of radial nerve

Abductor pollicis longus

Fig. 2.76a *Superficial structures on the dorsum of hand — lateral aspect.*

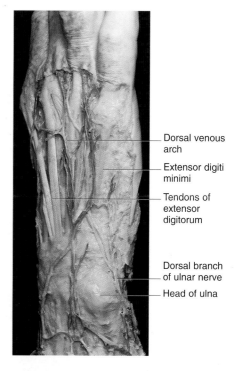

Dorsal venous arch

Extensor digiti minimi

Tendons of extensor digitorum

Dorsal branch of ulnar nerve

Head of ulna

Fig. 2.76b *Superficial structures on the dorsum of hand — medial aspect.*

round the lateral border of the wrist. From there it passes deep to the extensor pollicis longus tendon before piercing the first dorsal interosseous muscle to reach the palm of the hand to become the deep palmar arch.

Extensor tendons on the dorsum of the hand (Fig. 2.77)

The extensors of the carpus are inserted into the metacarpal bones; the radial (lateral) extensors into the bases of the first and second metacarpal bones and the ulnar extensor into the fifth metacarpal bone. The extensor digitorum forms the extensor expansion at the back of the fingers (see below) and the extensor digiti minimi which divides into two slips reinforces the extensor expansion at the back of the little finger. The extensor indicis is an additional extensor for the index finger. Its tendon joins the ulnar side of the extensor digitorum tendon on the index finger.

The tendons reaching the thumb are inserted as follows:

- Abductor pollicis longus to the lateral aspect of the base of the first metacarpal bone.
- Extensor pollicis brevis to the base of the first phalanx.
- Extensor pollicis longus to the base of the distal phalanx.

The extensor expansion (dorsal digital expansion) (Fig. 2.78)

At the wrist the extensor digitorum gives rise to four tendons which supply digits 2–5. Each slip forms an expanded hood over the dorsum of the digit. The expansion is attached to the base of the proximal phalanx before dividing into a central and two marginal slips. The central slip is inserted into the base of the middle phalanx. The marginal slips unite together and insert to the base of the distal phalanx. The interossei and the lumbricals are inserted into the proximal part of the extensor expansion.

THE JOINTS OF THE FOREARM AND HAND

Elbow joint (Fig. 2.79)

Osteology
At the elbow joint the upper surface of the head of radius articulates with the capitulum of the humerus and the trochlea of the humerus with the trochlear notch of the ulna. The capsule of the elbow encloses the superior radioulnar joint where the head of the radius articulates with the radial notch of the ulna.

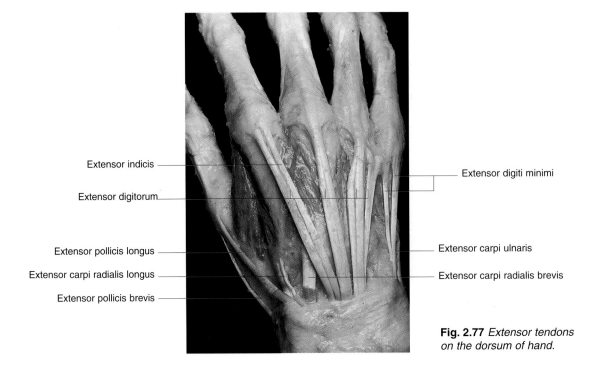

Extensor indicis

Extensor digitorum

Extensor pollicis longus

Extensor carpi radialis longus

Extensor pollicis brevis

Extensor digiti minimi

Extensor carpi ulnaris

Extensor carpi radialis brevis

Fig. 2.77 *Extensor tendons on the dorsum of hand.*

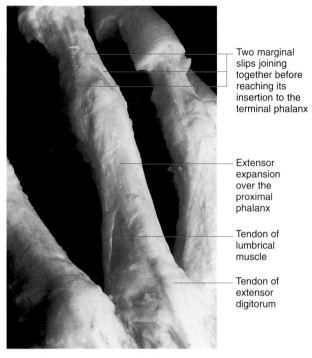

Two marginal slips joining together before reaching its insertion to the terminal phalanx

Extensor expansion over the proximal phalanx

Tendon of lumbrical muscle

Tendon of extensor digitorum

Fig. 2.78 *Extensor expansion or dorsal digital expansion.*

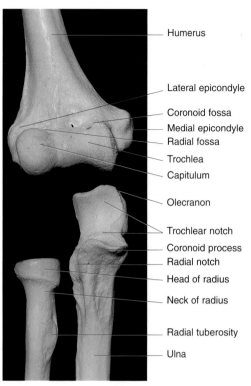

Humerus

Lateral epicondyle

Coronoid fossa

Medial epicondyle

Radial fossa

Trochlea

Capitulum

Olecranon

Trochlear notch

Coronoid process

Radial notch

Head of radius

Neck of radius

Radial tuberosity

Ulna

Fig. 2.79a *Lower end of humerus and upper ends of radius and ulna — anterior aspect.*

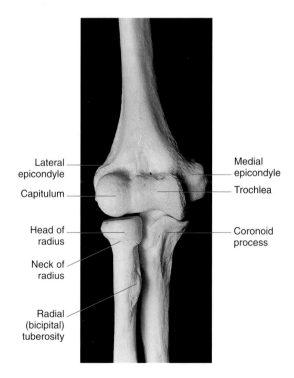

Lateral epicondyle

Capitulum

Head of radius

Neck of radius

Radial (bicipital) tuberosity

Medial epicondyle

Trochlea

Coronoid process

Fig. 2.79b *Bones of the elbow in the articulated position — anterior aspect.*

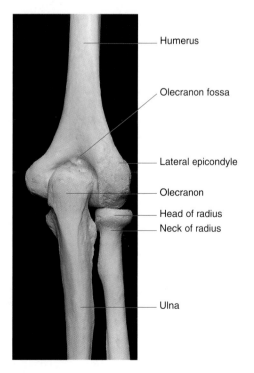

Humerus

Olecranon fossa

Lateral epicondyle

Olecranon

Head of radius

Neck of radius

Ulna

Fig. 2.79c *Bones of the elbow joint in the articulated position — posterior aspect.*

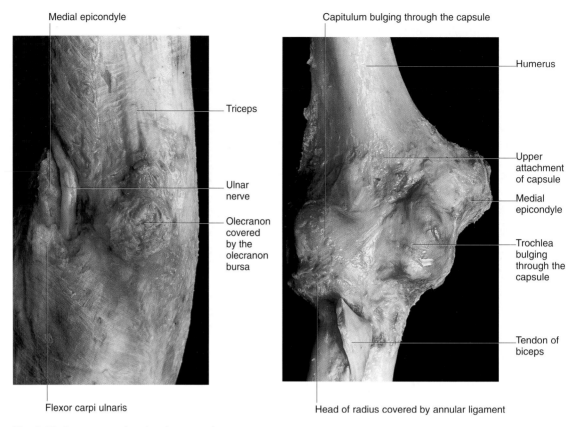

Fig. 2.80 *Structures related to the posterior aspect of the elbow joint.*

Fig. 2.81a *Capsule of the elbow joint — anterior aspect.*

Relations of the joint (Fig. 2.80)

Posteriorly there is the insertion of the triceps to the olecranon. The ulnar nerve lies on the back of the medial epicondyle and on the medial collateral ligament of the joint and may be damaged in a posterior dislocation. The brachial artery, the median and the radial nerves lie in front of the elbow joint. Also anteriorly there is the insertion of the tendon of the biceps to the radial tuberosity and that of the brachialis to the coronoid process of the ulna; the common flexor origin from the medial epicondyle and the common extensor origin from the lateral epicondyle are the other anterior relations of the joint.

The surgical approaches to the joint are usually from the medial or the lateral sides. In the medial approach the common flexor origin is detached after displacing the ulnar nerve to expose the capsule. In the lateral approach the common extensor origin is detached. The posterior interosseous nerve is vulnerable if the incision is extended below the level of the head of the radius.

Capsule and the interior of the joint (Fig. 2.81, 2.82, 2.83)

The elbow joint is a synovial joint. The capsular attachment on the humerus extends from the outer margins of the capitulum and trochlea upwards to enclose the olecranon fossa posteriorly and the coronoid fossa and radial fossa anteriorly. The medial and lateral epicondyles and the supracondylar ridges are extracapsular. Distally the capsule is attached to the margins of the trochlear notch. The capsule, and the olecranon, coronoid and radial fossae are all lined by synovial membrane.

Ligaments

The capsule is reinforced by extracapsular ligaments on either side. The triangular medial (ulnar) collateral ligament is attached to the medial epicondyle, coronoid process and the olecranon (Fig. 2.82). The ulnar nerve lies on this ligament. The lateral (radial) collateral ligament extends from the lateral epicondyle to the annular ligament. It is not attached to the radius.

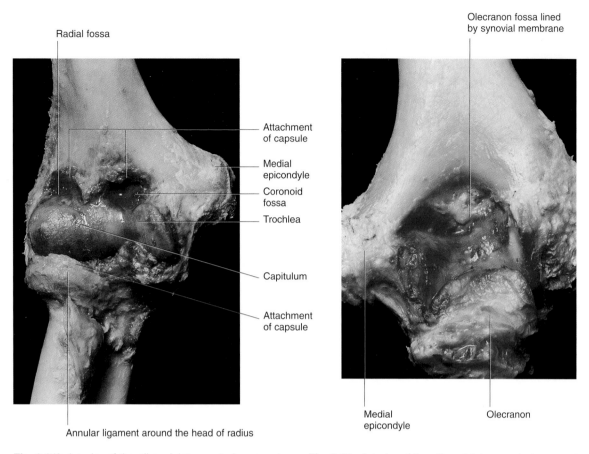

Radial fossa

Attachment
of capsule

Medial
epicondyle

Coronoid
fossa

Trochlea

Capitulum

Attachment
of capsule

Annular ligament around the head of radius

Olecranon fossa lined
by synovial membrane

Medial
epicondyle

Olecranon

Fig. 2.81b *Interior of the elbow joint — anterior aspect.*

Fig. 2.81c *Interior of the elbow joint — posterior aspect (elbow in semiflexed position).*

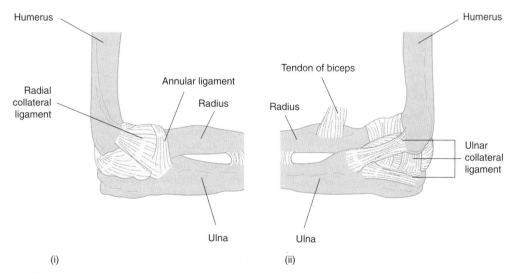

Humerus

Radial
collateral
ligament

Annular ligament

Radius

Ulna

(i)

Tendon of biceps

Radius

Humerus

Ulnar
collateral
ligament

Ulna

(ii)

Fig. 2.82 *Right elbow joint: (i) lateral view; (ii) medial view.*

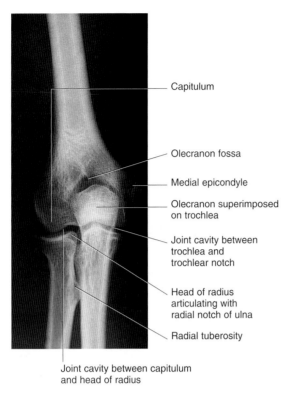

Capitulum

Olecranon fossa

Medial epicondyle

Olecranon superimposed on trochlea

Joint cavity between trochlea and trochlear notch

Head of radius articulating with radial notch of ulna

Radial tuberosity

Joint cavity between capitulum and head of radius

Fig. 2.83a *Anteroposterior radiograph of elbow joint.*

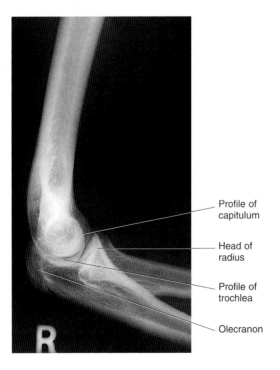

Profile of capitulum

Head of radius

Profile of trochlea

Olecranon

Fig. 2.83b *Lateral radiograph of the elbow joint — semi-flexed position.*

Movements

The long axis of the ulna is not in line with that of the humerus but is shifted outwards making the carrying angle about 170°. An increase of this valgus angle (cubitus valgus) due to fractures or epiphyseal injuries will stretch the ulnar nerve. The normal carrying angle of the elbow joint causes the axis of movements to be in an oblique plane. Flexion is about 140° and is done primarily by the brachialis and the biceps muscles and extension by the triceps muscle.

THE RADIOULNAR JOINTS: PRONATION AND SUPINATION

In the superior radioulnar joint, which shares the capsule of the elbow joint, the head of the radius articulates with the radial notch of the ulna. The two bones are held together by the annular ligament (Fig. 2.84a). The ligament is attached to the anterior and posterior margins of the radial notch of the ulna but is not attached to the radius. It circles round the head and neck of the radius. The upper end of the radius is totally free of ligamentous attachments enabling the radius to rotate freely inside the annular ligament. The inferior radioulnar joint between the head of the ulna is outside the capsule of the wrist joint. Here a triangular fibrocartilagenous disc extends from the ulnar notch of the radius to the fossa at the base of the ulnar styloid. The radius and ulna are also connected by the interosseous membrane (Fig. 2.84b).

At the superior and inferior radioulnar joints the radius rotates inwards to produce pronation (Fig. 2.84c). Pronation makes the palm of the hand face backwards in the anatomical position or downwards if the arm is flexed (Fig. 2.84d). This movement is produced by the pronator teres and the pronator quadratus. The opposite movement is supination in which the radius rotates outwards. In the flexed position of the elbow, the biceps acts as a powerful supinator. Supination is weak when the elbow is extended and is done by the supinator muscle. The axis of pronation and supination is across a line passing through the head of the radius to the styloid process of the ulna. However the ulna is not entirely stationary during these movements. Its distal end moves slightly posterolaterally during pronation and anteromedially in supination. About 140° of rotation of the forearm can take place during pronation and supination. It can however be further increased by rotation of the humerus and the scapula.

In a young child a sudden pull on the forearm may result in the head of the radius being pulled partly

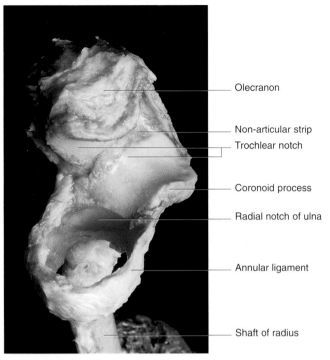

Olecranon

Non-articular strip

Trochlear notch

Coronoid process

Radial notch of ulna

Annular ligament

Shaft of radius

Fig. 2.84a *Annular ligament after removal of the upper end of radius. Viewed from above.*

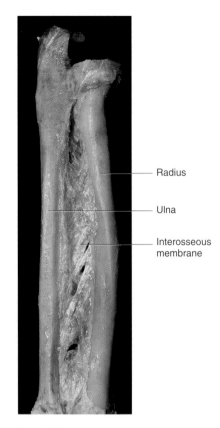

Radius

Ulna

Interosseous membrane

Fig. 2.84b *Interosseous membrane — posterior aspect (right side).*

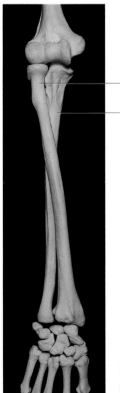

Radius

Ulna

Fig. 2.84c *Radius and ulna in pronation. Note that the radius crosses over the ulna carrying the hand with it.*

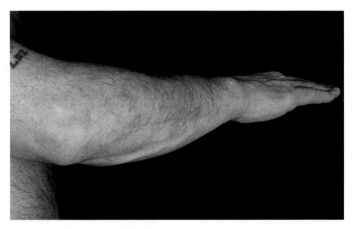

Fig. 2.84d *Pronation of forearm.*

outside the annular ligament. This injury is termed a 'pulled elbow'. In children the head of the radius is not fully formed and the annular ligament is circular. The annular ligament is of conical shape in the adult, facilitating a better grip on the radius.

THE WRIST JOINT (Fig. 2.85)

A number of synovial joints are present at the wrist region. The radiocarpal joint, also known as the wrist joint, is a biaxial joint. The midcarpal joint, between the two rows of carpal bones, and the intercarpal joint between the carpal bones are synovial joints with irregular joint cavities. These joint cavities communicate with each other and with those of the carpometacarpal joints and intermetacarpal joints (between the bases of the metacarpals).

At the wrist joint (radiocarpal joint) the scaphoid, lunate and triquetral bones articulate proximally with the distal end of the radius and the triangular fibrocartilagenous disc connecting the distal end of radius and ulna. The radius articulates with the scaphoid and the lunate. The head of ulna which does not take part in the formation of the joint is separated from the triquetral by the fibrocartilagenous disc which also separates the wrist joint from the inferior radioulnar joint. A capsule which is reinforced by palmar, dorsal and radial and ulnar collateral ligaments surrounds the joint.

Movements

Movements of the wrist joint are accompanied by similar movements at the midcarpal joint which is between the carpal bones. The range of movements and the muscles producing them are given below:

Movement	Muscles
Flexion — about 80° mostly at the midcarpal joint	Flexor carpi radialis and flexor carpi ulnaris aided by the long flexors of the digits and thumb and the abductor pollicis longus
Extension about 60° mostly at the wrist joint	Extensor carpi radialis longus and brevis and extensor carpi ulnaris assisted by extensors of the fingers and thumb
Abduction — limited to 15° due to radial styloid process projecting down	Flexor carpi radialis and extensor carpi radialis longus and brevis assisted by abductor pollicis longus
Adduction — about 45°	Flexor carpi ulnaris and extensor carpi ulnaris

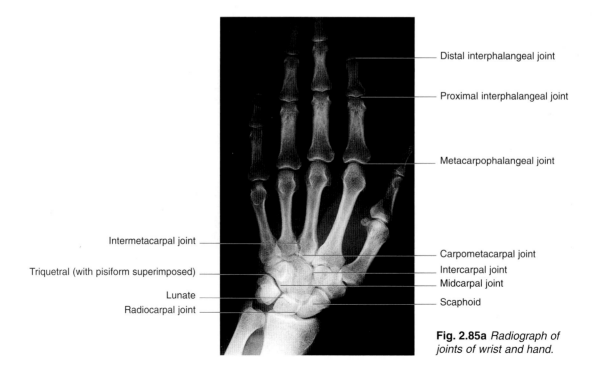

Distal interphalangeal joint

Proximal interphalangeal joint

Metacarpophalangeal joint

Intermetacarpal joint

Triquetral (with pisiform superimposed)

Lunate

Radiocarpal joint

Carpometacarpal joint

Intercarpal joint

Midcarpal joint

Scaphoid

Fig. 2.85a *Radiograph of joints of wrist and hand.*

Surgical approach to the joint is usually through the dorsal surface between the tendons of the extensor pollicis longus and the extensor digitorum and the indicis as this area has no major vessels or nerves.

Wrist drop

Paralysis of the radial nerve above the elbow will paralyse all the extensors of the wrist. The flexors of the wrist will overact and the wrist will adopt a flexed position, a condition known as wrist drop. Gripping with the hand is impossible in the flexed position of the wrist.

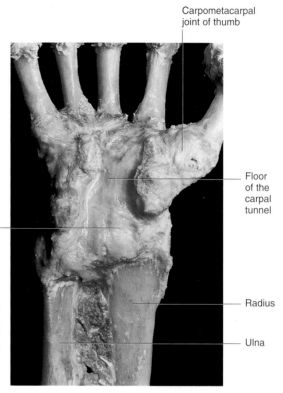

Carpometacarpal joint of thumb

Floor of the carpal tunnel

Capsule of the radiocarpal joint

Radius

Ulna

Fig. 2.85b *Capsule of radiocarpal joint and the floor of carpal tunnel formed by capsule of midcarpal and intercarpal joints.*

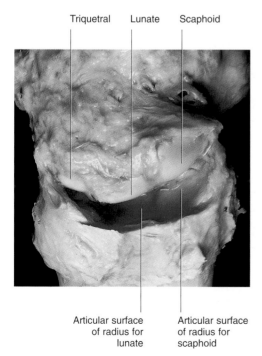

Triquetral   Lunate   Scaphoid

Articular surface of radius for lunate

Articular surface of radius for scaphoid

Fig. 2.85c *Interior of wrist joint — anterior view.*

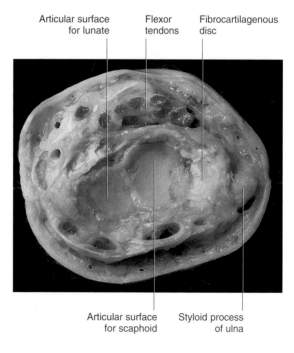

Articular surface for lunate   Flexor tendons   Fibrocartilagenous disc

Articular surface for scaphoid   Styloid process of ulna

Fig. 2.85d *Transverse section at the level of wrist joint showing the distal articular surface (for scaphoid and lunate) of the radius and the fibrocartilagenous disc connecting radius and ulna onto which the triquetral articulates.*

Carpometacarpal joint of the thumb
(Fig. 2.86)

The joint is between the trapezium and the first metacarpal bone and has a separate joint cavity. This is where most of the movements of the thumb take place. The articular surfaces are reciprocally saddle shaped to facilitate versatility of thumb movements including opposition.

Bennett's fracture

This is a fracture of the base of the first metacarpal bone involving the carpometacarpal joint of the thumb. This is usually sustained as a result of a blow to the point of the thumb as can occur in boxing.

The metacarpophalangeal joints
(Fig. 2.87)

These are synovial joints allowing flexion and extension as well as abduction and adduction. They lie along the distal skin crease of the palm where the prominence of the metacarpal heads can be easily felt. The joints are thus proximal to the interdigital webs. The palmar ligaments of these joints are strong fibrocartilagenous pads which are connected to each other by the deep transverse metacarpal ligament. These joints lie on the arc of a circle. Because of this when the fingers are extended they diverge from each other, whereas when they are flexed they crowd together in the palm. The collateral ligaments of the joints are taut in flexion and this limits abduction and adduction of the fixed joints.

The interphalangeal joints are hinge joints allowing only flexion and extension without any abduction and adduction. Their collateral ligaments are taut in all positions of the joints.

Trapezium   1st metacarpal bone

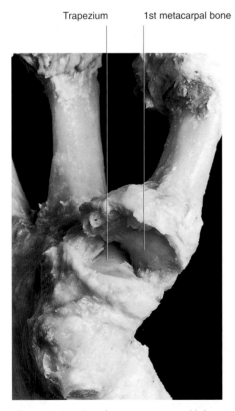

Fig. 2.86 *Interior of carpometacarpal joint of thumb.*

Base of proximal phalanx

Joint capsule   Head of metacarpal

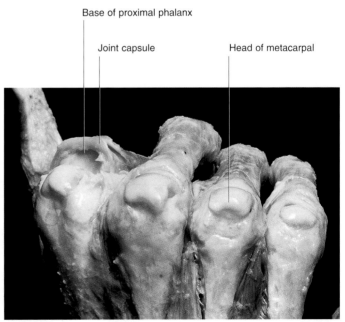

Fig. 2.87 *Metacarpophalangeal joints.*

THORAX

THE THORACIC CAGE AND THE INTERCOSTAL SPACE (Fig. 3.1)

The bony thoracic cage is formed by the 12 thoracic vertebrae at the back, the sternum in front and 12 pairs of ribs in between. The upper seven pairs of ribs articulate anteriorly direct with the sternum through their respective costal cartilages. The costal cartilage of ribs 8, 9 and 10 articulates with that of the rib above. These ribs with the xiphisternum form the lower costal margin. The lowermost point of the thoracic cage is the tenth costal cartilage.

The space between two adjacent ribs is known as the intercostal space. Thus there are 11 intercostal spaces on each side.

The junction between the manubrium and the body of the sternum is the sternal angle The second costal

cartilage articulates at the sternal angle. The seventh costal cartilage articulates at the junction between the body and the xiphisternum.

Surface anatomy

The sternal angle is palpable on the surface as a transverse ridge. This landmark is used to palpate the second costal cartilage and the second rib. It is possible to identify the other ribs as well as intercostal spaces by counting down from the second rib.

The first rib is not palpable as it is under the clavicle. Ribs 11 and 12 are rudimentary, confined to the back covered by muscles and hence are not palpable.

The intercostal space

The intercostal space contains the external intercostal, the internal intercostal and the innermost intercostal muscles arranged in three layers. The neurovascular bundle, consisting of the intercostal nerve and vessels,

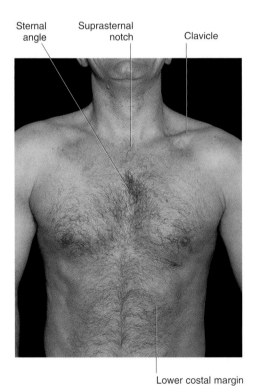

Fig. 3.1a *Surface anatomy of the chest wall.*

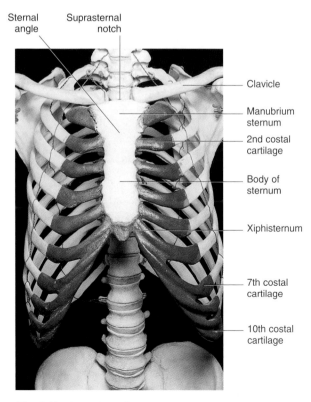

Fig. 3.1b *Bony thoracic cage.*

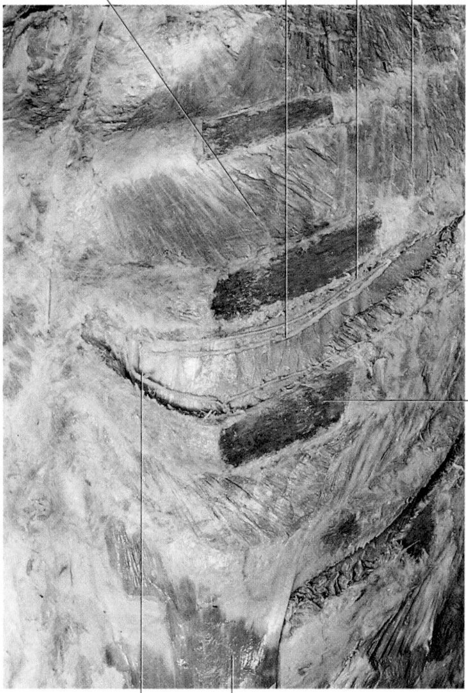

Intercostal nerve

Intercostal artery

Internal intercostal muscle

External intercostal muscle

Rib

Internal thoracic artery

Rectus abdominis

Fig. 3.1c *Intercostal spaces (left side).*

lies in between the internal and the innermost intercostals.

The external intercostal muscle fibres are directed downwards and forwards. In the anterior part the muscle fibres are replaced by a membrane. The internal intercostal fibres lie in the opposite direction to those of the external. The neurovascular bundle lies between the internal and the innermost intercostal muscles. If it is necessary to insert a chest drain or a needle into the intercostal space it is always placed in the lower part of the space to avoid damage to the neurovascular bundle (which lies along the lower border of the rib along the upper part of the space). The neurovascular bundle consists of, from above downwards, intercostal vein, artery and nerve.

The intercostal nerves are the anterior rami of the first eleven thoracic nerves.

The anterior intercostal arteries are branches of the internal thoracic artery or those of its musculophrenic branch. Most of the posterior intercostal arteries are derived from the descending thoracic aorta. Anastomoses between the anterior and posterior intercostal arteries are important collateral channels for circulation in cases of obstruction to the blood flow in the aorta anywhere beyond the origin of the left subclavian artery.

THE THORACIC CAVITY, LUNGS AND PLEURA

The thoracic cavity contains on either side the right and left lungs surrounded by the pleural cavities and the mediastinum in between.

The lungs and pleural cavities (Fig. 3.2)

The right lung is subdivided into superior, middle and inferior lobes by an oblique fissure and a horizontal fissure. The left lung usually has only two lobes, a superior and an inferior with an oblique fissure in between. Each lung has an apex which extends about 3 cm above the clavicle into the neck, a costal surface, a mediastinal surface and a base or diaphragmatic surface. The anterior border of the lung separates the costal and the mediastinal surfaces whereas the lower border is between the costal and the diaphragmatic surface.

The root of the lung connects the lung to the mediastinum and consists of, anterior to posterior, two pulmonary veins, the pulmonary artery and the bronchus. The pulmonary veins are at a lower level compared to the pulmonary artery (Fig. 3.2d, e). The right main bronchus gives off the superior lobar bronchus outside the lung. All the branches of the left bronchus are given off inside the lung. The root of the lung also contains the bronchial arteries supplying the bronchi and bronchioles as well as the lymph nodes draining the lung.

The right bronchus is shorter, wider and more vertical than the left. The angle between the two bronchi is about 70° in the adult; 25° to the right and 45° to the left from the midline. Therefore foreign bodies getting into the trachea tend to go to the right bronchus rather than into the left. At birth the bifurcation angle is about 110° with both bronchi angulating equally from the midline (55° each way).

The lung is surrounded by the pleural cavity, the potential space between the two layers of pleura. The outer parietal layer of pleura lines the thoracic cavity and the inner visceral or pulmonary layer closely fits on to the surface of the lung. The two layers become continuous with each other at the root of the lung. The parietal pleura lining the diaphragm is known as the diaphragmatic pleura and that lining the mediastinum as the mediastinal pleura.

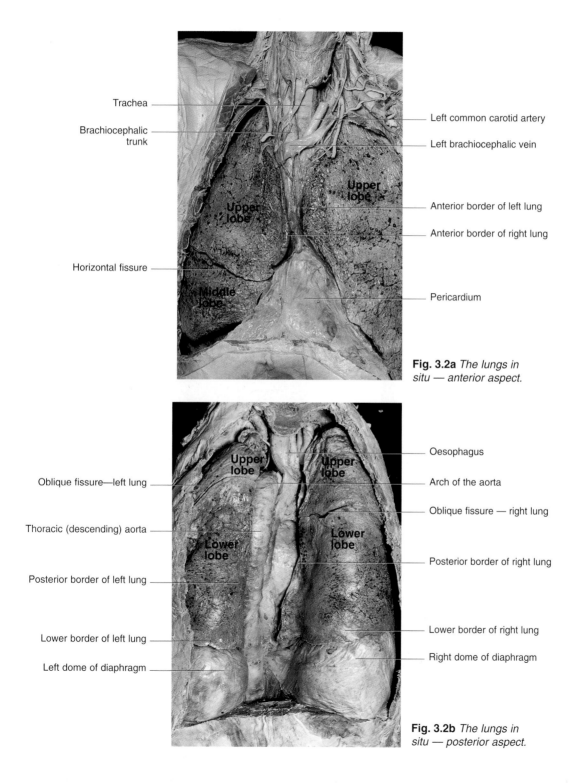

Fig. 3.2a *The lungs in situ — anterior aspect.*

Fig. 3.2b *The lungs in situ — posterior aspect.*

Surface anatomy (Fig 3.2f)

The apex of the lung and the surrounding pleural cavity extends about 3 cm above the medial part of the clavicle. The apical pleura is covered by a fascia, the suprapleural membrane (Sibson's fascia), which is attached to the inner border of the first rib (Fig. 3.2c). This fascia prevents the lung and pleura expanding too much into the neck during deep inspiration.

From the apex, the anterior border of the pleural cavity descends behind the sternoclavicular joint to reach the midline at the level of the sternal angle. (Here the two pleural cavities are close to each other.) The anterior limit of the right pleural cavity descends vertically downwards in the midline from the sternal angle to the level of the sixth costal cartilage. From there the lower border extends laterally, crossing the eighth rib in the midclavicular line, the tenth rib in the midaxillary line and then ascends to the middle of the twelfth rib at the back . The posterior border then ascends almost vertically upwards in the paravertebral region.

From the sternal angle the anterior border of the left pleural cavity deviates laterally to the lateral border of the sternum. The extent of the lower and the posterior margins are similar to those on the right.

The surface marking of the lung is the same as that of the pleura except for the lower margin and the cardiac notch (Fig. 3.2f). The lower margin of the lung is about two ribs higher than the lower margin of the pleura. Because of the bulge of the heart and pericardium, the anterior border of the left lung deviates laterally from the sternal angle to the apex of the heart (usually in the fifth intercostal space a little inside the midclavicular line) producing the cardiac notch. The oblique fissure lies along the sixth rib and the horizontal fissure on the right side extends from the midaxillary line along the fourth rib.

Knowledge of the extent of the lung and pleura is clinically important. Their lower parts overlap abdominal organs such as the liver, kidney and spleen. On the apical pleura lie the subclavian vessels and the brachial plexus. Procedures such as exposure of the

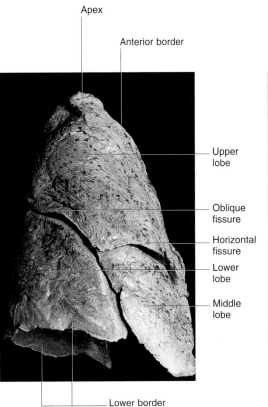

Fig. 3.2c *Costal surface of the right lung.*

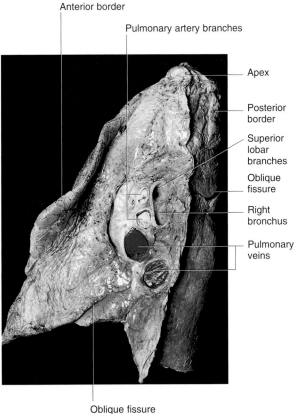

Fig. 3.2d *Mediastinal surface of the right lung.*

kidney, liver biopsy and cannulation of the subclavian vein may inadvertently produce a pneumothorax (air in the pleural cavity) resulting in collapse of the lung.

When the lung fields are markedly hyperinflated, the liver is pushed down by the diaphragm and may be palpable.

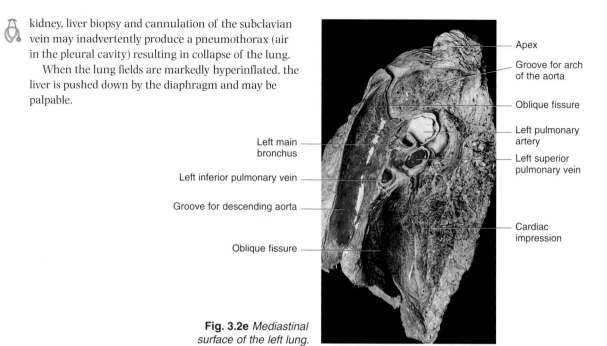

Fig. 3.2e *Mediastinal surface of the left lung.*

Labels: Apex; Groove for arch of the aorta; Oblique fissure; Left pulmonary artery; Left superior pulmonary vein; Left main bronchus; Left inferior pulmonary vein; Groove for descending aorta; Oblique fissure; Cardiac impression

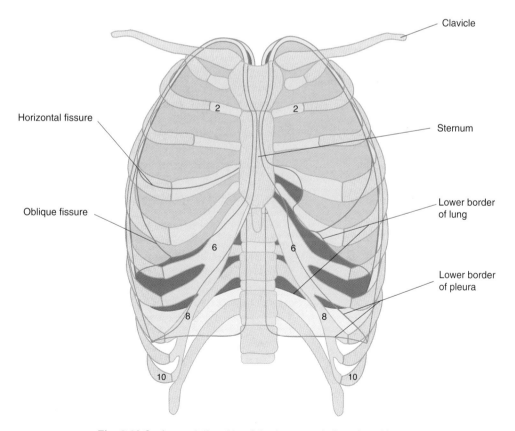

Fig. 3.2f *Surface relationship of the lungs and pleural cavities. The numbers indicate those of the ribs and costal cartilages.*

Labels: Clavicle; Horizontal fissure; Sternum; Oblique fissure; Lower border of lung; Lower border of pleura

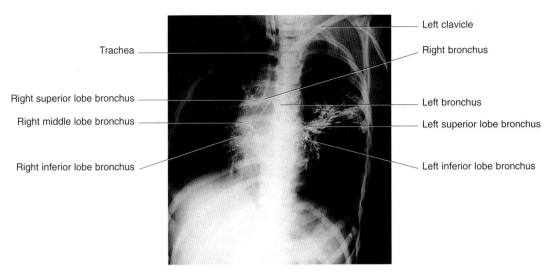

Trachea

Left clavicle

Right bronchus

Right superior lobe bronchus

Right middle lobe bronchus

Left bronchus

Left superior lobe bronchus

Right inferior lobe bronchus

Left inferior lobe bronchus

Fig. 3.2g *Bronchogram — left anterior oblique view.*

The trachea, bronchi and bronchioles

The trachea which is slightly to the right of the midline divides at the carina into right and left main bronchi. The right main bronchus is more vertical than the left and, hence, inhaled material is more likely to pass into it. The right main bronchus divides into three lobar bronchi (upper, middle and lower), whereas the left only into two (upper and lower) (Fig. 3.2g). Each lobar bronchus divides into segmental and subsegmental bronchi. There are about 25 generations of bronchi and bronchioles between trachea and the alveoli; the first 10 are bronchi and the rest bronchioles (Fig. 3.2h). The bronchi have walls consisting of cartilage and smooth muscle epithelial lining with cilia and goblet cells, submucosal mucous glands and endocrine cells containing 5-hydroxytryptamine. The bronchioles are tubes less than 2 mm in diameter and are also known as small airways. They have no cartilage or submucosal glands. Their epithelium has a single layer of ciliated cells but only few goblet cells and Clara cells secreting a surfactant-like substance

The alveolar ducts and alveoli

Each respiratory bronchiole supplies approximately 200 alveoli via alveolar ducts. There are about 300 million alveoli in each lung and their walls have type I and type II pneumocytes. Type II pneumocytes are the source of surfactant. The type I pneumocytes and the endothelial cells of adjoining capillaries constitute the blood–air barrier, the thickness of which is about 0.2–2 μm.

THE HEART (Fig 3.3)

Borders and surfaces of the heart

The heart has an anterior or sternocostal surface, formed mostly by the right ventricle, an inferior or

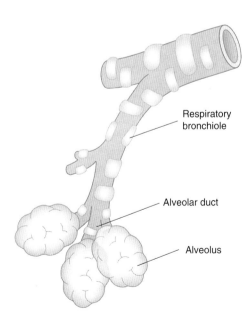

Respiratory bronchiole

Alveolar duct

Alveolus

Fig. 3.2h *The bronchioles and alveoli.*

diaphragmatic surface, formed mostly by the left ventricle, a base or posterior surface, formed by the left atrium, and an apex, formed entirely by the left ventricle. The borders of the heart (Fig. 3.3a) are the right border, formed by the right atrium, the inferior border, formed by the right ventricle, the left or obtuse border, formed mostly by the left ventricle with the left auricle at its superior end (Fig 3.3b).

The apex beat is defined as the lowermost and lateralmost cardiac pulsation in the precordium, normally felt inside the midclavicular line in the fifth left intercostal space (approximately 6 cm to the left of the midline) (Fig. 3.3b). However it is felt in the anterior axillary line when lying on the left side. The right border of the heart extends from the third to the sixth right costal cartilage approximately 3 cm to the right of the midline, the inferior border from the lower end of the right border to the apex and the left border from the apex to the second left intercostal space approximately 3 cm from the midline.

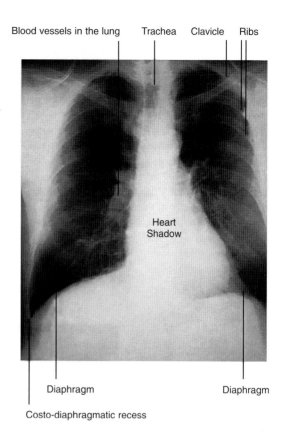

Blood vessels in the lung Trachea Clavicle Ribs

Heart Shadow

Diaphragm   Diaphragm

Costo-diaphragmatic recess

Fig. 3.3a *Posteroanterior radiograph of the chest.*

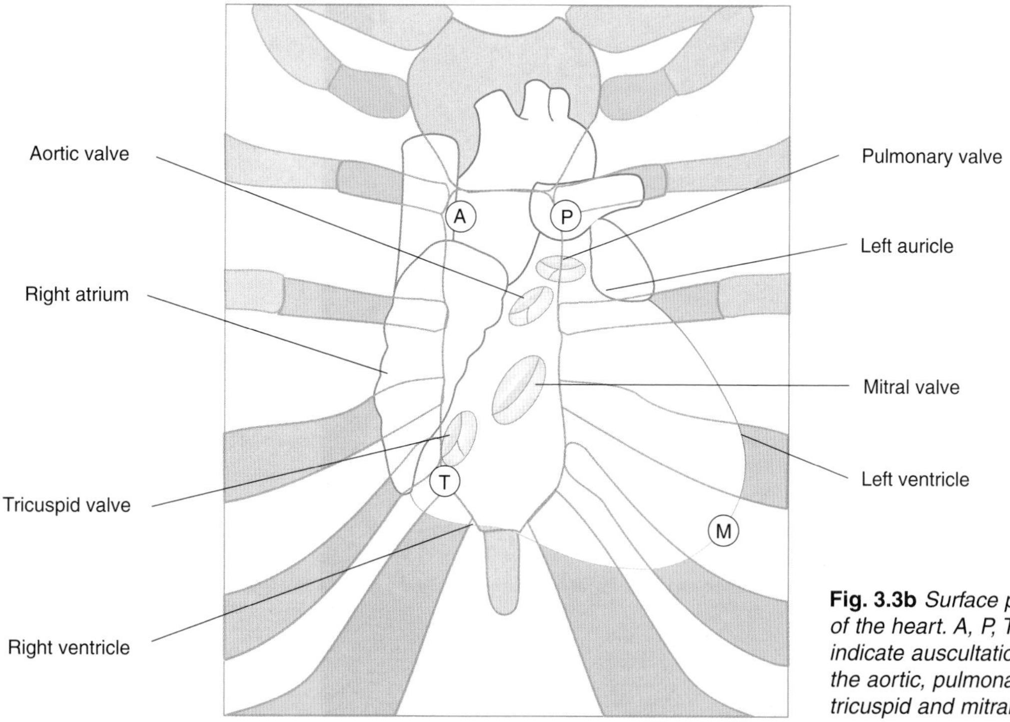

Aortic valve

Pulmonary valve

Left auricle

Right atrium

Mitral valve

Left ventricle

Tricuspid valve

Right ventricle

Fig. 3.3b *Surface projections of the heart. A, P, T and M indicate auscultation areas for the aortic, pulmonary, tricuspid and mitral valves.*

Blood supply of the heart (Fig. 3.3c–h)

The heart muscle is supplied by the right and left coronary arteries and is drained by the cardiac veins. The coronary arterial supply is of great clinical importance. Its occlusion is the chief cause of death in the western world.

The right coronary artery arises from the anterior aortic sinus. It passes between the pulmonary trunk and the right atrium to lie in the atrioventricular groove (Fig. 3.3c). It winds round the inferior border to reach the diaphragmatic surface where it anastomoses with the terminal part of the left coronary artery. It gives off an artery to the sinoatrial node, the right (acute) marginal artery and the posterior interventricular artery which is also known as the posterior descending artery.

The left coronary artery arises from the left posterior aortic sinus. It passes behind the pulmonary trunk and the left auricle to reach the atrioventricular groove where it divides into the circumflex and the anterior interventricular (anterior descending) arteries, both of equal size (Fig. 3.3d). The circumflex artery winds round the left margin where it gives off the left (obtuse) marginal artery and reaches the diaphragmatic surface to anastomose with the right coronary artery. The anterior descending artery (LAD), also known as the 'widow maker' because many men die of blockage of this artery, descends in the interventricular septum and gives off ventricular branches, septal branches as well as the diagonal artery. It then winds round the apex reaching the diaphragmatic surface to anastomose with the posterior descending artery. The main stem of the left coronary artery varies in length between 4 and 10 mm. In 10% of the population in whom the left coronary is larger and longer than usual — 'left

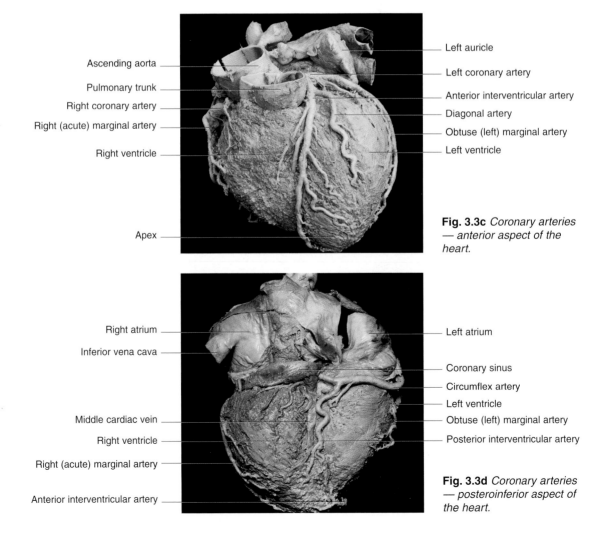

Fig. 3.3c *Coronary arteries — anterior aspect of the heart.*

Fig. 3.3d *Coronary arteries — posteroinferior aspect of the heart.*

dominance' — the posterior descending artery arises from it instead of from the right coronary. Another 10% have 'codominant' coronary circulation where both left and right coronaries contribute equally to the posterior interventricular artery. In a third of the population the left main stem divides into three branches instead of two, the third being a branch lying between the circumflex and the anterior descending the lateral aspect of the left ventricle.

The blood supply of the conducting system is of clinical importance. In about 60% of the population the sinoatrial node is supplied by the right coronary and in the rest by the circumflex branch of the left coronary. However occasionally (3%) it can have a dual

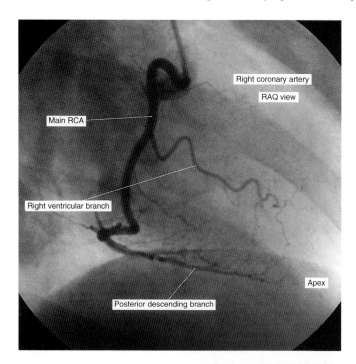

Fig. 3.3e *Right coronary arteriogram — right anterior oblique view.*

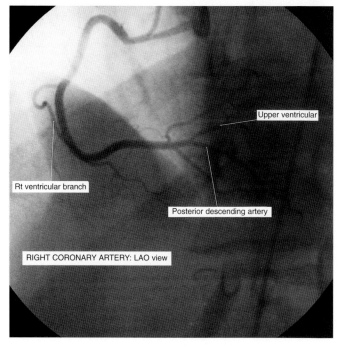

Fig. 3.3f *Right coronary arteriogram — left anterior oblique view.*

supply. The atrioventricular node is supplied by the right coronary in 90% and the circumflex in 10%.

Cardiac veins accompany the arteries. Most of them are tributaries of the coronary sinus, a sizable vein lying in the posterior part of the atrioventricular groove and opening into the right atrium. The great cardiac vein accompanies the anterior interventricular artery; the middle cardiac vein accompanies the

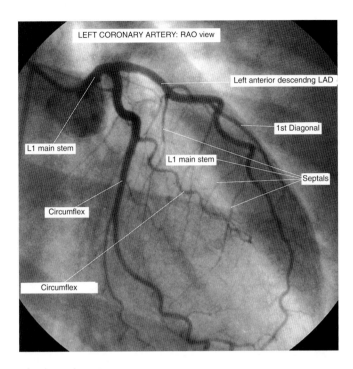

Fig. 3.3g *Left coronary arteriogram — right anterior oblique view.*

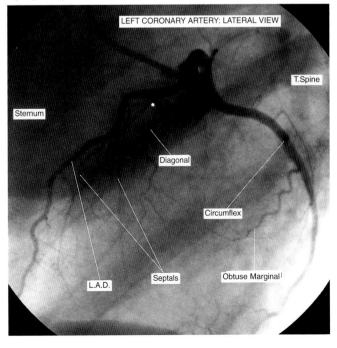

Fig. 3.3h *Left coronary arteriogram — lateral view.*

posterior interventricular artery and the small cardiac vein accompanies the marginal artery.

Right coronary artery occlusion leads to inferior myocardial infarction (necrosis of cardiac muscle), often associated with dysrhythmia (abnormal heart beats) due to ischaemia of SA node and/or AV node. Occlusion of the left coronary artery or its branches leads to anterior and/or lateral myocardial infarction, often with substantial ventricular damage and very poor prognosis.

The pericardium

The heart lies within the pericardial cavity, in the middle mediastinum. The pericardial cavity is similar in structure and function to the pleural cavity. The pericardium provides for the heart a friction-free surface to accommodate its sliding movements.

Components of the pericardium are the fibrous pericardium which is a collagenous outer layer fused with the central tendon of the diaphragm, the serous pericardium consisting of a parietal layer which lines the fibrous pericardium and a visceral layer which lines the outer surface of the heart and the commencement of the great vessels. The pericardial cavity is the space between the parietal and the visceral layers.

Two regions of the pericardial cavity have special names. The transverse sinus of the pericardial cavity lies between the ascending aorta and the pulmonary trunk in front and the venae cavae and the atria behind. The pericardial space behind the left atrium is the oblique sinus (Fig. 3.3i). The oblique sinus separates the left atrium from the oesophagus.

Anteriorly the pericardium is related to the sternum, third to sixth costal cartilages, lungs and the pleura. Posterior relations are oesophagus, descending aorta and T5–T8 vertebrae. Laterally on either side lie the root of the lung, mediastinal pleura and the phrenic nerve. Innervation of the fibrous and the parietal layer of serous pericardium is by the phrenic nerves. Pericardial pain originates in the parietal layer and is transmitted by the phrenic nerves. The pericardial cavity is closest to the surface at the level of the xiphoid process of sternum and the sixth costal cartilages.

Percardiocentesis
To remove fluid from the pericardial cavity a needle is inserted into the angle between the xiphoid process and the left seventh costal cartilage and is directed upwards at an angle of 45° towards the left shoulder. The needle passes through the central tendon of the diaphragm before entering the pericardial cavity.

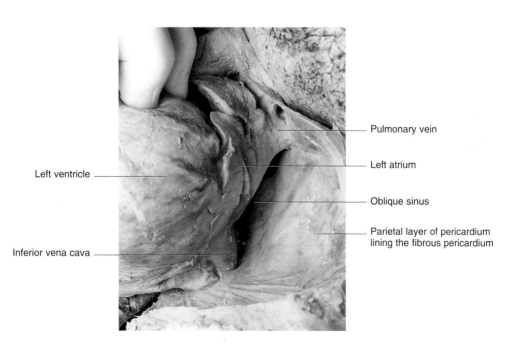

Pulmonary vein

Left atrium

Oblique sinus

Parietal layer of pericardium lining the fibrous pericardium

Left ventricle

Inferior vena cava

Fig. 3.3i *Pericardial cavity opened up and the heart lifted up to show the oblique sinus.*

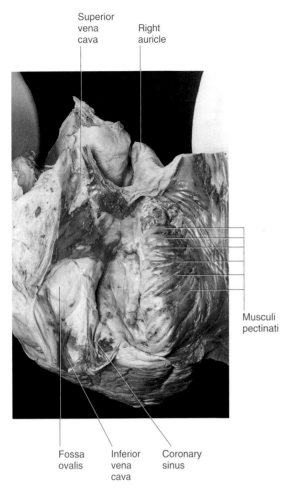

Superior vena cava

Right auricle

Musculi pectinati

Fossa ovalis

Inferior vena cava

Coronary sinus

Fig. 3.3j *Interior of the right atrium.*

Interior of the chambers of the heart

The right atrium (Fig. 3.3j)

The right atrium has a smooth and a rough part which are separated by a vertical ridge, the crista terminalis, extending between the superior and inferior venae cavae which bring systemic venous blood into the smooth part of the atrium. The coronary sinus opens anterior to the opening of the inferior vena cava. Developmentally the smooth part of the atrium is derived from the sinus venosus of the primitive cardiac tube and the rough part which has muscular ridges known as musculae pectinatae from the primitive atrium. The fossa ovalis, an oval depression on the interatrial wall, is the remnant of the foramen ovale in the fetus.

The right ventricle (Fig. 3.3k)

The right ventricular wall is thicker than that of the atrium. The tricuspid orifice is guarded by the tricuspid valve which has an anterior, posterior and a septal cusp. The interior of the ventricle has muscular ridges known as trabeculae carneae as well as the anterior, posterior and septal (small) papillary muscles and the chordae tendineae. The chordae tendineae connect the papillary muscles to the tricuspid valve cusps. These prevent the valve cusps being everted into the atrium during ventricular systole. The septomarginal trabecula (moderator band) is a muscular ridge extending from the interventricular septum to the base of the anterior papillary muscle of the heart. The moderator band is a part of the conducting system of the heart which

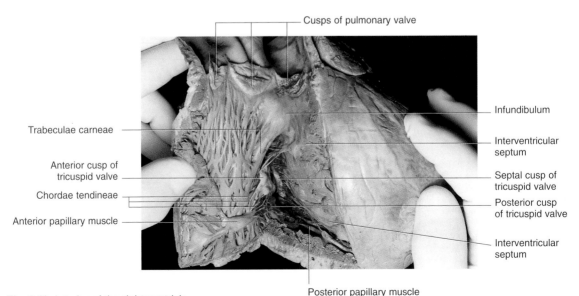

Cusps of pulmonary valve

Trabeculae carneae

Anterior cusp of tricuspid valve

Chordae tendineae

Anterior papillary muscle

Infundibulum

Interventricular septum

Septal cusp of tricuspid valve

Posterior cusp of tricuspid valve

Interventricular septum

Posterior papillary muscle

Fig. 3.3k *Interior of the right ventricle.*

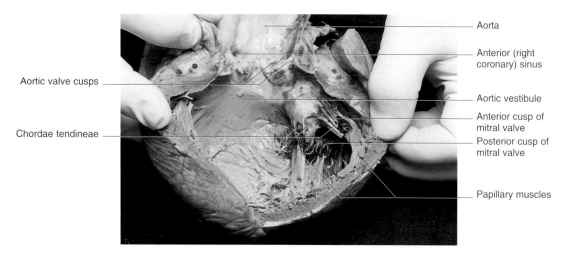

Fig. 3.3l *Interior of the left ventricle.*

regulates the cardiac cycle. The infundibulum leads on to the orifice of the pulmonary trunk. The pulmonary orifice has the pulmonary valve with three semilunar cusps. Each cusp has a thickening in the centre of its free edge.

The left atrium

The left atrium which develops by a combination of absorption of the pulmonary veins as well as from the primitive atrium has the openings of the four pulmonary veins. The mitral orifice separates the left atrium from the left ventricle.

The left ventricle (Fig. 3.3l)

The walls of the left ventricle are about three times thicker than those of the right ventricle because of the increased resistance of the systemic circulation compared to that of the pulmonary circulation. The mitral orifice is guarded by the mitral valve with an anterior and a posterior cusp. The large anterior cusp lies between the aortic and mitral orifices. The trabeculae carneae, papillary muscles and chordae tendineae are similar to those in the right ventricle. The aortic orifice has the aortic valve with the three semilunar aortic cusps, one anterior and two posterior in the anatomical position of the heart. These are thicker than those of the pulmonary valves to cope with the increased pressure. Alongside each cusp there is a dilation, the aortic sinus. The coronary arteries originate from the sinuses, the right from the anterior and the left from the left posterior aortic sinus. The interventricular septum which has the muscular and the membranous parts bulges into the right ventricle and separates the left ventricle from the right.

The conducting system of the heart
(Fig. 3.3m)

The sinoatrial node (SA node) or 'pacemaker of the heart' is situated in the right atrium at the upper end of the crista terminalis. From there the cardiac impulse spreads through the atrial musculature to reach the AV node (atrioventricular node) which is situated in the interatrial septum near the opening of the coronary sinus. From there the atrioventricular bundle of His

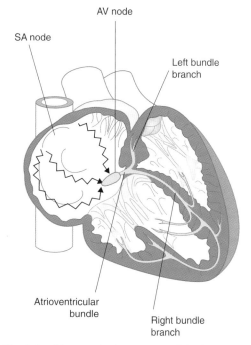

Fig. 3.3m *The conducting system of the heart.*

(AV bundle) passes through the fibrous ring at the atrioventricular junction to reach the membranous part of the interventricular septum where it divides into a right and left bundle branch. The atrioventricular bundle is the only pathway through which impulses can reach the ventricles from the

atrium. The left and right bundles descend towards the apex and break up into Purkinje fibres which activate the musculature of the ventricle in such a way that the papillary muscles contract first followed by the simultaneous contraction of both the ventricles from apex towards the base.

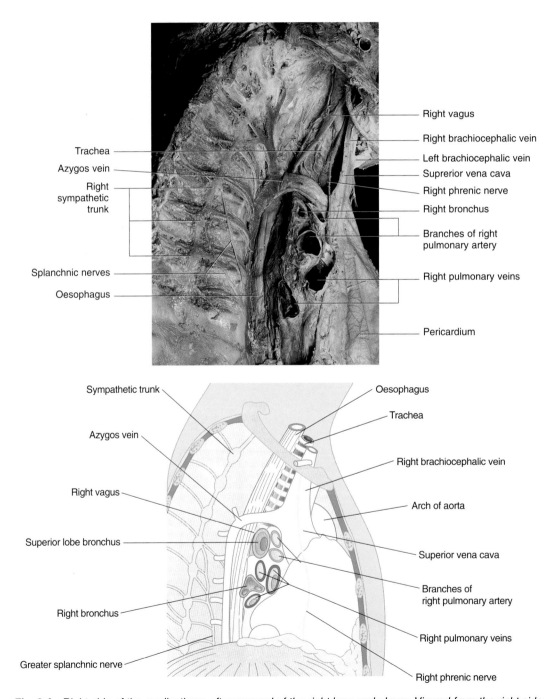

Fig. 3.4a *Right side of the mediastinum after removal of the right lung and pleura. Viewed from the right side.*

The mediastinum (Fig. 3.4)

The mediastinum is the region between the two pleural cavities. It contains the heart, great vessels, trachea, oesophagus and many other structures. The mediastinum is divided into four parts for descriptive purposes. The superior mediastinum lies above an imaginary line joining the sternal angle to the lower border of T4. The middle mediastinum contains the

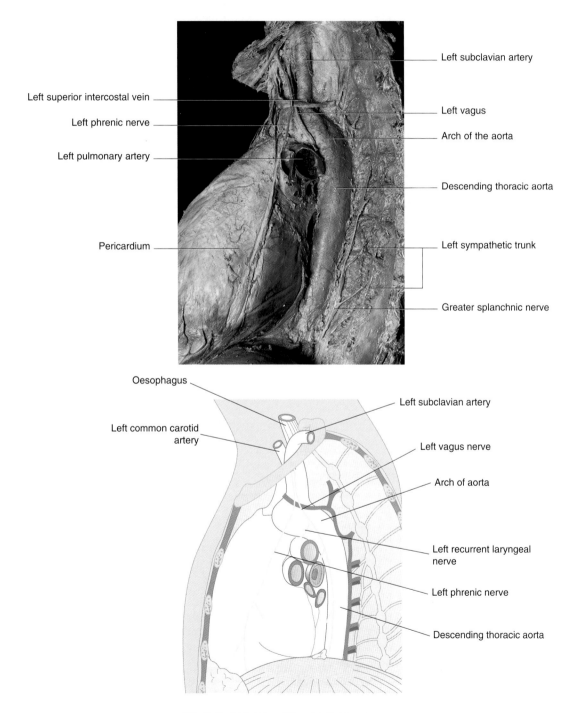

Fig. 3.4b *Left side of the mediastinum.*

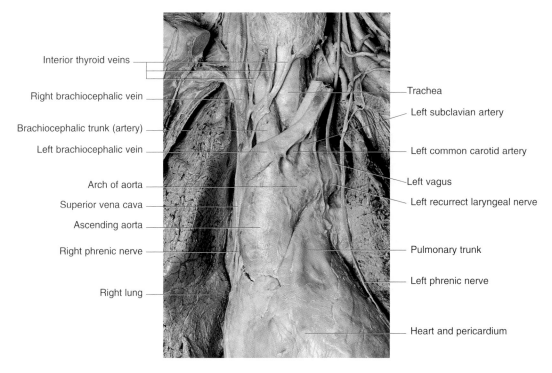

Interior thyroid veins

Right brachiocephalic vein

Brachiocephalic trunk (artery)

Left brachiocephalic vein

Arch of aorta

Superior vena cava

Ascending aorta

Right phrenic nerve

Right lung

Trachea

Left subclavian artery

Left common carotid artery

Left vagus

Left recurrect laryngeal nerve

Pulmonary trunk

Left phrenic nerve

Heart and pericardium

Fig. 3.4c *Structures in the superior mediastinum seen after removal of the thoracic cage and the parietal pleura. The lungs have been retracted to expose the structures.*

heart and pericardium; the anterior mediastinum is in front of this and the posterior mediastinum behind.

The brachiocephalic vein and the superior vena cava (Fig. 3.4a)

The brachiocephalic vein, one on each side, is formed by the union of the subclavian and the internal jugular veins. The right and left brachiocephalic veins join together to form the superior vena cava which drains into the right atrium. The azygos vein which receives segmental veins from the thoracic and posterior abdominal walls (intercostal and lumbar veins) joins the superior vena cava.

The right phrenic nerve (Fig. 3.4a)

The right and left phrenic nerves are formed in the cervical plexus (C3,4,5). Besides supplying the diaphragm they give sensory innervation to pleura, pericardium and peritoneum. The thoracic part of the right phrenic nerve reaches the diaphragm lying on the surface of the right brachiocephalic vein, the superior vena cava, the right side of the heart and pericardium

(where it lies in front of the root of the lung) and the inferior vena cava.

The right vagus nerve (Fig. 3.4a)

The right vagus nerve lies on the trachea and crosses behind the root of the lung and breaks up into branches on the oesophagus. It leaves the thorax by passing along with the oesophagus through the diaphragm as the posterior gastric nerve.

The left vagus and the left phrenic nerves (Fig. 3.4b, 3.4c)

Both nerves cross the arch of the aorta. The phrenic nerve descends in front of the root of the lung whereas the vagus crosses behind it. The left vagus gives off an important branch, the left recurrent laryngeal nerve, as it crosses the arch of the aorta. The left recurrent laryngeal nerve winds round the ligamentum arteriosum, a fibrous connection between the left pulmonary artery and the arch of the aorta. The ligamentum arteriosum is the remnant of the ductus arteriosus which shunts blood from the pulmonary

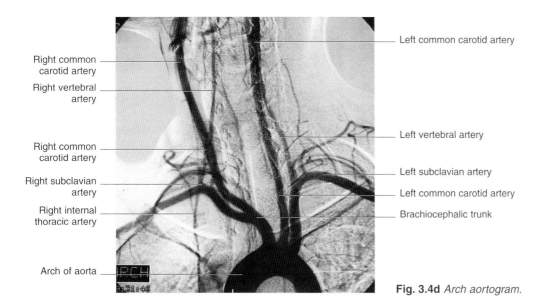

Right common carotid artery

Right vertebral artery

Right common carotid artery

Right subclavian artery

Right internal thoracic artery

Arch of aorta

Left common carotid artery

Left vertebral artery

Left subclavian artery

Left common carotid artery

Brachiocephalic trunk

Fig. 3.4d *Arch aortogram.*

trunk to the aorta in the fetus. The recurrent laryngeal nerve ascends to the neck lying in the groove between the trachea and the oesophagus and supplies the muscles and mucous membrane of the larynx.

 Carcinoma of the oesophagus, mediastinal lymph node enlargement and aortic arch aneurysm may compress the left recurrent laryngeal nerve to cause change in voice.

Arch of the aorta (Fig. 3.4b–d)

The ascending aorta commencing from the left ventricle continues upwards and to the left over the root of the left lung as the arch of the aorta. It then descends down to become the descending thoracic aorta. The arch of the aorta is entirely confined to the superior mediastinum. It has three branches: the

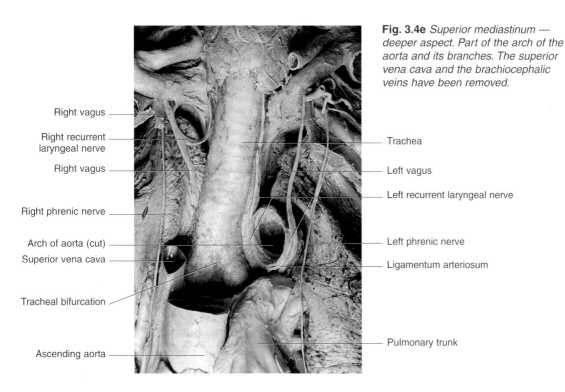

Fig. 3.4e *Superior mediastinum — deeper aspect. Part of the arch of the aorta and its branches. The superior vena cava and the brachiocephalic veins have been removed.*

Right vagus

Right recurrent laryngeal nerve

Right vagus

Right phrenic nerve

Arch of aorta (cut)

Superior vena cava

Tracheal bifurcation

Ascending aorta

Trachea

Left vagus

Left recurrent laryngeal nerve

Left phrenic nerve

Ligamentum arteriosum

Pulmonary trunk

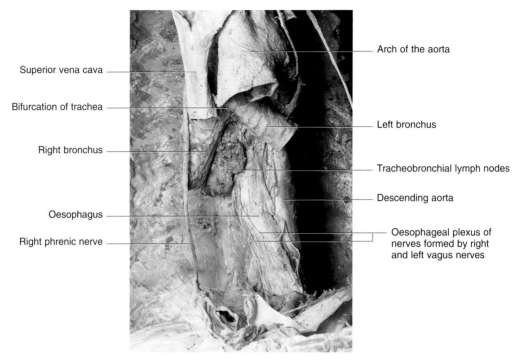

Superior vena cava

Bifurcation of trachea

Right bronchus

Oesophagus

Right phrenic nerve

Arch of the aorta

Left bronchus

Tracheobronchial lymph nodes

Descending aorta

Oesophageal plexus of nerves formed by right and left vagus nerves

Fig. 3.4f *The superior and posterior mediastinum seen after removal of the heart, pericardium, lungs and pleura.*

brachiocephalic trunk which divides into the right common carotid and the right subclavian arteries, the left common carotid artery and the left subclavian artery (Fig. 3.4d). The left vagus and the left phrenic nerves cross the arch of the aorta. The small vein lying across the arch of the aorta is the left superior intercostal vein. This drains the second and third left intercostal spaces and in turn drains into the left brachiocephalic vein (Fig. 3.4b).

The trachea (Fig. 3,4e, f)

The trachea extends from the lower border of the cricoid cartilage in the neck to the tracheal bifurcation at the level of the lower border of the T4 vertebra. In the living, in the erect posture, the tracheal bifurcation is at a lower level. The trachea is made up of a series of C-shaped cartilages closed posteriorly by the trachealis muscle. It is elastic enabling it to stretch during swallowing and its diameter changes during coughing and sneezing. The cervical part of the trachea lies in the midline and is easily palpable

The angle of bifurcation of the trachea in the adult is such that the right main bronchus is more vertical than the left. The cartilage at the tracheal bifurcation is the keel-shaped carina which projects into the lumen

as a vertical ridge. Flattening of this ridge is a sign of alteration of the bifurcation angle, often due to enlargement of the tracheobronchial group of lymph nodes. The angle of bifurcation of the trachea is normally wider in children, with no difference in the angulation of the right and left main bronchi.

The descending (thoracic) aorta (Fig. 3,4b, f)

The descending aorta commences where the arch of the aorta ends at the lower border of T4 vertebra. It leaves the posterior mediastinum in the midline at the level of T12 vertebra by passing between the crura of the diaphragm. The descending aorta gives off nine pairs of posterior intercostal arteries, a pair of subcostal arteries, two bronchial arteries for the left lung and small branches to the oesophagus.

Radicular arteries arise from the posterior intercostal arteries and supply the spinal cord. One such artery (usually from the tenth or eleventh intercostal space) is large and is known as the great radicular artery or artery of Adamkiewicz. Blood flow through radicular arteries may be interfered with during aortic surgery producing ischaemia of the spinal cord resulting in paraplegia.

The oesophagus

The oesophagus starts as a continuation of the pharynx at the level of C6 vertebra and ends by entering the stomach at the cardiac orifice. The thoracic part of the oesophagus lies in the superior and posterior mediastinum and enters the abdomen by piercing the diaphragm at the level of T10 vertebra. In the superior mediastinum it lies behind the trachea with the arch of the aorta lying on its left side. The left recurrent laryngeal nerve lies in the groove between the trachea and the oesophagus. The left main bronchus crosses in front of the oesophagus and the part below that is related to the left atrium. The arch of the aorta, the left main bronchus and the left atrium produce indentations on the oesophagus which can be seen clearly on radiograph taken after barium swallow (Fig. 3.4g).

The close relationship of the oesophagus and the left atrium is made use of in determining left atrial enlargement in mitral stenosis. Barium swallow may show displacement of the oesophagus by the enlarged atrium. The lumen of the oesophagus is narrower at its commencement, where the left bronchus crosses it and where it passes through the diaphragm to enter the stomach. These are sites where foreign bodies swallowed are usually impacted and where strictures develop after swallowing caustic fluids. They are also common sites for carcinoma of the oesophagus.

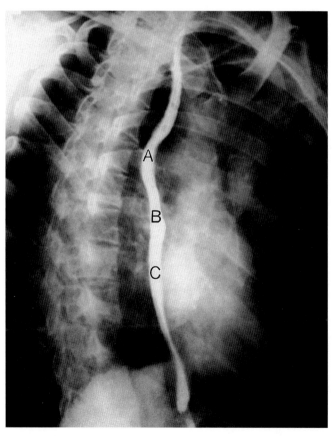

Fig. 3.4g *Oblique radiograph of the thorax during a 'barium swallow' outlining the oesophagus. The three indentations produced by the arch of the aorta (A), left bronchus (B) and the left atrium (C) are seen well.*

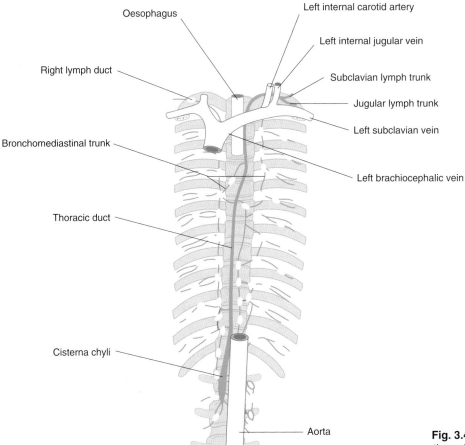

Oesophagus

Left internal carotid artery

Left internal jugular vein

Right lymph duct

Subclavian lymph trunk

Jugular lymph trunk

Left subclavian vein

Bronchomediastinal trunk

Left brachiocephalic vein

Thoracic duct

Cisterna chyli

Aorta

Fig. 3.4h *Cisterna chyli, thoracic duct and right lymph duct.*

Thoracic duct

The thoracic duct starts as the continuation of the cysterna chyli in the abdomen, passes through the thorax and enters the neck lying on the left border of the oesophagus (Fig. 3.4h). In the neck it arches to the left, lying in the plane between the carotid sheath and vertebral arteries, to enter the junction between the subclavian and internal jugular veins. It carries lymph from the whole body except that from the right side of thorax, right upper limb, right side of head and neck and the lower lobe of right lung.

The azygos vein

The azygos vein enters the thorax through the aortic opening of the diaphragm and passes upwards lying on the vertebral bodies and arches over the root of the right lung to drain into the superior vena cava. The azygos vein receives the lower eight posterior intercostal veins of the right side and the right superior intercostal vein (Fig. 3.4i). The hemiazygos veins which receive the intercostal veins of the left side drain into the azygos vein.

The sympathetic trunk

The sympathetic trunks lie on each side of the vertebral column, extending from the base of the skull to the coccyx where the two chains fuse together. Each trunk contains a number of sympathetic ganglia, the thoracic region having about 11 ganglia which lie on the neck of the ribs. The ganglia are closely related to the intercostal nerves from which they receive pre-ganglionic fibres as white rami communicantes. The post-ganglionic fibres from the ganglia go back to the intercostal nerves as grey rami communicantes. The

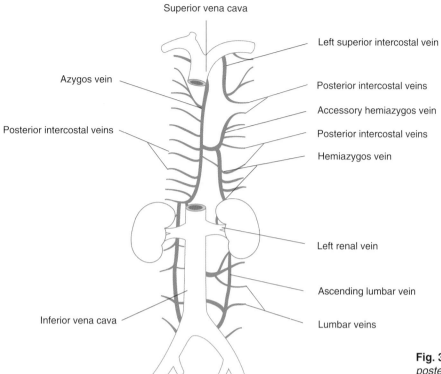

Superior vena cava

Left superior intercostal vein

Azygos vein

Posterior intercostal veins

Accessory hemiazygos vein

Posterior intercostal veins

Posterior intercostal veins

Hemiazygos vein

Left renal vein

Ascending lumbar vein

Inferior vena cava

Lumbar veins

Fig. 3.4i *Veins of the posterior chest and abdominal wall.*

thoracic ganglia give off the greater, lesser and least splanchnic nerves to supply the abdominal viscera. The splanchnic nerves are pre-ganglionic fibres which will synapse in collateral ganglia displaced from the sympathetic trunk (e.g. coeliac ganglion) in the abdomen.

Diaphragm (Fig. 3.4j, k)

The diaphragm separates the thoracic and abdominal cavities. It transmits the inferior vena cava, the oesophagus, the sympathetic trunk and the splanchnic nerves. The aorta passes behind the diaphragm between its two crura. The peripheral part of the diaphragm is muscular whereas its central part, the central tendon, is fibrous. Its upper surface fuses with

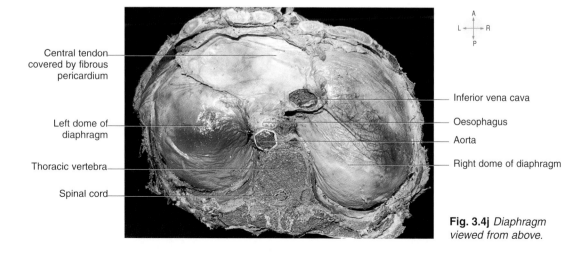

Central tendon covered by fibrous pericardium

Left dome of diaphragm

Thoracic vertebra

Spinal cord

Inferior vena cava

Oesophagus

Aorta

Right dome of diaphragm

Fig. 3.4j *Diaphragm viewed from above.*

the fibrous pericardium. The muscular part is attached to the upper lumbar vertebrae and the intervertebral discs through the right and left crura. Fibres of the diaphragm also take origin from the medial and lateral arcuate ligaments which are thickenings of the fascia overlying the psoas major and the quadratus lumborum muscles on the posterior abdominal wall. Besides these vertebral attachments the diaphragm is attached to the inner aspects of the lower six ribs, and costal cartilages as well as to the xiphoid process of the sternum. The aortic opening lies at the level of T12 and transmits the abdominal aorta, thoracic duct and the azygos vein. The oesophagus passes through the left crus with the fibres of the right crus looping around it at the level of T10. The oesophageal orifice also transmits the vagus nerves and the left gastric vessels. The inferior vena caval opening which lies more anteriorly in the central tendon of the diaphragm at the level of T8 also transmits the right phrenic nerve. The sympathetic trunk enters the abdomen by passing

under the medial arcuate ligament and the splanchnic nerves by piercing the crura.

The nerve supply of the diaphragm, both sensory and motor, is by the phrenic nerve and hence pain due to diaphragmatic irritation is felt in the shoulder region as a referred pain. There is additional supply of sensory nerves to the peripheral aspect by the intercostal nerves. On contraction the diaphragm descends down to increase the vertical diameter of the thoracic cavity. It thus acts as the major muscle of inspiration. The abdominal pressure is increased by contraction of the diaphragm and hence it contributes importantly to functions such as defecation, micturition and parturition.

Injury to the phrenic nerve will paralyse the corresponding half of the diaphragm resulting in paradoxical movement during respiration. Instead of descending during inspiration the paralysed side gets pushed upwards by the abdominal viscera. This can be detected radiographically.

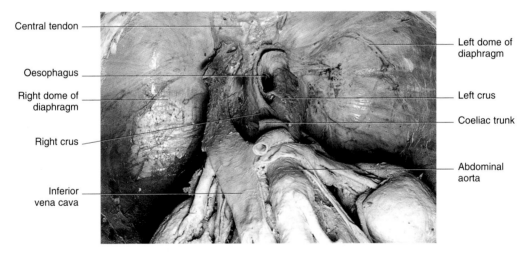

Fig. 3.4k *Diaphragm viewed from below. Liver, stomach, spleen and the small and large intestines have all been removed.*

ABDOMEN

SURFACE ANATOMY, REGIONS OF THE ABDOMEN (Fig. 4.1)

The lower costal margin extends from the xiphoid process of the sternum to the tenth costal cartilage. The transpyloric plane passing across the lower border of L1 vertebra lies halfway between the suprasternal notch and the pubic symphysis. This plane passes through the pylorus, the neck of the pancreas, the duodenojejunal flexure, the fundus of the gall bladder and the hila of the kidneys. It can also be drawn by connecting the tips of the ninth costal cartilages. The subcostal plane passing through the lower margin of the tenth costal cartilage cuts across the L3 vertebra.

The abdominal muscles and the skin are segmentally innervated by spinal nerves T7 to L1. The distribution can be remembered by knowing that T7 supplies the region near the xiphoid, T10 the region of the umbilicus and L1 the suprapubic region.

For descriptive purposes the abdomen is divided into nine regions by two horizontal and two vertical planes. The transpyloric and transtubercular (connecting the tubercles of the iliac crest) are the horizontal planes, the two midclavicular lines the vertical. The nine regions are the epigastrium, the right and left hypochondrium, the umbilical region, the right and left lumbar region, the hypogastrium (or the suprapubic region) and the right and left iliac fossa. Reference to these regions are made in relation to location of viscera, localisation of pain and location of an abdominal mass.

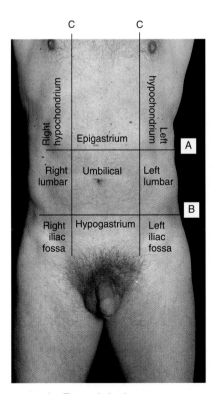

A = Transpyloric plane
B = Transtubercular plane
C = Midclavicular line

Fig. 4.1a *Regions of the abdomen.*

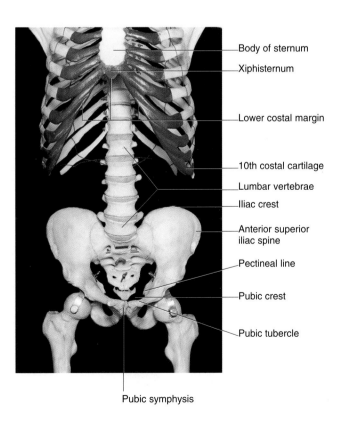

Body of sternum
Xiphisternum
Lower costal margin
10th costal cartilage
Lumbar vertebrae
Iliac crest
Anterior superior iliac spine
Pectineal line
Pubic crest
Pubic tubercle
Pubic symphysis

Fig. 4.1b *Bony thoracic cage and pelvis.*

MUSCLES OF THE ANTERIOR ABDOMINAL WALL (Fig. 4.2)

The anterior abdominal wall has three flat muscles, i.e. external oblique, internal oblique and transversus, which are fleshy laterally and aponeurotic in front. The aponeuroses ensheath the rectus abdominis muscle and fuse in the midline to form the linea alba. The linea alba extends from the pubic symphysis to the xiphoid process of the sternum.

External oblique

This arises from the lower eight ribs and is inserted to the iliac crest, pubic tubercle and pubic crest. Between the anterior superior iliac spine and the pubic tubercle its lower curved free border forms the inguinal ligament. The anterior part of the aponeurosis contributes to the anterior wall of the rectus sheath.

Internal oblique

This arises from the lumbar fascia, the iliac crest and the lateral two-thirds of the inguinal ligament. The majority of its fibres run upwards and medially at right angles to the fibres of the external oblique. The fibres arising from the inguinal ligament arch over the spermatic cord to fuse with the aponeurosis of the transversus to form the conjoint tendon which extends behind the cord to be attached to the pubic crest.

Transversus abdominis

This arises from the inner surface of the lower six ribs, the lumbar fascia, the iliac crest and the lateral third of the inguinal ligament. The major part of the muscle is inserted to the linea alba via an aponeurosis which contributes to the posterior wall of the rectus sheath. The fibres from the inguinal ligament fuse with similar fibres from the internal oblique to form the conjoint tendon.

Rectus abdominis

This muscle lying on either side of the midline arises from the pubic symphysis and pubic crest to be inserted to the fifth, sixth and seventh costal cartilages. The anterior surface of the muscle has three tendinous

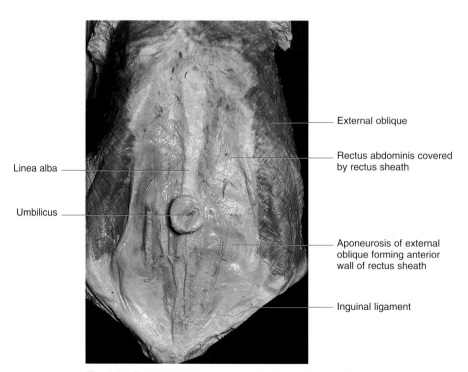

Linea alba

Umbilicus

External oblique

Rectus abdominis covered by rectus sheath

Aponeurosis of external oblique forming anterior wall of rectus sheath

Inguinal ligament

Fig. 4.2a *External oblique, rectus sheath and linea alba.*

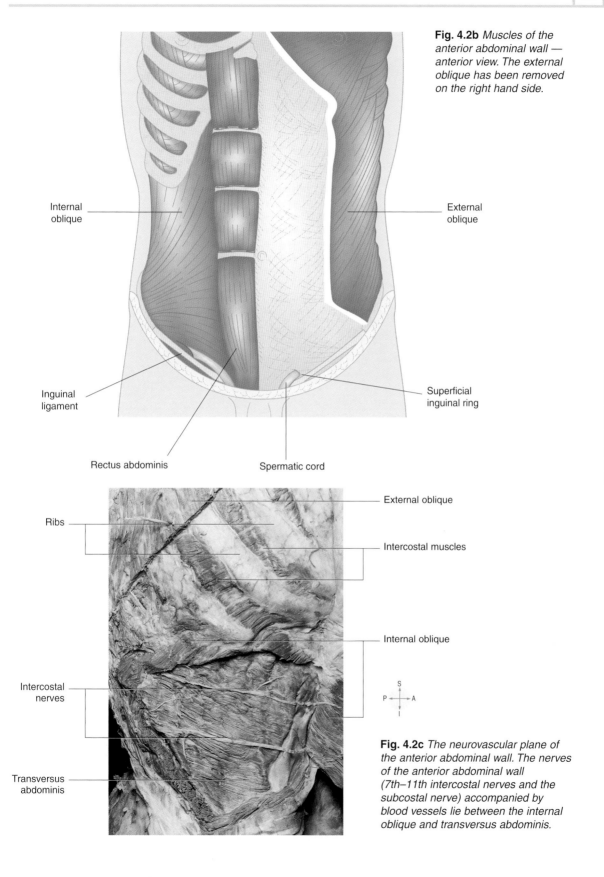

Fig. 4.2b *Muscles of the anterior abdominal wall — anterior view. The external oblique has been removed on the right hand side.*

Internal oblique

External oblique

Inguinal ligament

Superficial inguinal ring

Rectus abdominis

Spermatic cord

External oblique

Ribs

Intercostal muscles

Internal oblique

Intercostal nerves

Transversus abdominis

Fig. 4.2c *The neurovascular plane of the anterior abdominal wall. The nerves of the anterior abdominal wall (7th–11th intercostal nerves and the subcostal nerve) accompanied by blood vessels lie between the internal oblique and transversus abdominis.*

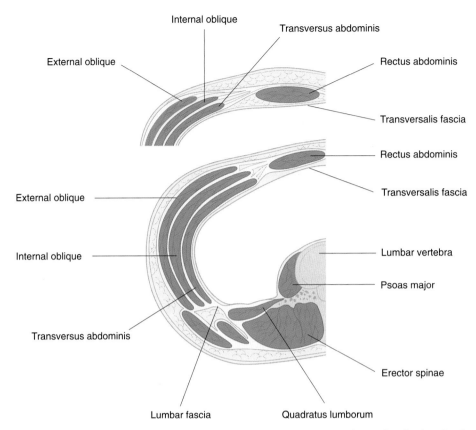

Fig. 4.2d *Transverse section of the abdominal wall, showing the arrangement of muscles, lumbar fascia and rectus sheath. The upper figure shows the rectus abdominis and the formation of the rectus sheath below the arcuate line.*

intersections, one at the level of the xiphoid, one at the umbilicus and the third halfway between these two levels. The intersections are adherent to the anterior wall of the rectus sheath but not to the posterior.

The rectus sheath (Fig. 4.2d)

The arrangement of the rectus sheath which strengthens the rectus and gives additional support to this region of the abdomen is as follows:

- Above the costal margin where the muscle is attached to the costal cartilages the sheath's anterior wall is by external oblique aponeurosis only.
- From the costal margin to a point midway between the pubic crest and umbilicus the internal oblique aponeurosis splits to enclose the rectus. The anterior aspect of the sheath thus formed is reinforced by the external oblique aponeurosis and the posterior aspect by the transversus.

- Below the point halfway between the umbilicus and the pubic crest the aponeurosis of the external oblique, internal oblique and transversus pass in front of the rectus. Thus the sheath is deficient posteriorly in this region. The posterior wall of the rectus sheath thus has a free border halfway between the umbilicus and the pubic crest. This is known as the arcuate line of Douglas. The inferior epigastric artery enters the rectus sheath at this point to anastomose with the superior epigastric artery.

THE INGUINAL CANAL (Fig. 4.3)

The inguinal canal is a slit-like space in between the muscles of the anterior abdominal wall, above the medial half of the inguinal ligament. It contains the spermatic cord and the ilioinguinal nerve in the male

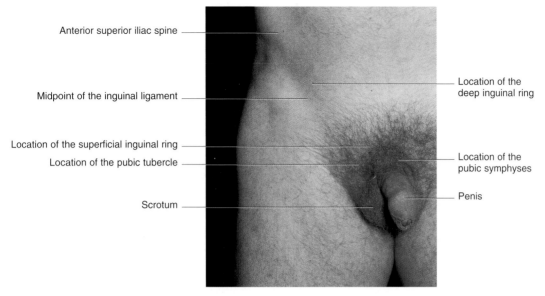

Fig. 4.3a *Surface anatomy of the groin.*

and the round ligament of the uterus and the ilioinguinal nerve in the female. It is about 6 cm long and extends from the deep inguinal ring to the superficial inguinal ring. The deep inguinal ring is a defect in the transversalis fascia about 1 cm above the midpoint of the inguinal ligament. The superficial inguinal ring which is above and medial to the pubic tubercle is a defect in the external oblique aponeurosis.

Walls of the inguinal canal

The anterior wall (i.e. structures in front of the spermatic cord) is formed by the external oblique aponeurosis reinforced laterally by fibres of the internal oblique. The posterior wall (structures behind the spermatic cord) throughout is formed by the transversalis fascia and is reinforced medially by the conjoint tendon.

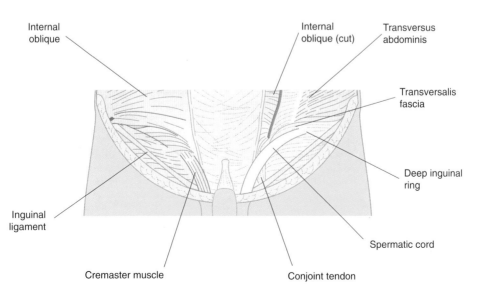

Fig. 4.3b *Inguinal region in the male. On the right-hand side of the inguinal region the external oblique has been removed; on the left-hand side the external oblique and internal oblique have been partially removed.*

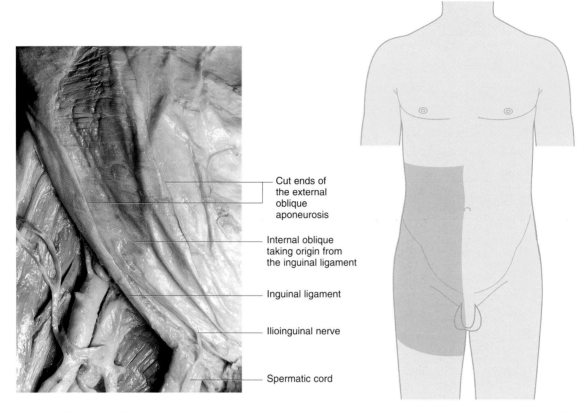

Cut ends of
the external
oblique
aponeurosis

Internal oblique
taking origin from
the inguinal ligament

Inguinal ligament

Ilioinguinal nerve

Spermatic cord

Fig. 4.3c *External oblique aponeurosis cut to show the internal oblique fibres arching over the spermatic cord. Also seen is the ilioinguinal nerve between the external oblique aponeurosis and the internal oblique.*

Roof and floor of the inguinal canal

The roof of the canal (structures above the cord) is formed by the arched fibres of the transversus and the internal oblique. The floor is formed by the inguinal ligament. The lacunar ligament (pectineal part of the inguinal ligament or Gimbernat's ligament) which is the continuation of the attachment of the inguinal ligament to the pubic ramus is an additional structure on the floor in the medial part of the canal.

Inguinal hernias

Part of the intestine or peritoneal fold can herniate through the inguinal canal as an inguinal hernia. These hernias are more common in the male as the canal is bigger. An indirect inguinal hernia comes through the deep inguinal ring and hence traverses the whole extent of the canal. It is contained inside the coverings of the spermatic cord. A direct inguinal hernia on the other hand invaginates the posterior wall of the canal.

TESTIS, EPIDIDYMIS AND THE SPERMATIC CORD (Fig. 4.4)

The testis which lies within the scrotum has the following coverings:

- scrotal skin
- dartos muscle (muscle developed in the superficial fascia)
- external spermatic fascia
- cremaster muscle and fascia
- internal spermatic fascia
- tunica vaginalis.

The testis measures about 4 cm from its upper pole to the lower pole, 3 cm from anterior border to posterior border and about 2.5 cm from its medial to lateral surface. The left testis is at a lower level than the right. The testis has a fibrous capsule, the tunica albuginea, which in turn is surrounded by a double-layered serous membrane, the tunica vaginalis. The internal structure consists of a large number of lobules separated by

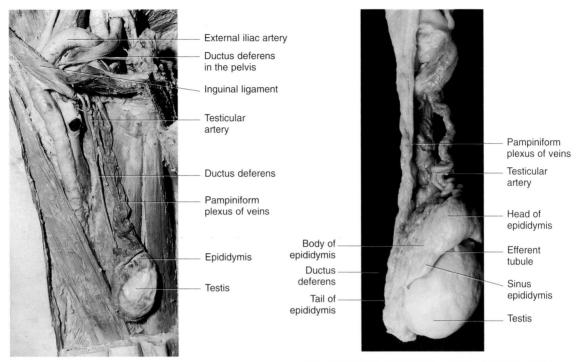

Fig. 4.4a External iliac artery / Ductus deferens in the pelvis / Inguinal ligament / Testicular artery / Ductus deferens / Pampiniform plexus of veins / Epididymis / Testis

Fig. 4.4a *Contents of the scrotum and spermatic cord dissected and displaced on to the front of the thigh.*

Fig. 4.4b Pampiniform plexus of veins / Testicular artery / Head of epididymis / Efferent tubule / Sinus epididymis / Testis / Body of epididymis / Ductus deferens / Tail of epididymis

Fig. 4.4b *Testis, epididymis and the contents of the spermatic cord after removal of their coverings.*

septae, each lobule containing between one and three seminiferous tubules within which the sperms are produced.

The epididymis lies on the posterolateral aspect of the testis. The groove between the testis and epididymis is the sinus epididymis. The epididymis has an upper part or head and a lower part which continues as the ductus deferens. The epididymis is also covered by tunica vaginalis except along its posterior border. The seminiferous tubules drain into an irregular series of ducts known as the rete testis from which efferent tubules enter the head of the epididymis. Sperm produced in the seminiferous tubules of the testis are stored in the epididymis and the ductus before ejaculation. The ductus deferens which joins the duct of the seminal vesicle to form the ejaculatory duct in turn enters the prostatic part of the urethra and transports sperm to the urethra.

The testis and the epididymis at their upper ends may have embryological remnants known as appendix testis and appendix epididymis respectively. These small pedunculated bodies may undergo torsion.

The testis lies outside the body cavity in the scrotum where it is maintained at a temperature 2–3°C lower than the body temperature. Failure to descend into the scrotum causes failure of spermatogenesis.

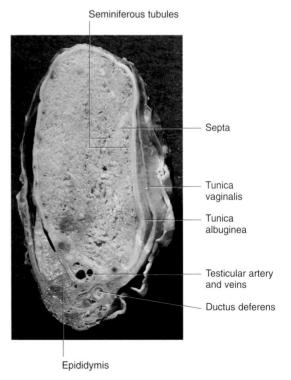

Seminiferous tubules / Septa / Tunica vaginalis / Tunica albuginea / Testicular artery and veins / Ductus deferens / Epididymis

Fig. 4.4c *Transverse section of left testis and epididymis.*

Blood supply

The testis and epididymis are suspended by the spermatic cord containing their arterial supply, venous and lymphatic drainage and nerve supply. The testis develops in the L2/L3 vertebral region and drags its vascular, lymphatic and nerve supply from this region to the scrotum. Testicular pain hence may radiate to the loin and renal pain often is referred to the scrotum.

The arterial supply is via the testicular artery which is a branch of the abdominal aorta given off just below the level of origin of the renal arteries. The venous drainage is via the pampiniform plexus of veins which become a single testicular vein before terminating in the inferior vena cava on the right side and the left renal vein on the left side. The lymphatics of the testis and epididymis accompany the blood vessels and drain into the paraaortic lymph nodes. Upper abdomen must therefore be palpated when searching for secondary lymphatic spread from a carcinoma of the testis.

The spermatic cord (Fig. 4.4a, b, d)

The spermatic cord contains the ductus deferens (vas deferens), the testicular artery and the pampiniform plexus of veins. Other structures in the cord are the cremasteric artery, the artery to the vas, nerve to the cremaster, sympathetic nerves and the lymphatics of the testis and epididymis. Because of its passage through the inguinal canal the spermatic cord acquires three coverings, i.e. the external spermatic fascia from the external oblique aponeurosis at the superficial inguinal ring, the cremasteric muscle and fascia from the internal oblique, and the internal spermatic fascia from the transversalis fascia at the deep inguinal ring.

THE PERITONEAL CAVITY (Fig. 4.5)

The peritoneal cavity of the abdomen is a potential space between the parietal and the visceral layers of peritoneum. The parietal peritoneum lines the inner surface of the abdominal and pelvic wall. The visceral peritoneum is the continuation of the parietal

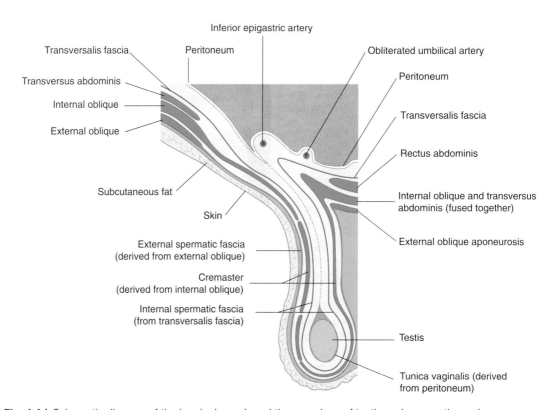

Fig. 4.4d *Schematic diagram of the inguinal canal, and the coverings of testis and spermatic cord.*

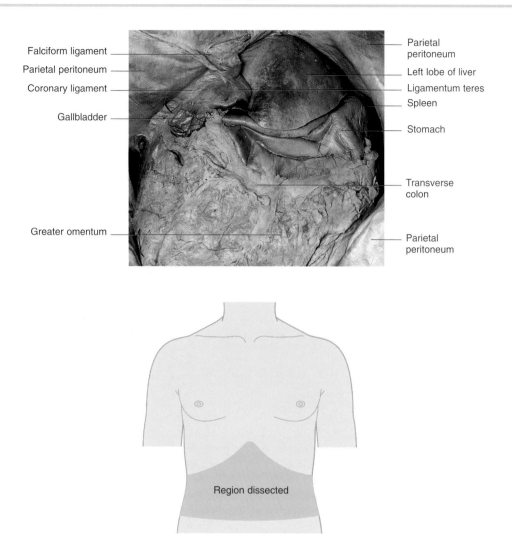

Falciform ligament

Parietal peritoneum

Coronary ligament

Gallbladder

Greater omentum

Parietal peritoneum

Left lobe of liver

Ligamentum teres

Spleen

Stomach

Transverse colon

Parietal peritoneum

Region dissected

Fig. 4.5a *Abdomen opened up to show the upper part of the peritoneal cavity and related organs.*

peritoneum and it invests many of the abdominal organs. In some such as duodenum, ascending and descending colon and kidneys only the anterior surfaces of the organs are covered by the peritoneum making them retroperitoneal organs. Peritoneal membranes connecting the parietal peritoneum to the visceral peritoneum has different names in different regions. The mesentery connects the small intestine, mesocolon the large intestine, omentum is attached to the stomach, and the peritoneal ligaments connect the liver.

In the male the peritoneal cavity is a closed sac, but in the female the ends of the uterine tubes open into the peritoneal cavity resulting in a communication with the exterior via the cavity of the tube, the uterus and the vagina. This is a potential source of infection of the peritoneal cavity from the exterior.

The peritoneal cavity is subdivided into a greater sac and a smaller lesser sac or the omental bursa. The greater sac is connected to the lesser sac through the epiploic foramen or the foramen of Winslow. The greater sac is subdivided into a supracolic and an infracolic compartments by the transverse colon and the transverse mesocolon.

The falciform ligament, a double-layered fold of peritoneum, extends from the umbilicus onto the liver holding a cord-like ligamentum teres (which is the obliterated umbilical vein) in its free edge (Fig. 4.5a).

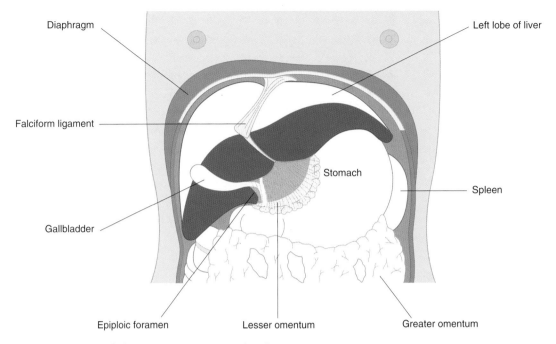

Fig. 4.5b *Liver, stomach, lesser omentum — anterior view.*

The right layer of the falciform ligament covers the right lobe of the liver and gets reflected onto the diaphragm as the coronary ligament. The left layer of the falciform ligament after enclosing the left lobe is reflected onto the diaphragm as the left triangular ligament.

After enclosing the liver the peritoneum extends from the liver to the lesser curvature of the stomach and to the first part of the duodenum as the lesser omentum. The two-layered lesser omentum has a right free border (Fig. 4.5a,b,c) which contains the common bile duct, the hepatic artery and the portal vein.

Along the lesser curvature the lesser omentum splits to enclose the stomach. Along the greater curvature of the stomach it reforms again as the greater omentum. The greater omentum hangs down like an apron from the greater curvature. Two layers from the greater curvature pass down as the anterior two layers of the greater omentum and fold on themselves to go upwards and backwards as its two posterior layers. The posterior layers split to enclose the transverse colon and continue on to the anterior aspect of the pancreas as the transverse mesocolon (Fig. 4.5d). From this attachment the upper layer continues as the parietal peritoneum of

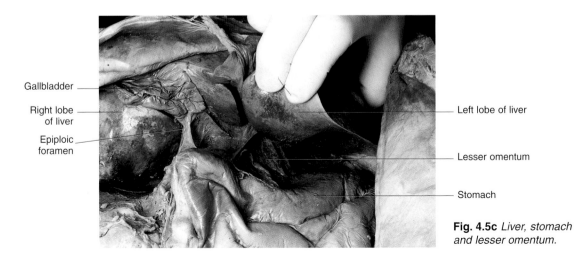

Fig. 4.5c *Liver, stomach and lesser omentum.*

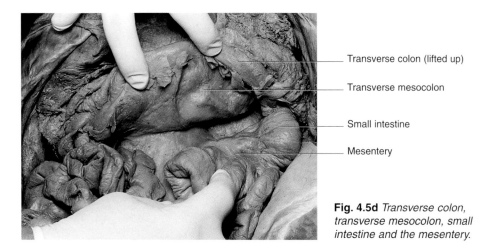

Fig. 4.5d *Transverse colon, transverse mesocolon, small intestine and the mesentery.*

- Transverse colon (lifted up)
- Transverse mesocolon
- Small intestine
- Mesentery

the posterior abdominal wall and that lining the diaphragm to be reflected back onto the liver. The lower layer from the attachment of the transverse mesocolon similarly continues downwards as the parietal peritoneum of the lower part of the posterior abdominal wall and then onto the pelvic viscera, ultimately becoming the parietal peritoneum of the anterior abdominal wall

(FIg. 4.5e). The parietal peritoneum of the posterior abdominal wall, however, is interrupted in two places. It is reflected to enclose the jejunum and ileum forming the mesentery of the small intestine and also further down it is interrupted where it is reflected to enclose the sigmoid colon forming the sigmoid mesocolon, the peritoneal membrane connecting the sigmoid colon to

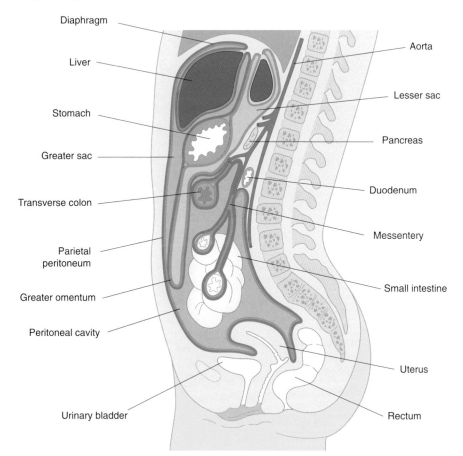

- Diaphragm
- Liver
- Stomach
- Greater sac
- Transverse colon
- Parietal peritoneum
- Greater omentum
- Peritoneal cavity
- Urinary bladder
- Aorta
- Lesser sac
- Pancreas
- Duodenum
- Messentery
- Small intestine
- Uterus
- Rectum

Fig. 4.5e *Peritoneum and peritoneal cavity — midline sagittal section.*

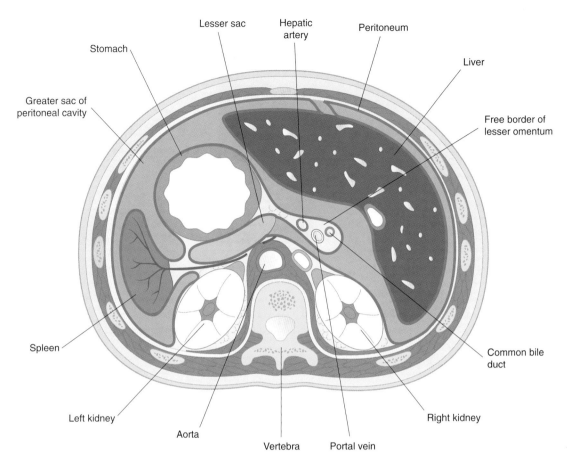

Fig. 4.5f *Peritoneum and peritoneal cavity — transverse section at the level of vertebra T12.*

the abdominal and pelvic wall. The line of attachment of the mesentery to the posterior abdominal wall is known as the root of the mesentery.

From the greater curvature of the stomach the greater omentum extends to the left as the gastrosplenic ligament which splits to invest the spleen and continues onto the left kidney as the lienorenal ligament (Fig. 4.5f).

In the pelvis the peritoneum covers the front and sides of the upper third of the rectum and only the front of its middle third. In the male, from the rectum it is reflected on to the upper surface of the urinary bladder and from there to the anterior abdominal wall.

The peritoneal space between the rectum and the bladder is the rectovesical pouch. In the female the reflection is onto the posterior wall of the vagina and then over the posterior upper and anterior surfaces of the uterus to the bladder. Between the uterus and the rectum is the rectouterine pouch and between the uterus and the bladder is the uterovesical pouch.

The lesser sac is a part of the peritoneal cavity that

lies behind the lesser omentum and the stomach and it also extends into the greater omentum. (The rest of the peritoneal cavity is known as the greater sac.) The lesser sac extends to the left up to the spleen where the sac is bounded by the gastrosplenic and lienorenal ligaments. To the right aspect of the lesser sac is the epiploic foramen through which it communicates with the greater sac of peritoneum.

The epiploic foramen has the following important boundaries:

- Anteriorly—the free border of the lesser omentum containing the bile duct, hepatic artery and the portal vein (Fig. 4.5f). The hepatic artery can be compressed here between the finger and thumb to stop haemorrhage from a torn cystic artery during cholecystectomy. This is known as Pringle's manoeuvre.
- Posteriorly—the inferior vena cava.
- Inferiorly—the first part of the duodenum.
- Superiorly—the caudate process of the liver.

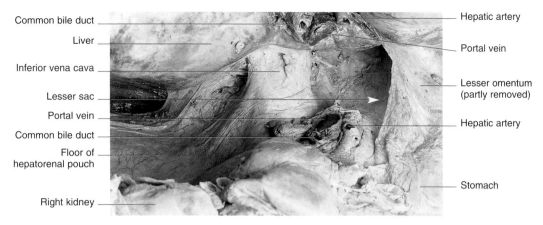

Common bile duct — Hepatic artery

Liver — Portal vein

Inferior vena cava

Lesser sac — Lesser omentum (partly removed)

Portal vein — Hepatic artery

Common bile duct

Floor of hepatorenal pouch

Right kidney — Stomach

Fig. 4.5g *Lesser sac seen after partial removal of the lesser omentum. Transverse colon and the right side of the lesser omentum were removed to obtain this dissection.*

OESOPHAGUS AND STOMACH
(Fig. 4.6)

Abdominal part of the oesophagus

The oesophagus extends from the pharynx in the neck via the thorax to the cardiac end of the stomach. Its abdominal part which is about 2.5 cm long lies behind the left lobe of the liver and the left triangular ligament. The oesophagus enters the abdominal cavity by passing through the right crus of the diaphragm at the level of the tenth thoracic vertebra.

The lower oesophageal sphincter and the external 'sphincter' formed by crural fibres of the diaphragm are the two major anatomical sphincter mechanisms to prevent gastrooesophageal reflux. The lower oesophageal sphincter is formed by specialised circular muscle fibres in the region passing through diaphragm, the abdominal part kept closed by tonic contraction of muscle. The sphincter which relaxes only during swallowing and during vomiting is controlled by intramural plexuses of enteric nervous system. The neural release of nitric oxide may aid relaxation. The tone of the diaphragm, the phrenooesophageal membrane which connects the oesophagus to the surrounding right crus of diaphragm and the intraabdominal pressure also exert a sphincteric effect.

Stomach

The stomach has two borders — the greater and lesser curvatures, two surfaces, the anterior and posterior surfaces, and two orifices, the cardia and pylorus. It is approximately J shaped but its shape and its size are very variable. It can lie transversely as the 'steer-horn'

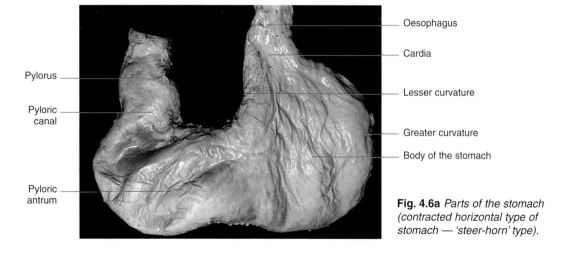

Pylorus

Pyloric canal

Pyloric antrum

Oesophagus

Cardia

Lesser curvature

Greater curvature

Body of the stomach

Fig. 4.6a *Parts of the stomach (contracted horizontal type of stomach — 'steer-horn' type).*

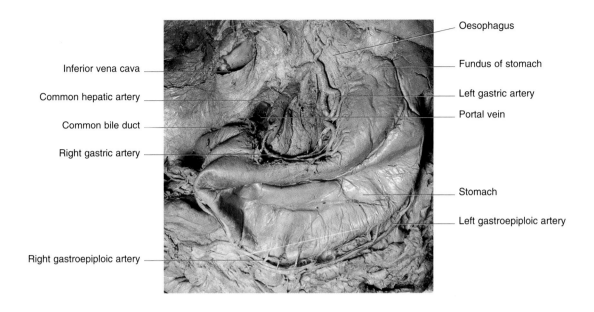

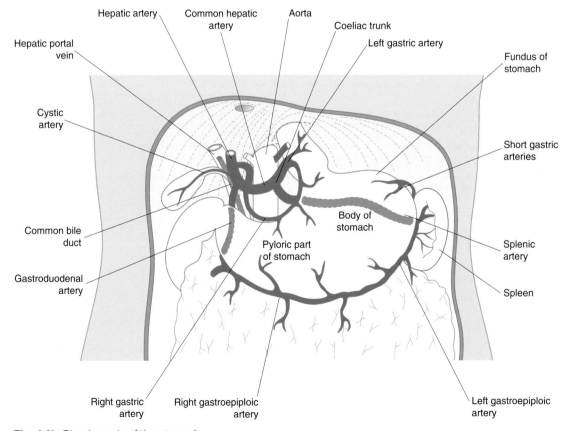

Fig. 4.6b *Blood supply of the stomach.*

type. Between the cardia and the pylorus lies the body and the pyloric part of the stomach, the latter having an expanded pyloric antrum which is proximal to the narrow pyloric canal. At the junction between the pyloric canal and the first part of the duodenum is the pyloric sphincter. This is a well-marked sphincter and is palpable at operation. Its position corresponds to a vertical vein on the surface — the pre-pyloric vein of Mayo. The part of the stomach projecting upwards from the cardia is the fundus.

Anteriorly the stomach is related to the anterior abdominal wall and the left lobe of the liver. Posteriorly it is related to the diaphragm, aorta, pancreas, left kidney, and suprarenal gland and the spleen with the lesser sac of peritoneum intervening between these and its posterior surface (Fig. 4.5e, f).

Blood supply of the stomach (Fig. 4.6b)
Rich arterial anastomoses are present along the greater and lesser curvatures. The left and right gastric arteries anastomose along the lesser curvature, the right and left gastroepiploic arteries and the short gastric arteries along the greater curvature of the stomach. The gastroduodenal artery, a branch of the common hepatic artery, lies behind the first part of the duodenum and can bleed when a peptic ulcer on the posterior wall erodes into it.

Lymphatic drainage
The lymphatics accompany the blood vessels. Lymphatics accompanying the splenic artery branches drain to the nodes along the upper border of the pancreas, nodes at the hilum of the spleen and then into the coeliac group of lymph nodes. Similarly branches of the hepatic artery are also accompanied by lymphatic vessels which too eventually reach the coeliac nodes. When the stomach is affected by carcinoma secondaries can also spread in a retrograde manner and affect the lymph nodes at the porta hepatis. These may block the bile duct to cause obstructive jaundice.

Nerve supply
The stomach is supplied by the two vagus nerves as the anterior and posterior gastric nerves. These nerves are related to the oesophagus. The anterior gastric nerves (from the left vagus) lie on the anterior surface of the oesophagus and the posterior gastric nerves (right vagus) behind. The vagus constitutes the motor and secretory nerve supply of the stomach. Vagotomy (division of vagus) reduces acid secretion from the stomach.

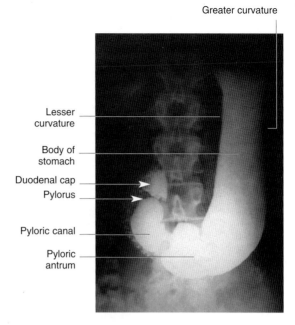

Fig. 4.6c *Radiograph of the stomach after barium meal where barium sulphate is used as a contrast medium. The fundus is filled with gas (air) as the patient is in the erect position. Pylorus is seen as a gap in the barium proximal to the duodenal cap which is the first part of the duodenum.*

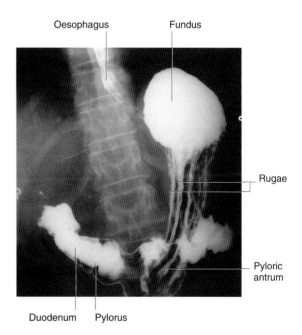

Fig. 4.6d *Radiograph of the stomach after barium meal. The patient is in the recumbent position. The fundus is well outlined. Rugae, the longitudinal folds of mucosa are also well seen.*

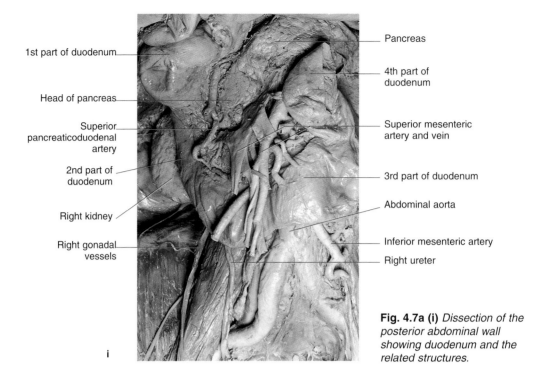

1st part of duodenum

Head of pancreas

Superior
pancreaticoduodenal
artery

2nd part of
duodenum

Right kidney

Right gonadal
vessels

Pancreas

4th part of
duodenum

Superior mesenteric
artery and vein

3rd part of duodenum

Abdominal aorta

Inferior mesenteric artery

Right ureter

Fig. 4.7a (i) *Dissection of the
posterior abdominal wall
showing duodenum and the
related structures.*

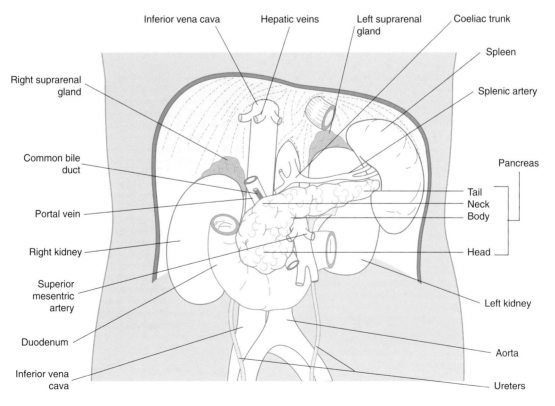

Inferior vena cava　　Hepatic veins　　Left suprarenal
gland　　Coeliac trunk

Spleen

Right suprarenal
gland

Splenic artery

Common bile
duct

Pancreas

Tail
Neck
Body

Portal vein

Right kidney

Head

Superior
mesentric
artery

Left kidney

Duodenum

Inferior vena
cava

Aorta

Ureters

Fig. 4.7a (ii) *Pancreas, duodenum and the related structures.*

THE DUODENUM (Fig. 4.7a, b, c)

The small intestine, the major site of digestion and absorption, extends from the pylorus of the stomach to the ileocaecal junction. It is 2–7 m long. The first 25 cm is the duodenum, the next two-fifths is the jejunum and the distal three-fifths is the ileum.

The duodenum is C-shaped and it curves around the head of the pancreas. It is divided into four parts. Except for the first 2–3 cm the entire duodenum is retroperitoneal.

The first part

The first part is about 5 cm long. Posteriorly it is related to the gastroduodenal artery, bile duct and the portal vein (Fig. 4.6b, 4.7b). A duodenal ulcer on the posterior wall can erode into the artery causing haematemesis (vomiting of blood) and melaena (altered blood in stool). Anteriorly this part of the duodenum is related to the liver and gall bladder.

The second part

The bile duct (Fig. 4.7b) and the pancreatic duct enter the major duodenal papilla on the posteromedial wall about 10 cm from the pylorus. This point also is the junction between the foregut and midgut components of the developing gastrointestinal tract

The accessory pancreatic duct of Santorini opens a little above. The second part of the duodenum is related posteriorly to the hilum of the right kidney and the ureter and anteriorly it is crossed by the transverse colon.

The third part

As this part runs horizontally to the left it crosses the inferior vena cave and the aorta. It is crossed anteriorly by the root of the mesentery and the superior mesenteric vessels.

The fourth part

This part ascends vertically and turns abruptly to end as the duodenojejunal flexure. A peritoneal fold, the

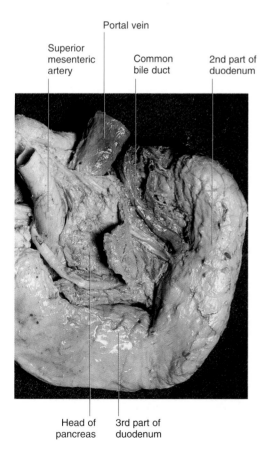

Fig. 4.7b *Posterior aspect of the duodenum and the head of pancreas.*

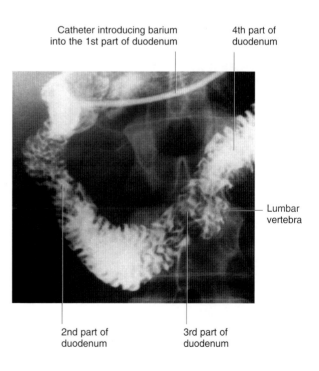

Fig. 4.7c *Radiograph of the duodenum outlined by barium sulphate. Barium is broken up by circular folds in the duodenum.*

ligament of Treves from the right crus of diaphragm, is an identification point for the duodenojejunal flexure at operation.

Blood supply

The duodenum is supplied by the superior and the inferior pancreaticoduodenal arteries. The former is a branch of the gastroduodenal artery and the latter that of the superior mesenteric. Along the curved border of the duodenum these arteries anastomose and supply the duodenum and the head of the pancreas.

JEJUNUM AND ILEUM (Fig. 4.7d, e)

Unlike the duodenum, the jejunum and ileum are very mobile because of the mesentery by which they are anchored to the posterior abdominal wall. The root of the mesentery which is about 15 cm long extends from the duodenojejunal flexure obliquely downwards and

to the right to the ileocaecal junction. It crosses the third part of the duodenum, the aorta, the inferior vena cava, the right ureter and the right gonadal arteries. The superior mesenteric artery, a branch of the abdominal aorta, enters the mesentery as it crosses the third part of the duodenum. The mesentery also contains the superior mesenteric vein, lymphatics and lymph nodes as well as autonomic nerves.

Transition between the jejunum and ileum is gradual. There is no landmark between the two. Yet it is important for the surgeon to distinguish a loop of the jejunum from that of the ileum. The jejunum has a thicker wall due to circular folds or valvulae conniventes or plicae circulares. These are more numerous in the jejunum than in the ileum. The jejunal and ileal branches from the superior mesenteric artery form arcades from which terminal vessels — vasae rectae — supply the gut wall. The jejunum has only one or two arcades making the vasa rectae longer than that of the ileum. The number of arcades are more in the ileal mesentery which have relatively short vasae rectae.

The veins corresponding to the arterial branches drain into the superior mesenteric vein and then into the hepatic portal vein.

Loops of small intestine may get twisted around

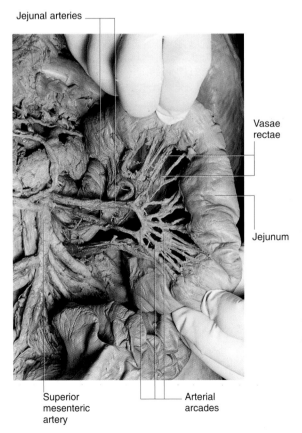

Jejunal arteries

Vasae rectae

Jejunum

Superior mesenteric artery

Arterial arcades

Fig. 4.7d *Jejunal arteries, arterial arcades and vasae rectae.*

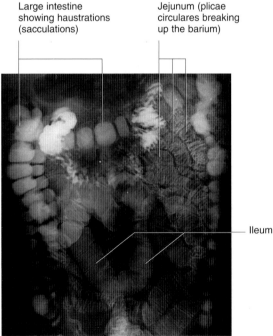

Large intestine showing haustrations (sacculations)

Jejunum (plicae circulares breaking up the barium)

Ileum

Fig. 4.7e *Radiograph of the abdomen after barium meal showing jejunum, ileum and parts of the large intestine.*

abnormal peritoneal bands or adhesions, producing a volvulus. A volvulus can result in intestinal obstruction and strangulation of its blood supply. Malrotation of the gut during development may result in a very short root of the mesentery and this may also produce a volvulus.

Meckel's (ileal) diverticulum is a remnant of the vitellointestinal duct (connection between the midgut and the yolk sac) of the developing gut. It is present only in 2% of individuals. This may be seen about 2 feet (60 cm) proximal to the ileocaecal junction in the ante-mesenteric border of the ileum. The Meckel's diverticulum may often have pancreatic or gastric mucosa as a lining, resulting in ulceration and bleeding.

LARGE INTESTINE (Fig. 4.8)

The large intestine consists of the caecum, ascending colon, transverse colon, descending colon and the sigmoid colon. The transverse and sigmoid colon have their own mesentery (the transverse and sigmoid mesocolon) and hence are mobile. The ascending and the descending colon are retroperitoneal structures. The caecum often has peritoneum reflected on to its posterior wall forming a retrocaecal recess and hence may be mobile.

The presence of taenia coli, haustrations and appendices epiploicae distinguish the large intestine from the small intestine. Taenia coli are longitudinal bands of muscle. There are three of them and they

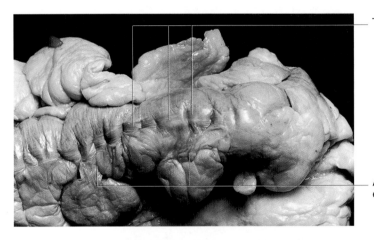

Taenia coli

Appendices epiploicae

Fig. 4.8a *Large intestine — taenia coli and appendices epiploicae.*

Right colic (hepatic) flexure

Ascending colon

Caecum

Appendix

Rectum

Left colic (splenic) flexure

Transverse colon

Descending colon

Haustrations (sacculations)

Sigmoid colon

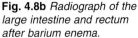

Fig. 4.8b *Radiograph of the large intestine and rectum after barium enema.*

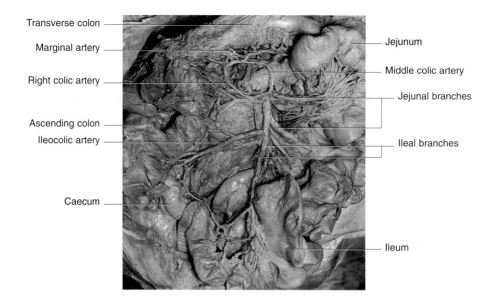

Transverse colon

Marginal artery

Right colic artery

Ascending colon

Ileocolic artery

Caecum

Jejunum

Middle colic artery

Jejunal branches

Ileal branches

Ileum

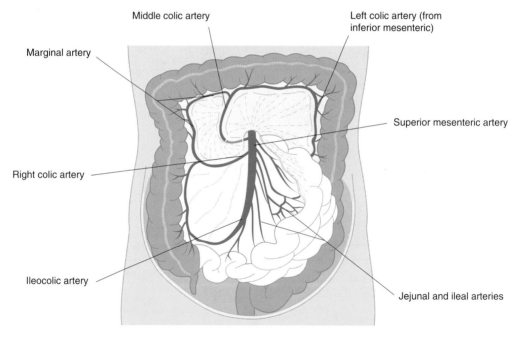

Middle colic artery

Left colic artery (from inferior mesenteric)

Marginal artery

Superior mesenteric artery

Right colic artery

Ileocolic artery

Jejunal and ileal arteries

Fig. 4.8c *The distribution of the superior mesenteric artery.*

converge together at the root of the appendix (root of the appendix can be identified at operation by tracing the taenia coli). Sacculations caused by the pull of the taenia coli are known as haustrations. Appendices epiploicae are fat lobules covered by peritoneum. They are more abundant in the sigmoid colon.

The caecum (Fig. 4.8c, g, h, i)

The caecum which is the dilated blind-ending commencement of the large intestine is located in the right iliac fossa. The ileocaecal valve is located on the left side at the junction between the caecum and the ascending colon. Although the lips of the valve may to a certain extent prevent colonic content getting into the ileum, the sphincteric action of the valve is thought to be poor. Tumours in the caecum may grow to a large size without causing obstruction until they involve the ileocaecal junction. Appendices epiploicae are not present on the caecum.

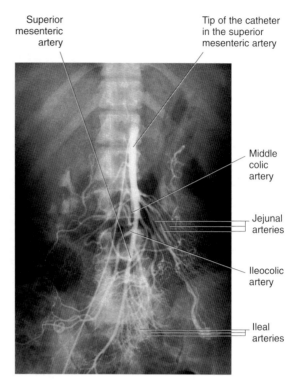

Fig. 4.8d *Superior mesenteric arteriogram.*

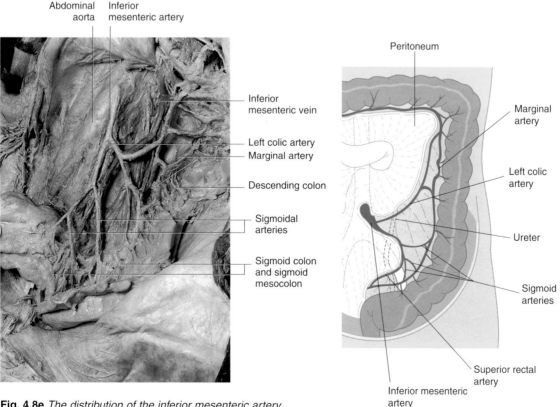

Fig. 4.8e *The distribution of the inferior mesenteric artery.*

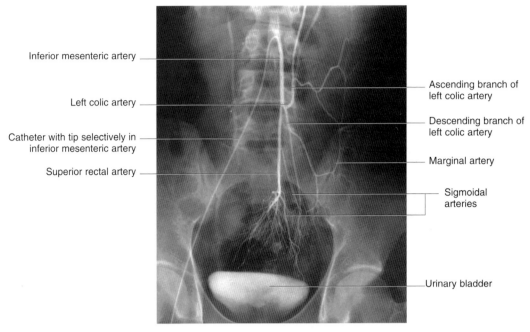

Inferior mesenteric artery

Left colic artery

Catheter with tip selectively in
inferior mesenteric artery

Superior rectal artery

Ascending branch of
left colic artery

Descending branch of
left colic artery

Marginal artery

Sigmoidal
arteries

Urinary bladder

Fig. 4.8f *The inferior mesenteric artery angiogram.*

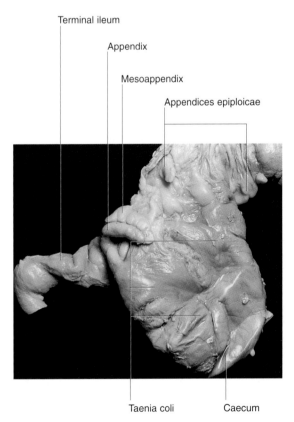

Terminal ileum

Appendix

Mesoappendix

Appendices epiploicae

Taenia coli   Caecum

Fig. 4.8g *Posterior aspect of the caecum with a
retrocalceal appendix.*

The appendix (Fig. 4.8g, h)

The appendix is attached to the posteromedial aspect of
the caecum. Its size and position are variable. In about
75% of cases it is retrocaecal, whereas in about 20% it
hangs into the pelvis. The three taenia coli merge at the
root of the appendix. However the appendix itself is
devoid of taenia and appendices epiploicae. It has a
mesentery which contains the appendicular artery,
which is a branch of the ileocolic artery or that of one
of its caecal branches. The artery is functionally an end
artery, thrombosis of which in appendicitis causes
gangrene of the appendix leading to perforation.

The surface marking of the appendix is the
McBurney's point which is the junction between the
lower third and the upper two-thirds of the line
connecting the anterior superior iliac spine to the
umbilicus.

Sigmoid colon (Fig. 4.8b, also 4.15l)

The sigmoid colon extends from the pelvic brim to the
rectosigmoid junction. It has a mesentery which makes
it hang down into the pelvic cavity where it is closely
related to the urinary bladder in the male and the
uterus and vagina in the female. Diverticulitis of the

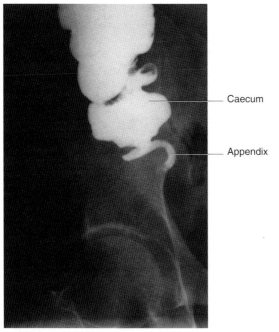

Caecum

Appendix

Fig. 4.8h *Radiograph of caecum and appendix following barium enema.*

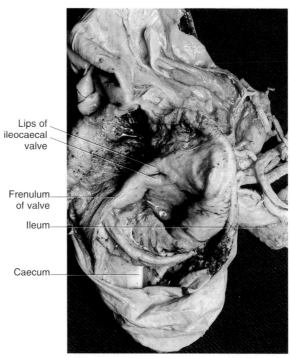

Lips of
ileocaecal
valve

Frenulum
of valve

Ileum

Caecum

Fig. 4.8i *Interior of the caecum showing the ileocaecal valve.*

sigmoid colon can give rise to vesicocolic or vaginocolic fistulae. The appendices epiploicae are most numerous in the sigmoid colon.

Blood supply and lymphatic drainage of the large intestine

The large intestine is supplied by the superior and inferior mesenteric arteries. The branches of the superior mesenteric artery are the ileocolic, right colic and the middle colic arteries. The ileocolic also gives off the anterior and posterior caecal arteries and the appendicular artery. The superior mesenteric artery supplies the region up to the splenic flexure and the inferior mesenteric branches supply the region beyond. The inferior mesenteric artery gives off the left colic and the sigmoidal arteries and continues into the pelvis as the superior rectal artery. The colic arteries form a series of anastomoses giving rise to the marginal artery of Drummond which extends from the ileocolic to the colorectal junction. A good blood supply to the colon is maintained through the marginal artery even if one or two colic arteries are ligated. The weakest part of the anastomosis is near the splenic flexure where the

superior and inferior mesenteric branches meet. Deficiency of blood supply can lead to ischaemic colitis.

Lymphatic drainage of the large intestine follows the course of the arteries. The primary nodes lie along the wall of the gut from where efferents go to the nodes along the branches of the superior and inferior mesenteric vessels and finally into the nodes around the superior mesenteric artery.

RECTUM AND ANAL CANAL
(Fig. 4.8j, k, l, m)

The rectum starts at the level of the third piece of sacrum and ends in front of the coccyx. The lower part of the rectum is expanded to form the ampulla of the rectum. Unlike the sigmoid colon the rectum has no mesentery, appendices epiploicae or taenia coli. Peritoneum covers the anterior and lateral aspect of the upper third but only the anterior aspect of the middle third.

The lower third of the rectum lying below the pelvic peritoneum is completely extraperitoneal. The rectum follows the curvature of the sacrum and also has three lateral flexures. Its upper part is convex to the left, middle part convex to the right and lower part again convex to the left.

Relations

The upper part of the rectum is related to the rectovesical pouch containing coils of ileum and sigmoid colon. In the male the lower part is related anteriorly to the seminal vesicles ductus and bladder and the ends of the ureters and the rectouterine pouch, whereas in the female the vagina and the posterior fornix and the uterine cervix form the immediate relations. A layer of fascia, Denonvillier's fascia separates these anterior structures from the rectum. In surgical mobilisation of rectum during abdominoperineal resection the plane of dissection should be on the rectal side of the fascia to avoid injury to anterior structures

Posteriorly the rectum is related to the sacrum, coccyx, the sacral nerves, the median sacral artery and the sacral veins. A fascia known as the Waldeyer's

fascia separates the rectum from these structures and contains the plexus of veins draining the rectum.

During surgery dissection on the rectal side of Waldeyer's fascia should be done to avoid bleeding from sacral veins. Rectal cancer spreading posteriorly causes sciatic pain. On the lateral aspect of the rectum there is a lateral ligament formed by condensation of fascia around middle rectal vessels. Also related are the ureter, sympathetic chain and the superior and inferior hypogastric plexuses. During rectal surgery damage to ureters should be avoided and both the superior and inferior hypogastric plexuses which are autonomic nerve plexuses in the pelvis should also be kept intact to avoid sexual dysfunction.

Anal canal

The space below the pelvic diaphragm is defined as the perineum. The rectum passes through the pelvic diaphragm to become the anal canal in the perineum. The anal canal which is about 4 cm long passes downwards and backwards from the anorectal junction

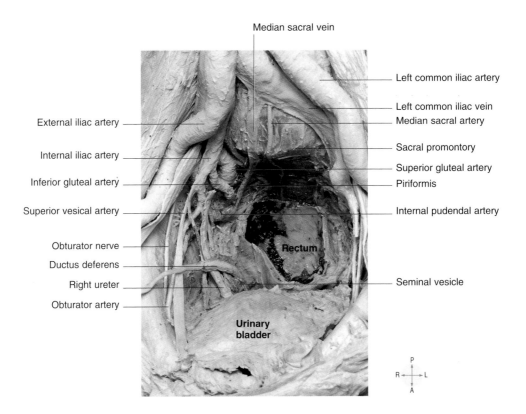

Fig. 4.8j *Dissection of the male pelvis after removal of the sigmoid colon. The rectum, urinary bladder and the related structures are viewed from above.*

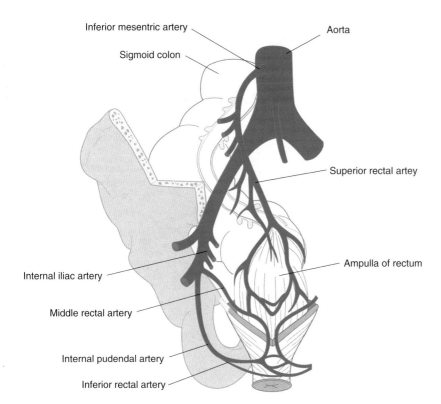

Fig. 4.8k *Arterial supply of the rectum and anal canal — posterior view.*

to the anus, the external opening. It is surrounded by the internal sphincter which is the continuation of the circular muscle fibres of the rest of the gut (smooth muscle) and an external sphincter which is a striated muscle. The lining mucosa show vertical columns, anal columns or columns of Morgagni. Their lower ends are connected by folds forming the anal valves or valves of Ball. Behind the valves are small anal sinuses into which the anal glands open. The line along which the anal valves are arranged is the dentate or pectinate line. It represents the function between endoderm and ectoderm. The anal canal above the dentate line is lined by columnar epithelium and the part below derived from the ectoderm is lined by stratified squamous

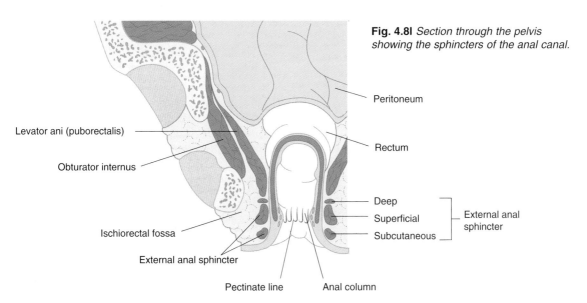

Fig. 4.8l *Section through the pelvis showing the sphincters of the anal canal.*

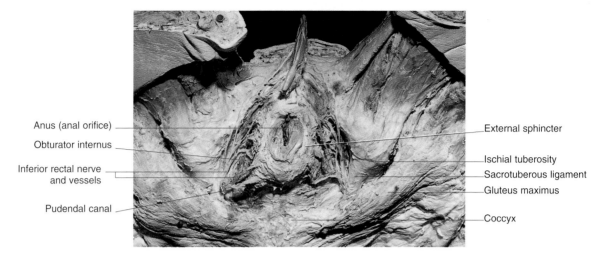

Anus (anal orifice)

Obturator internus

Inferior rectal nerve
and vessels

Pudendal canal

External sphincter

Ischial tuberosity

Sacrotuberous ligament

Gluteus maximus

Coccyx

Fig. 4.8m *The anal canal and the two ischiorectal fossae. The anococcygeal body is removed to show the continuity of one fossa to the other.*

epithelium. A carcinoma of the upper anal canal therefore is an adenocarcinoma and that of the lower anal canal is a squamous cell carcinoma. Also due to the developmental differences the part above the dentate line is supplied by autonomic nerves and is insensitive to ordinary pain stimuli, whereas the lower part is supplied by somatic nerves making it painful to ulceration, to injections and instrumentations.

Blood supply of the rectum and anal canal (Fig. 4.8k)

The superior rectal artery supplies the whole of the rectum and the upper part of the anal canal up to the dentate line, and the inferior rectal artery supplies the lower part of the anal canal and its supply may extend up to the peritoneal reflection. The small middle rectal artery may supply only the muscle coats of the rectum. The arteries are accompanied by veins. The tributaries of the superior rectal vein drain into the portal vein whereas the middle and inferior rectal veins drain into the internal iliac vein.

Ischiorectal fossa (Fig. 8.8l, m)

The ischiorectal fossa is a fat-containing space which allows expansion of the anal canal. The ischiorectal fossa can get infected, forming an ischiorectal abscess which may need surgical intervention. It is a wedge-shaped space bounded laterally by the obturator internus muscle and medially by the levator ani and the anal canal. The anal canal here is surrounded by its

external sphincter. The obturator internus takes origin from the inner aspect of the obturator membrane covering the obturator foramen. The ischiorectal fossa is crossed by the inferior rectal nerves and vessels from lateral to medial side. These are branches of the internal pudendal nerves and vessels which lie on the lateral wall of the fossa in the pudendal canal (Alcock's canal) in the fascia covering the obturator internus.

The two ischiorectal fossae are separated in the midline behind the anal canal, by a fibromuscular partition, the anococcygeal body which has an opening in its upper portion through which the two ischiorectal fossae communicate with each other. Infection from one fossa can readily pass on to the other side through this communication.

LIVER (Fig. 4.9)

The liver occupies a major part of the upper abdominal cavity. It is supplied by the hepatic artery and the hepatic portal vein and is drained by the hepatic veins which join the inferior vena cava. Bile produced by the liver drains into the second part of the duodenum via the biliary duct system. Normal liver is not palpable except in small children and in patients with emphysema where the diaphragm is at a lower level. On palpation the sharp inferior border is felt as the liver moves down on deep inspiration. The movement is due to the attachment of the liver to the diaphragm via the hepatic veins and the inferior vena cava.

The liver has diaphragmatic and visceral surfaces,

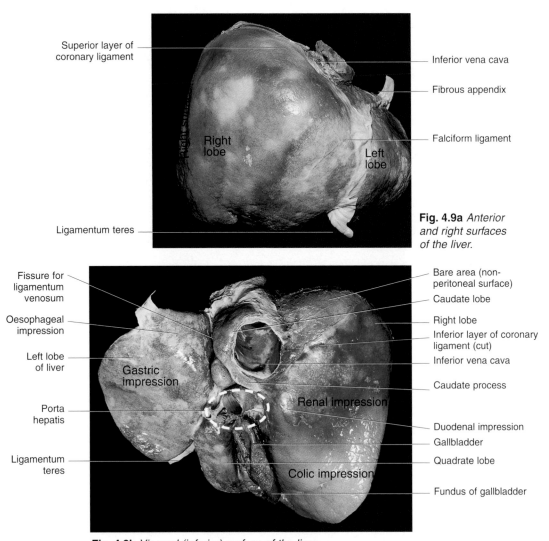

Superior layer of coronary ligament

Inferior vena cava

Fibrous appendix

Falciform ligament

Right lobe

Left lobe

Ligamentum teres

Fig. 4.9a *Anterior and right surfaces of the liver.*

Fissure for ligamentum venosum

Oesophageal impression

Left lobe of liver

Gastric impression

Porta hepatis

Ligamentum teres

Bare area (non-peritoneal surface)

Caudate lobe

Right lobe

Inferior layer of coronary ligament (cut)

Inferior vena cava

Caudate process

Renal impression

Duodenal impression

Gallbladder

Quadrate lobe

Colic impression

Fundus of gallbladder

Fig. 4.9b *Visceral (inferior) surface of the liver.*

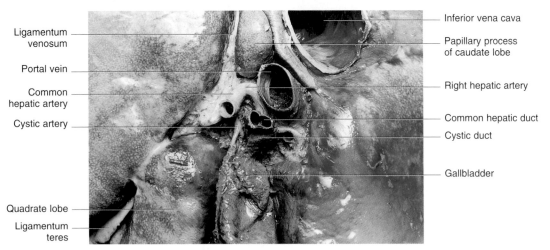

Ligamentum venosum

Portal vein

Common hepatic artery

Cystic artery

Quadrate lobe

Ligamentum teres

Inferior vena cava

Papillary process of caudate lobe

Right hepatic artery

Common hepatic duct

Cystic duct

Gallbladder

Fig. 4.9c *Inferior surface of the liver. Structures at the porta hepatis.*

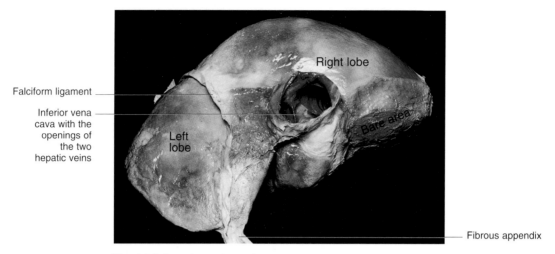

Falciform ligament

Inferior vena cava with the openings of the two hepatic veins

Right lobe

Left lobe

Bare area

Fibrous appendix

Fig. 4.9d *Superior surface of the liver.*

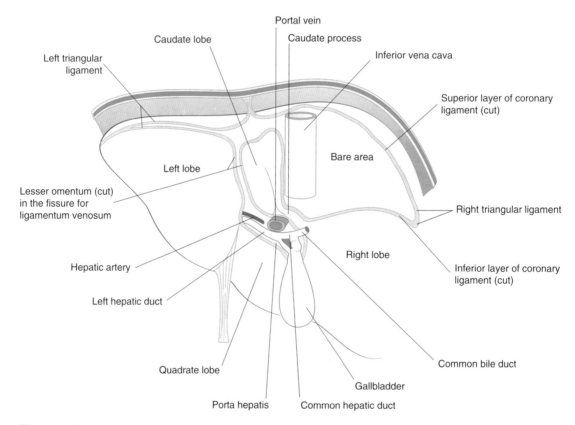

Portal vein

Caudate lobe

Caudate process

Left triangular ligament

Inferior vena cava

Superior layer of coronary ligament (cut)

Left lobe

Bare area

Lesser omentum (cut) in the fissure for ligamentum venosum

Right triangular ligament

Hepatic artery

Right lobe

Inferior layer of coronary ligament (cut)

Left hepatic duct

Common bile duct

Quadrate lobe

Gallbladder

Porta hepatis

Common hepatic duct

Fig. 4.9e *Liver — posterior view.*

the former subdivided into posterior superior, right and anterior surfaces which are not demarcated by sharp borders. The sharp inferior border of the liver separates the anterior and right surfaces from the visceral surface. Most main vessels and ducts enter or leave the liver at the porta hepatis on the visceral surface. The hepatic veins however leave the liver to enter the inferior vena cava at the posterior surface.

Peritoneal relations (Fig. 4.9a, b, d, e, f)

The liver is completely covered by peritoneum except in the bare area which is bounded by the two layers of the coronary ligament and the inferior vena cava. The liver (Fig. 4.9e) is divided into right and left lobes by the falciform ligament. The right layer of the falciform ligament covers the right lobe of the liver and gets reflected onto the diaphragm as the coronary ligament. The gap between the upper and lower layers of the coronary ligament is the bare area. The right end of the coronary ligament is known as the right triangular ligament. Besides continuing on to the diaphragm the peritoneum covering the right lobe of the liver also continues downwards onto the stomach as the posterior layer of the lesser omentum. The left layer of the falciform ligament after enclosing the left lobe is reflected onto the diaphragm as the left triangular ligament. It also extends downwards as the anterior layer of the lesser omentum.

Subphrenic and subhepatic spaces (Fig. 4.9f, 4.5g)

These spaces between the liver and the diaphragm are clinically important as they are sites of subphrenic abscess formation. The right and left subphrenic spaces lie on either side of the falciform ligament between the anterior surface of the liver and the diaphragm. The right subhepatic space or the hepatorenal pouch (of Rutherford Morrison) is the one of the most dependent parts of the peritoneal cavity in the recumbent position (the other being the rectovesical or rectouterine pouch). The space is between the peritoneum covering the liver and the right kidney. Intestinal content can easily gravitate into it as a sequelae of perforated appendix, duodenal ulcer or perforated diverticulitis and get infected giving rise to subphrenic abscess. The left subhepatic space is the lesser sac.

Lobes of the liver (Fig. 4.9b, e)

The liver is divided into right and left lobes by the

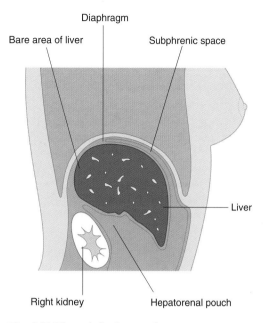

Fig. 4.9f *The subdiaphragmatic spaces.*

falciform ligament. The larger right lobe has two well-defined small lobes, the caudate lobe and a quadrate lobe on its posterior and inferior aspect respectively. The former is bounded by the inferior vena cava and a fissure which holds the ligamentum venosum (remnant of the ductus venosus) and the latter by the gall bladder and the groove for the ligamentum teres (remnant of the left umbilical vein). The liver also has functional divisions. The demarcation between the functional left and right lobes is a plane connecting the gall bladder fossa to the inferior vena cava, making the caudate and quadrate lobes as parts of the functional left lobe. The right branch of the common hepatic artery and the right branch of the portal vein supply the right functional lobe whereas the left functional lobe is supplied by the left branch of the vessels. Similarly the right and left hepatic ducts drain the corresponding functional lobes. Each functional lobe thus has its own arterial and portal venous blood supply and drainage system. Each lobe is further divided into segments based on the intrahepatic branching pattern of the vessels and ducts.

Visceral and posterior surfaces of the liver (Fig. 4.9b, c, e)

The porta hepatis on the visceral surface of the liver is where major vessels and ducts enter or leave the liver.

From anterior to posterior the porta hepatis has the right and left hepatic ducts, the right and left hepatic arteries and the portal vein (i.e. vein, artery and duct — VAD). The ducts being in front make them more accessible to surgery. It also contains lymph nodes and nerves.

The gall bladder lies in a shallow fossa on the visceral surface. The visceral surface is also related to the stomach, duodenum, right kidney and right colic flexure (hepatic flexure) (Fig. 4.9b). The left of the liver is related to the oesophagus which can be exposed by cutting the left triangular ligament and mobilising the left lobe. The right adrenal gland is related to the bare area which also has the inferior vena cava as one of its boundaries.

Blood supply of the liver

About 25% of the total blood supply of the liver reaches it via the hepatic artery and the remaining 75% through the low pressure portal vein. Blood leaves the liver through the hepatic veins which join the inferior vena cava. Besides the three major hepatic veins there are a number of small veins draining the right lobe which enter the inferior vena cava directly. These may be the only veins draining the liver when the main veins are thrombosed as in Budd–Chiari syndrome.

ANATOMY OF THE BILIARY TRACT
(Fig. 4.10)

For descriptive purposes the gallbladder is divided into fundus, body and neck, the latter continuing as the cystic duct. The fundus which projects out from the inferior border of the liver is located at the level of the ninth costal cartilage in the midclavicular line. The right and left hepatic ducts which collect the bile from the liver join to form the common hepatic duct which in turn is joined by the cystic duct to form the common bile duct. The common bile duct lies in the free border of the lesser omentum along with the hepatic artery and the portal vein.

Lower down it passes behind the duodenum and the head of the pancreas, and hence a tumour of the head of the pancreas can block the common bile duct to produce obstructive jaundice.

Before its termination the common bile duct is joined by the pancreatic duct to form the ampulla of Vater. The ampulla and the ends of the two ducts are surrounded by sphincteric muscles, the whole constituting the sphincter of Oddi. The hepatopancreatic ampulla terminates at the papilla of Vater on the posteromedial wall of the second part of the duodenum about 10 cm distal to the pylorus.

The gallbladder is supplied by the cystic artery, usually a branch of the right hepatic artery and by small arteries from its liver bed. The artery lies in the Calot's triangle bounded by the cystic duct, common hepatic duct and the liver. Variations in the origin of

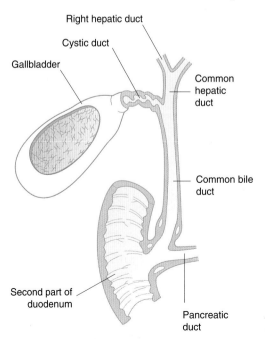

Fig. 4.10a *Biliary system.*

the artery are common. The presence of a cystic vein accompanying the artery is uncommon. The venous return is by small veins in the gallbladder bed entering the substance of the liver and then into the hepatic veins.

The common bile duct is supplied by branches from the cystic artery and the gastroduodenal artery. There is a good anastomosis between these two sets of arteries.

Variation to the pattern of the biliary duct system is common. The cystic duct may join the right hepatic duct or the common bile duct. Failure to appreciate these variations may result in errors in gallbladder surgery.

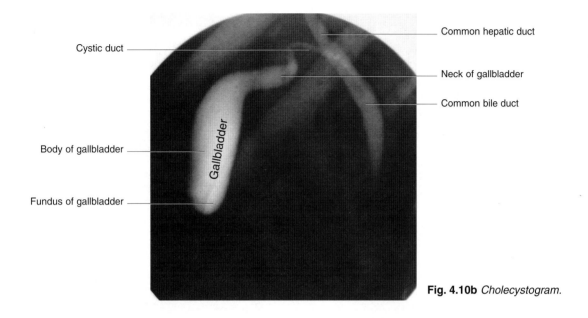

Cystic duct

Common hepatic duct

Neck of gallbladder

Common bile duct

Body of gallbladder

Gallbladder

Fundus of gallbladder

Fig. 4.10b *Cholecystogram.*

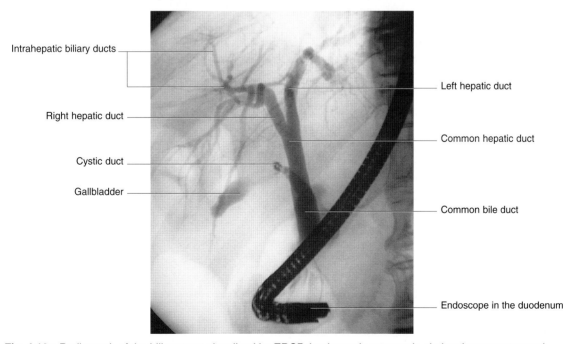

Intrahepatic biliary ducts

Left hepatic duct

Right hepatic duct

Common hepatic duct

Cystic duct

Gallbladder

Common bile duct

Endoscope in the duodenum

Fig. 4.10c *Radiograph of the biliary tract visualized by ERCP (endoscopic retrograde cholangiopancreatogram).*

PANCREAS (Fig. 4.11)

The pancreas, lying transversely across the posterior abdominal wall, has four parts: head, neck, body and the tail (Fig. 4.11a). The head of the pancreas is moulded to the C-shaped concavity of the duodenum. Its posterior surface is related to the inferior vena cava, and the right and left renal veins, and is indented or

even tunnelled by the common bile duct (Fig 4.11b). As the bile duct is intimately related to the head of the pancreas, carcinoma of the head of pancreas blocks the bile duct and produces obstructive jaundice. This may be an early manifestation of the disease. The lower part of the head hooks behind the superior mesenteric vessels as the uncinate process of the pancreas.

The hepatic portal vein is formed behind the neck of

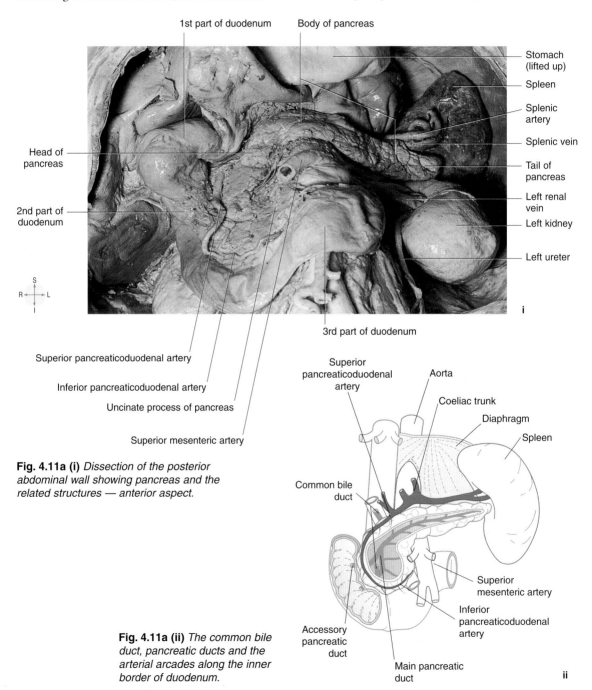

Fig. 4.11a (i) *Dissection of the posterior abdominal wall showing pancreas and the related structures — anterior aspect.*

Fig. 4.11a (ii) *The common bile duct, pancreatic ducts and the arterial arcades along the inner border of duodenum.*

the pancreas which lies in the transpyloric plane. The body of the pancreas crosses the abdominal aorta and the left kidney. The tail of the pancreas which is in the lienorenal ligament reaches the hilum of the spleen. The head of the pancreas is supplied by branches from the arterial arcade formed by the superior and inferior pancreaticoduodenal arteries. The body and tail of the pancreas is supplied by the splenic artery and is drained by the splenic vein. The splenic artery runs along its upper border whereas the splenic vein which is slightly at a lower level is related to its posterior surface.

The main pancreatic duct extends from the tail of the pancreas to where it terminates at the hepatopancreatic ampulla in the second part of the duodenum (Fig. 4.11a, c). Interlobular ducts join the main duct almost vertically, giving it a 'herring bone'

appearance. The main pancreatic duct (of Wirsung) in about 80% of the population joins the bile duct and together they form the hepatopancreatic ampulla of Vater which opens at the major duodenal papilla in the second part of the duodenum approximately 10 cm distal to the pylorus. The accessory pancreatic duct opens at the minor duodenal papilla about 2 cm proximal to the major papilla. The accessory duct drains the uncinate process and lower part of the head. There are communications between the two ducts.

In the condition known as pseudopancreatic cyst, collection of pancreatic juice and debris develops in the lesser sac of peritoneum following rupture of pancreatic duct in acute pancreatitis. The pancreas lies behind the lesser sac. Only a layer of parietal peritoneum intervenes between the lesser sac and the pancreas.

Inferior mesenteric vein   Superior mesenteric artery

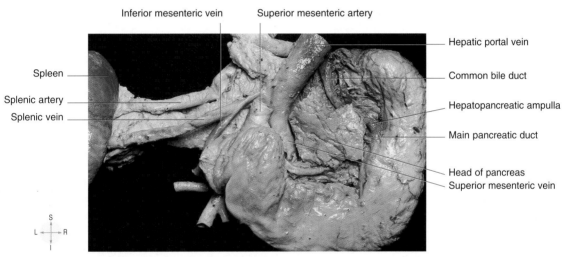

Spleen

Splenic artery
Splenic vein

Hepatic portal vein

Common bile duct

Hepatopancreatic ampulla

Main pancreatic duct

Head of pancreas
Superior mesenteric vein

Fig. 4.11b *Posterior aspect of the pancreas with the related structures.*

Main pancreatic duct   Common bile duct

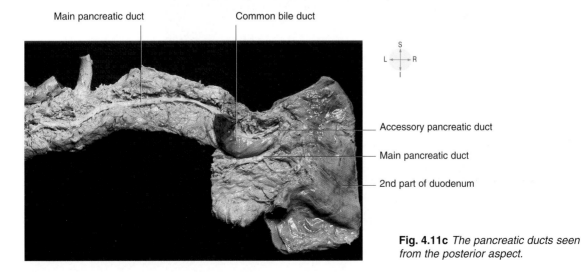

Accessory pancreatic duct

Main pancreatic duct

2nd part of duodenum

Fig. 4.11c *The pancreatic ducts seen from the posterior aspect.*

SPLEEN (Fig. 4.11d)

The spleen has diaphragmatic and visceral surfaces. The diaphragm separates the spleen from ribs 9–11 as well as the left lung and pleura. The visceral surface is related to the stomach, the splenic flexure of the colon and the left kidney. The hilum of the spleen is related to the tail of the pancreas, the splenic vessels and the lymph nodes. The spleen is almost completely invested by peritoneum and is connected to the stomach and the left kidney by gastrosplenic and lienorenal ligaments respectively.

Normal spleen is not palpable. It has to enlarge two to three times its normal size before it is palpable. The spleen may be enlarged in many conditions. It is sometime difficult to distinguish it from an enlarged left kidney. It is palpated under the left costal margin. The direction of the splenic enlargement from the subcostal region is downwards and towards the right iliac fossa. It is felt as a firm swelling with rounded borders. A notch may often (not always) be felt in the lower medial border of the spleen. The upper border of the enlarged spleen cannot be felt (it is not possible to reach above the swelling). The swelling descends on inspiration because of its intimate relation to the diaphragm. It is dull on percussion as it is not overlapped by coils of the gut.

THE COELIAC TRUNK (Fig. 4.12a, b)

The coeliac trunk is the first major branch of the abdominal aorta and arises immediately below the aortic opening in the diaphragm. Its branches supply the lower part of the oesophagus, the stomach and the first half of the duodenum as well as the liver, pancreas and the spleen.

The coeliac trunk divides into three branches: the common hepatic artery, the splenic artery and the left gastric artery. The common hepatic artery ascends to the porta hepatis in the free border of the lesser omentum lying to the left of the common bile duct in front of the portal vein (Fig. 4,6b) It gives off the right gastric artery and the gastroduodenal artery. The coeliac trunk is the artery of the foregut and hence the supply by its branches extends up to the region of the entrance of the bile duct in the duodenum which is the junction between the foregut and midgut.

THE COELIAC PLEXUS (Fig. 4.12c)

The coeliac plexus is the largest sympathetic plexus and surrounds the coeliac trunk. The plexus receives the greater and lesser splanchnic nerves (p. 81) and also a branch from the right vagus. The two coeliac ganglia, in which the preganglionic fibres of the splanchnic nerves synapse, lie on the crura of the diaphragm. Each ganglion is about 2 cm in diameter. A large contribution of preganglionic fibres from the plexus supply the adrenal medulla. The rest of the plexus descends over the abdominal aorta and is distributed to

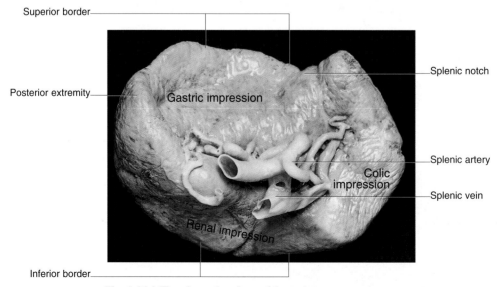

Fig. 4.11d *The visceral surface of the spleen.*

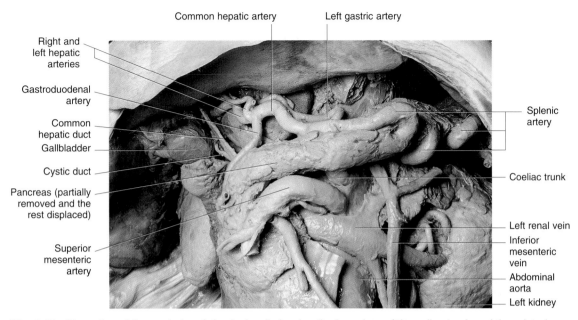

Fig. 4.12a *Dissection of the posterior abdominal wall showing the branches of the celiac trunk and the related structures. Stomach, small intestine, large intestine and the associated peritoneal membranes have been removed.*

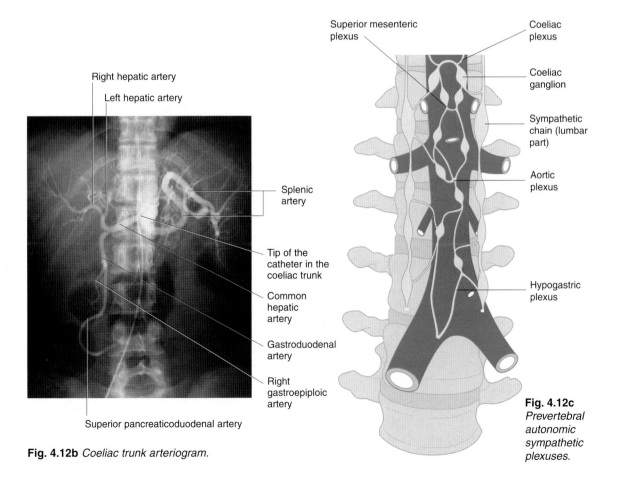

Fig. 4.12b *Coeliac trunk arteriogram.*

Fig. 4.12c *Prevertebral autonomic sympathetic plexuses.*

the abdominal viscera as plexuses accompanying the branches of the aorta.

Pain from the abdominal viscera is transmitted through the afferent sympathetic fibres in the coeliac plexus. Coeliac plexus block obtained with an anaesthetic drug is therapeutically used to relieve intractable abdominal pain produced by conditions such as chronic pancreatitis and carcinoma of the pancreas.

THE HEPATIC PORTAL VEIN (Fig. 4.12d, e)

The hepatic portal vein is formed by the union of the superior mesenteric and the splenic veins behind the neck of the pancreas. The inferior mesenteric vein may join the splenic vein or the superior mesenteric vein. In its course towards the porta hepatis the portal vein lies behind the first part of the duodenum and the free border of the lesser omentum.

The portal vein tributaries anastomose with those of the systemic veins forming portosystemic anastomoses. When the portal venous pressure rises above 10–12 mmHg (normal 5–8 mmHg) as in cirrhosis of the liver the sites of portosystemic anastomoses dilate. It also causes splenomegaly. The main sites of anastomoses are those under the mucosa of the lower

end of oesophagus, rectum, retroperitoneal region and the umbilical area via the paraumbilical vein. The most important are the oesophageal veins, as the oesophageal varices can produce life-threatening haematemesis.

THE ADRENAL (SUPRARENAL) GLANDS (Fig. 4.13)

The adrenal (suprarenal) glands lie on the upper poles of the kidneys overlapping on to the anterior surface. The right gland lies behind the bare area of the liver and its lower part is behind the hepatorenal pouch. The inferior vena cava overlaps it medially. Posteriorly lies the diaphragm. The left adrenal gland lies on the left crus of diaphragm and its upper part is anteriorly related to the stomach separated by the lesser sac whereas the lower part lies behind the pancreas and the splenic artery.

Each gland is supplied by three arteries and drained by one vein. The arterial supply is derived by branches from the aorta, renal artery and the inferior phrenic artery. The right adrenal vein joins the inferior vena cava whereas the left adrenal vein drains into the left renal vein.

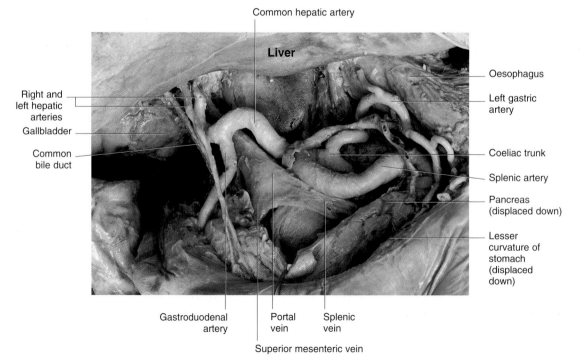

Fig. 4.12d *Formation of the portal vein and the branches of the coeliac trunk seen after the removal of the lesser omentum. Stomach and pancreas have been displaced downwards.*

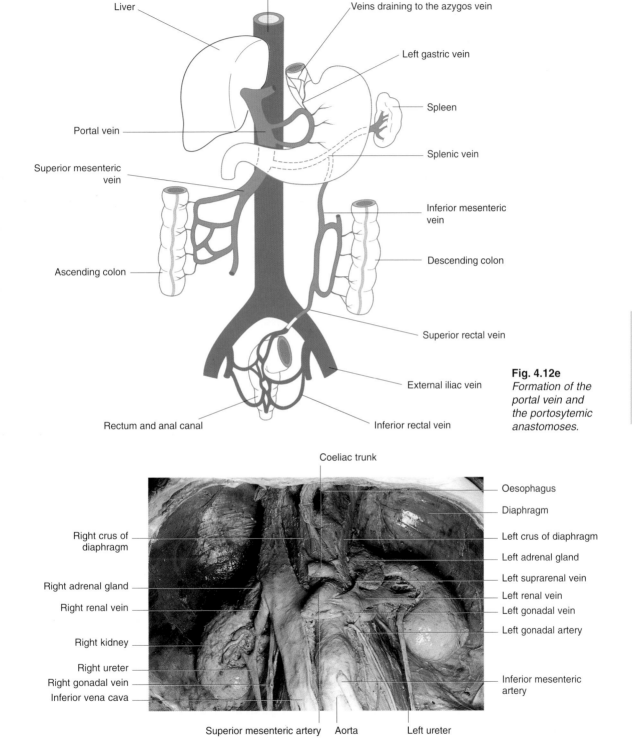

Inferior vena cava

Liver

Veins draining to the azygos vein

Left gastric vein

Portal vein

Spleen

Splenic vein

Superior mesenteric vein

Inferior mesenteric vein

Ascending colon

Descending colon

Superior rectal vein

External iliac vein

Rectum and anal canal

Inferior rectal vein

Fig. 4.12e *Formation of the portal vein and the portosytemic anastomoses.*

Coeliac trunk

Oesophagus

Diaphragm

Right crus of diaphragm

Left crus of diaphragm

Left adrenal gland

Right adrenal gland

Left suprarenal vein

Right renal vein

Left renal vein

Left gonadal vein

Left gonadal artery

Right kidney

Right ureter

Right gonadal vein

Inferior mesenteric artery

Inferior vena cava

Superior mesenteric artery   Aorta   Left ureter

Fig. 4.13 *Structures in the upper part of the posterior abdominal wall. Stomach, intestines, liver, pancreas and spleen have all been removed.*

THE ABDOMINAL AORTA (Fig. 4.14)

The thoracic aorta enters the abdomen by passing between the two crura of the diaphragm behind the median arcuate ligament to become the abdominal aorta. It lies on the bodies of the lumbar vertebrae and inclines slightly to the left as it descends. The abdominal aorta bifurcates into two common iliac arteries in front of the body of the fourth lumbar vertebra (Fig. 4.14a, b, c, d, e).

The surface marking of the aorta extends from a point just above the transpyloric plane in the midline to a point just to the left of the midline in a plane connecting the highest points of the iliac crest.

Branches can be grouped into three categories. The unpaired visceral branches are the three gut arteries — coeliac trunk, superior mesenteric artery and the inferior mesenteric artery. The paired visceral branches are the suprarenal, renal and gonadal arteries. The branches to the abdominal wall are the paired inferior phrenic and the lumbar arteries as well as the unpaired median sacral artery. The lumbar arteries (usually four in number) branching off from the sides of the aorta accompany the lumbar veins. The median sacral artery arising from the bifurcation of the aorta enters the pelvis, anastomoses with the sacral arteries and supplies the pelvic wall.

Relations (Fig. 4.7a, 4.11a, 4.12a, 4.14d, e, f, g)

The pancreas and the splenic vein cross the aorta in between the origin of the coeliac trunk and the superior mesenteric arteries. Between the origins of the superior and inferior mesenteric arteries the aorta is crossed by the third part of the duodenum and the left renal vein. The third and fourth left lumbar veins cross behind the aorta.

A tumour of the pancreas or mass of paraaortic lymph nodes transmitting aortic pulsation can be mistaken for an aneurysm of the aorta.

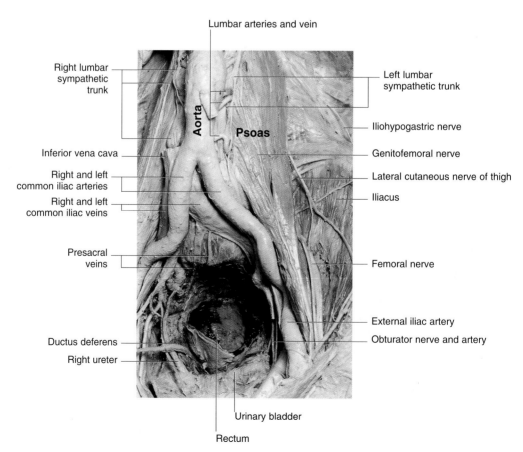

Lumbar arteries and vein

Right lumbar sympathetic trunk

Left lumbar sympathetic trunk

Aorta

Psoas

Iliohypogastric nerve

Inferior vena cava

Genitofemoral nerve

Right and left common iliac arteries

Lateral cutaneous nerve of thigh

Right and left common iliac veins

Iliacus

Presacral veins

Femoral nerve

External iliac artery

Ductus deferens

Obturator nerve and artery

Right ureter

Urinary bladder

Rectum

Fig. 4.14a *Lower part of the posterior abdominal wall and pelvis.*

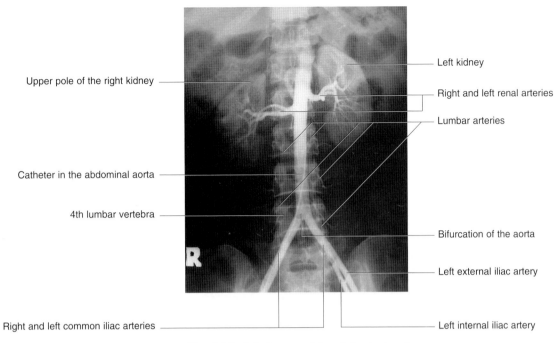

Upper pole of the right kidney

Catheter in the abdominal aorta

4th lumbar vertebra

Right and left common iliac arteries

Left kidney

Right and left renal arteries

Lumbar arteries

Bifurcation of the aorta

Left external iliac artery

Left internal iliac artery

Fig. 4.14b *Arteriogram of the abdominal aorta.*

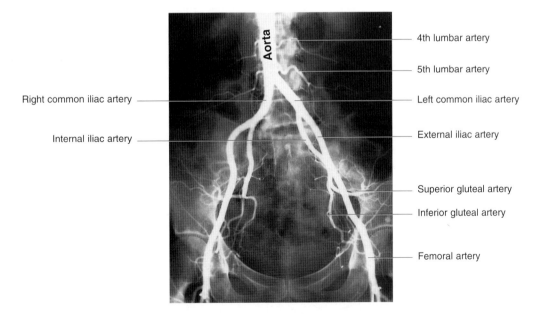

Aorta

Right common iliac artery

Internal iliac artery

4th lumbar artery

5th lumbar artery

Left common iliac artery

External iliac artery

Superior gluteal artery

Inferior gluteal artery

Femoral artery

Fig. 4.14c *Arteriogram of the lower part of abdominal aorta and the iliac arteries.*

THE INFERIOR VENA CAVA
(Fig. 4.14a, f, g; Fig. 4.15a, b; also Fig. 4.7a)

The inferior vena cava lying close to the abdominal aorta on its right side is longer than the aorta. It commences in front of the fifth lumbar vertebra by the union of two common iliac veins. It lies on the lumbar vertebrae and the right crus of the diaphragm and enters the thorax by piercing the central tendon of the diaphragm at the level of T8 vertebra. It crosses the right gonadal, the right renal and the right inferior phrenic arteries and overlaps the right lumbar sympathetic trunk. In the infracolic compartment the inferior vena cava, lying behind the parietal peritoneum, is crossed by the root of the mesentery, the right gonadal artery and the third part of the duodenum. In the supracolic compartment the peritoneum covering the inferior vena cava forms the posterior wall of the epiploic foramen and above that level it lies behind the bare area of the liver. The vein–artery relationship alters as the inferior vena cava ascends. At its commencement the inferior vena cava lies behind the common iliac artery, whereas in the upper part it lies in a plane anterior to that of the aorta. The surface marking is by a vertical line 2.5 cm to the right of the midline extending from the intertubercular plane to the right sixth costal cartilage.

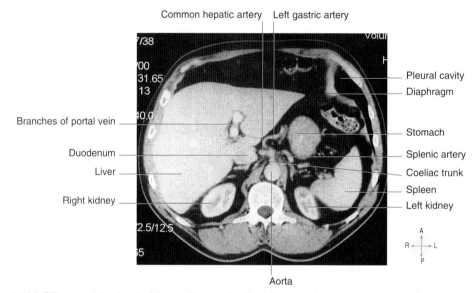

Fig. 4.14d *CT scan at the level of the coeliac trunk after injection of intravenous contrast medium.*

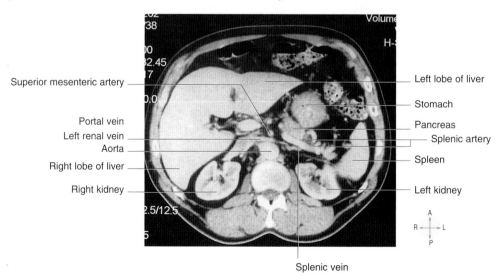

Fig. 4.14e *CT scan at the level of the splenic artery after injection of intravenous contrast medium.*

Tributaries

Besides the two common iliac veins, the lumbar veins, the right gonadal veins, the renal veins, the right suprarenal vein, the right inferior phrenic vein and the three hepatic veins and several accessory hepatic veins drain into the vena cava. The left gonadal veins, the left adrenal vein and the left inferior phrenic vein are tributaries of the left renal vein. As the left renal vein crosses in front of the aorta it may have to be ligated and divided during surgery for aortic aneurysm. If this is done to the right of where its tributaries enter, the left kidney may survive. The inferior vena cava and its tributaries with the exception of the gonadal veins do not have valves.

THE COMMON ILIAC ARTERIES AND VEINS (Fig. 4.14a, b)

The common iliac artery from the bifurcation of the aorta passes downwards and laterally and bifurcates in front of the sacroiliac joint into external and internal iliac arteries, the former continues into the lower limb as the femoral artery and the latter divides into branches to supply the pelvis and perineum. The ureter crosses in front of the bifurcation of the artery. The apex of the sigmoid mesocolon also is related to this point. The common iliac and the external iliac arteries can be marked on the surface by extending the point of bifurcation of the abdominal aorta to a point midway

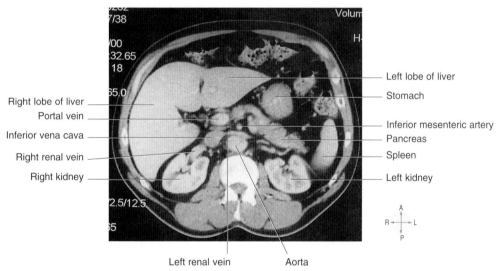

Fig. 4.14f *CT scan at the level of the renal veins after injection of intravenous contrast medium.*

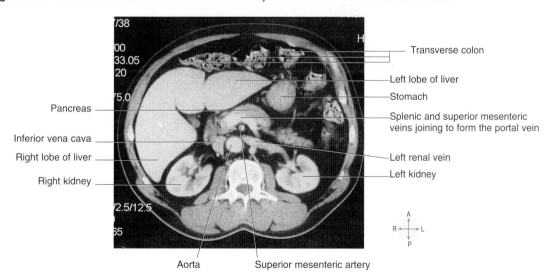

Fig. 4.14g *CT scan at the level of the formation of the portal vein after injection of intravenous contrast medium.*

between the anterior superior iliac spine and the pubic symphysis (the midinguinal point).

The common iliac veins formed by the union of external and internal iliac veins lie medial to the corresponding arteries at a deeper plane. The left vein is longer than the right as the inferior vena cava lies on the right side of the aorta. It crosses behind the right common iliac artery before joining the right vein to form the inferior vena cava.

THE LUMBAR SYMPATHETIC TRUNK
(Fig. 4.14a)

The lumbar part of the sympathetic chain lies along the anterolateral surface of the bodies of the lumbar vertebrae and along the medial border of the psoas. There are usually four ganglia in the lumbar region. The left lumbar sympathetic chain is overlapped by the aorta and the right by the inferior vena cava. Postganglionic fibres from the lumbar ganglia (grey rami) are distributed to the lumbar spinal nerves. The lumbar splanchnic nerves are preganglionic fibres connecting the ganglia to the aortic plexus (Fig. 4.12c). Lumbar sympathectomy is undertaken surgically or by producing neurolysis by injection of chemical agents such as phenol or alcohol. The procedure interrupts

vasoconstrictor fibres and is undertaken in cases of peripheral vascular diseases of the lower limb.

KIDNEYS (Fig. 4.15)

The kidneys lie on the posterior abdominal wall behind the parietal peritoneum mostly covered by the costal margin. The right kidney is at a lower level compared to the left.

The kidney is covered by renal fascia and the perirenal fat. These coverings along with the renal vessels anchor the kidney on the posterior abdominal wall. The hilum of the kidney is in the transpyloric plane about 5 cm from the midline, its upper pole lies 2.5 cm and the lower pole 7.5 cm away from the midline. Posteriorly, the kidneys lie on the diaphragm, the psoas major, the quadratus lumborum and the transversus abdominis. The costodiaphragmatic recess of the pleura which is separated by the diaphragm is an important posterior relation of the kidney.

The suprarenal gland on both sides sits on the upper pole of the kidney and overlaps onto its anterior surface (Fig. 4.15a). Both kidneys are related to important regions of the peritoneal cavity. The right kidney lies behind the hepatorenal pouch whereas the left kidney lies behind the lesser sac. The anterior relations of the

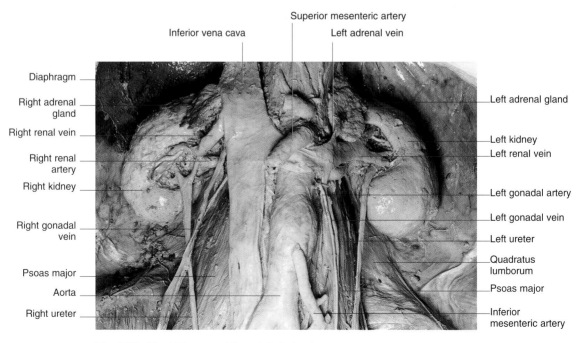

Fig. 4.15a *The kidneys and the related structures.*

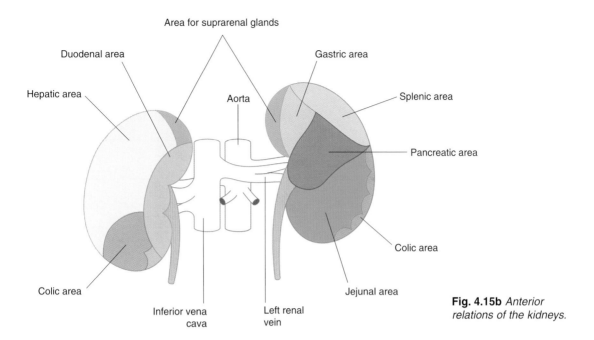

Fig. 4.15b *Anterior relations of the kidneys.*

right kidney are the liver, the right suprarenal gland, the duodenum and the hepatic flexure of the colon. Similarly the stomach, spleen and the splenic flexure of the colon lie in front of the left kidney (Fig. 4.15b).

The hilum of the kidney has the renal vein, the renal artery and the renal pelvis (also called the pelvis of the ureter) from before backwards (VAD). The renal pelvis which is the commencement of the ureter may be bifid.

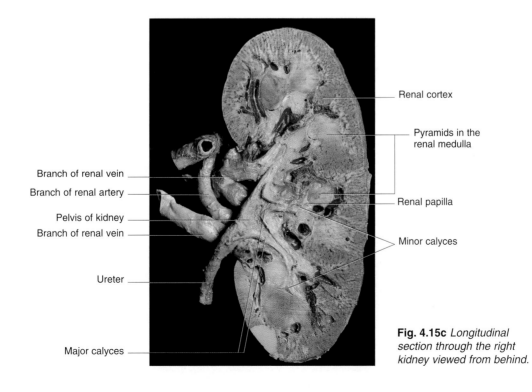

Fig. 4.15c *Longitudinal section through the right kidney viewed from behind.*

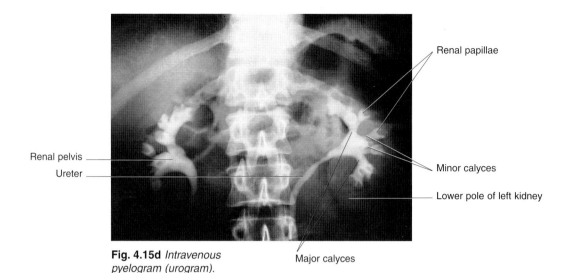

Renal papillae

Renal pelvis

Ureter

Minor calyces

Lower pole of left kidney

Major calyces

Fig. 4.15d *Intravenous pyelogram (urogram).*

Also the renal artery may give off branches and the renal vein may receive tributaries. These variations may create problems for the surgeon during dissection of the hilum.

In a longitudinal section of the kidney the renal cortex which contains the glomeruli and the convoluted tubules can be distinguished from the medullary pyramids, which has the loops of Henle, collecting ducts and collecting tubules. The apex of the pyramid projects into the minor calyx as renal papillae, one to three papillae opening into one minor calyx. The minor calyces unite together to form two or three major calyces which open into the renal pelvis (Fig 4.15c, d).

At the hilum the renal artery typically divides into anterior and posterior branches from which five segmental arteries arise viz. apical, upper, middle, lower, and posterior. Each further divides into lobar arteries, one for each pyramid and the adjoining cortex.

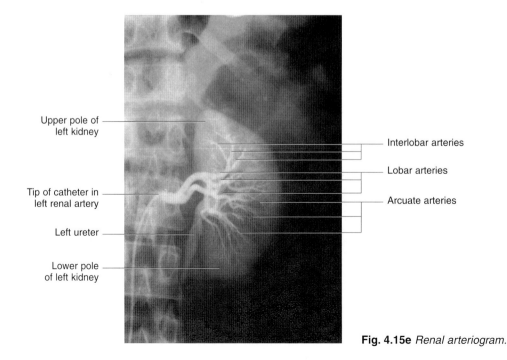

Upper pole of left kidney

Interlobar arteries

Lobar arteries

Tip of catheter in left renal artery

Arcuate arteries

Left ureter

Lower pole of left kidney

Fig. 4.15e *Renal arteriogram.*

The lobar arteries divide into interlobar branches which give rise to arcuate arteries. There is virtually no anastomosis between branches of adjacent segmental arteries (Fig. 4.15e, f).

A normal kidney is not usually palpable. When enlarged, the swelling descends on inspiration. It is bimanually palpable. The upper border of the swelling can be felt (can reach above the swelling). Unlike the spleen, a notch is not felt on the renal swelling. These points are of importance to distinguish an enlarged left kidney from an enlarged spleen.

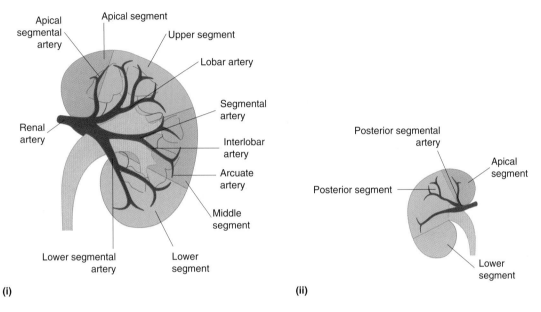

(i)

(ii)

Fig. 4.15f *The arterial supply of the kidney and the vascular segments:* **(i)** *anterior segments;* **(ii)** *posterior segments.*

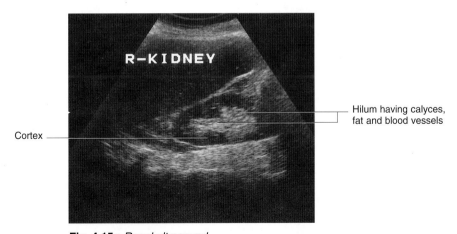

Fig. 4.15g *Renal ultrasound.*

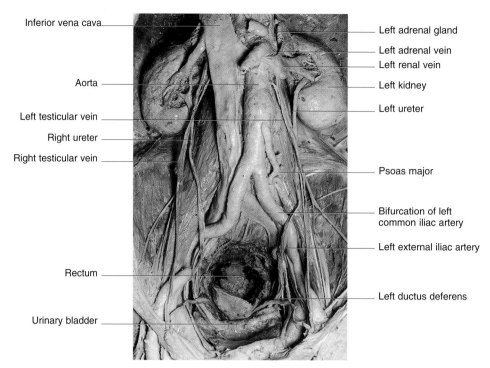

Inferior vena cava

Aorta

Left testicular vein

Right ureter

Right testicular vein

Rectum

Urinary bladder

Left adrenal gland

Left adrenal vein

Left renal vein

Left kidney

Left ureter

Psoas major

Bifurcation of left common iliac artery

Left external iliac artery

Left ductus deferens

Fig. 4.15h *The kidneys, ureters and the urinary bladder with the related structures. Dissection of the posterior abdominal wall.*

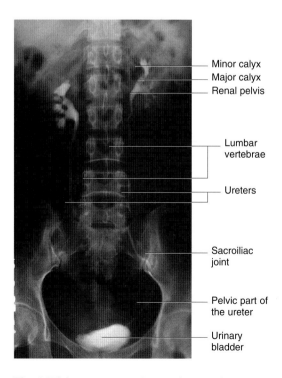

Minor calyx

Major calyx

Renal pelvis

Lumbar vertebrae

Ureters

Sacroiliac joint

Pelvic part of the ureter

Urinary bladder

Fig. 4.15i *Intravenous pyelogram (urogram) showing kidney, ureter and urinary bladder.*

THE URETERS (Fig. 4.15h, i, j)

The ureter lies on the psoas major muscle behind the parietal peritoneum to which it is adherent. On both sides the ureters cross the genitofemoral nerves and are crossed by the gonadal vessels. The right ureter lies behind the third part of the duodenum and as it descends is crossed by the ileocolic vessels and the root of the mesentery. The left ureter is crossed by the left colic vessels and at the pelvic brim by the apex of the sigmoid mesocolon. The psoas major separates the ureter from the transverse processes of the lumbar vertebrae. On a radiograph the ureter can be seen lying along the tips of the transverse processes and then in front of the sacroiliac joint. At operation it can be distinguished from nerves and vessels as a whitish non-pulsatile cord which is adherent to the peritoneum and showing peristaltic activity when gently pinched with a forceps.

The ureter enters the pelvis by crossing anterior to the termination of the common iliac artery. The pelvic part of the ureter lies on the side wall of the pelvis where it is related to the obturator nerve, obturator artery and other branches of the internal iliac artery. In the male the ductus deferens crosses the ureter before reaching the posterior surface of the bladder, whereas in the female the uterine artery crosses above the ureter very near to the lateral fornix of the vagina (see Fig. 4.17d). During hysterectomy (removal of uterus), while the surgeon ligates and cuts the uterine arteries, the ureters are in danger of being clamped or cut inadvertently.

The lumen of the ureter is not uniform throughout. It is narrower at the pelviureteric junction, where it crosses the bifurcation of the common iliac artery and where it enters the bladder. A renal stone passing through the ureter can be arrested at any of these sites. Pain sensation from the ureter is transmitted via sympathetic nerves to T11 to L1 segments and hence radiates from loin to groin and onto the medial part of the thigh.

The blood supply of the ureter is segmental by branches from the renal, gonadal, vesical and uterine arteries which anastomose on the adventitia covering its wall. The blood supply is therefore compromised if the ureter is stripped clean of its adventitia.

URINARY BLADDER (Fig. 4.15j, k, l, m)

The empty bladder has a superior surface, two inferolateral surfaces and a base. The base faces posteriorly. The lower part of the bladder which is continuous with the urethra is known as the bladder neck. Only the superior surface is covered by peritoneum.

The sigmoid colon rests on the superior surface of the bladder. Because of this relationship a colovesical fistula can occur in diverticular disease. The body of the uterus lies superior to the bladder in the female and the supravaginal cervix and the vagina separates the posterior surface from the rectouterine pouch and the rectum. The posterior surface of the bladder in the male is related to the seminal vesicle and the ductus deferens (lying below the rectovesical pouch), behind which lies the rectum.

The mucosa of the empty bladder is thrown into folds. These flatten as the bladder distends. The inner aspect of the posterior wall however is smooth. This is known as the trigone of the bladder and is bounded laterally by the opening of the two ureters and below by the urethra. In the male the trigone overlies the median part of the central zone of the prostate which,

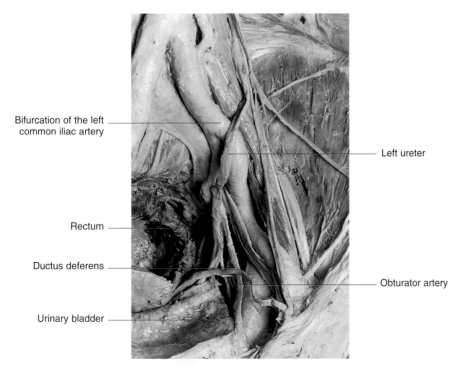

Fig. 4.15j *Dissection of the lower part of the posterior abdominal wall and pelvis in the male to show the course of the left ureter. Sigmoid colon and the sigmoid mesocolon have been removed.*

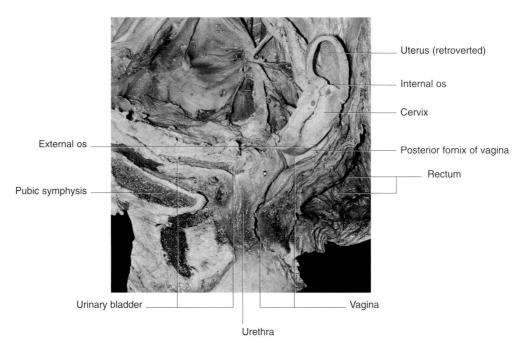

Uterus (retroverted)

Internal os

Cervix

External os

Posterior fornix of vagina

Rectum

Pubic symphysis

Urinary bladder

Vagina

Urethra

Fig. 4.15k *Female pelvis and perineum — sagittal section, urinary bladder and the urethra.*

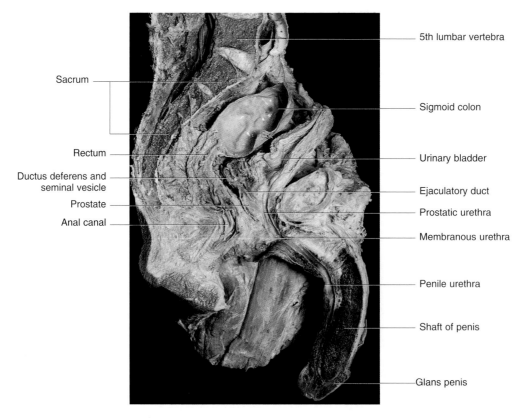

5th lumbar vertebra

Sacrum

Sigmoid colon

Rectum

Urinary bladder

Ductus deferens and
seminal vesicle

Ejaculatory duct

Prostate

Prostatic urethra

Anal canal

Membranous urethra

Penile urethra

Shaft of penis

Glans penis

Fig. 4.15l *Male pelvis and perineum — sagittal section, urinary bladder and the urethra.*

after middle age, projects above the internal orifice of the urethra as the uvula of the bladder. In the upper border of the trigone is the interureteric crest (interureteric ridge or bar) which extends between the two ureteric orifices. The interureteric crest can be seen during cystoscopy (examination of the interior of the bladder). The two ureters will be seen discharging urine at its two ends. The ureters lie obliquely in the bladder wall before their termination and have a valve-like mechanism which prevents reflux of urine into them during contraction of the bladder.

The mucosa of the bladder is lined by transitional epithelium which will not absorb urine. The underlying muscle is the detrusor muscle, the fibres of which run in different directions and interlace with each other.

In urinary obstruction the detrusor muscle hypertrophies and the spaces in between the muscle fibres deepen to give rise to bladder diverticulae. Urine will collect in the diverticulae without draining and lead on to infection of the bladder.

The muscle of the trigone is different from the detrusor. It extends into the lower part of the ureters and also into the urethra. At the bladder neck the trigonal muscle is circular in the male and forms the internal sphincter of the bladder. This prevents regurgitation of semen into the bladder during ejaculation. In the female urinary bladder, these fibres are longitudinal in direction and hence do not form a sphincter at the bladder neck.

The bladder is innervated by sympathetic and parasympathetic nerves. The motor innervation of the bladder is by the parasympathetic nerves from S2, 3, 4

segments of the spinal cord (pelvic splanchnic nerves) except the trigonal muscle and the internal sphincter which are supplied by the sympathetics. Sensation of bladder distension travels via the parasympathetic nerves whereas pain is transmitted by both para-sympathetics and sympathetics.

THE MALE URETHRA (Fig. 4.15l, n)

The male urethra is about 20 cm long having three parts. It passes through the prostate (prostatic urethra), deep perineal pouch (membranous urethra) and then through the corpus spongiosum of the penis (penile urethra).

The prostatic urethra which is about 2.5 cm long is the widest and the most dilatable part of the urethra. The posterior wall of this part has a linear bulge, the urethral crest, the widest part of which is the colliculus seminalis or verumontanum. Into the urethral crest opens the prostatic utricle, a small blind-ending sac which is the remnant of the paramesonephric duct. The two ejaculatory ducts, each formed by the union of the ductus deferens and the duct of the seminal vesicle, also open here. The gutter on either side of the urethral crest has the openings of the prostatic ducts from the peripheral zone of the prostate, whereas the central zone ducts open into the verumontanum around the orifices of the ejaculatory ducts.

The membranous part which is 1.5 cm long is short and narrow and is the least dilatable part of the male urethra. This part lying in the deep perineal pouch is

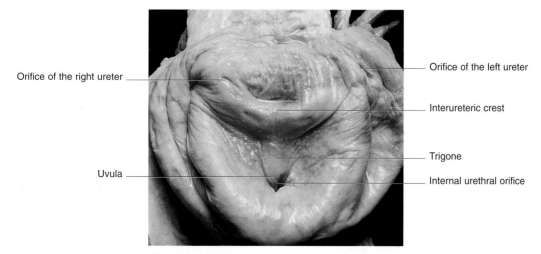

Orifice of the right ureter

Uvula

Orifice of the left ureter

Interureteric crest

Trigone

Internal urethral orifice

Fig. 4.15m *The interior of the urinary bladder.*

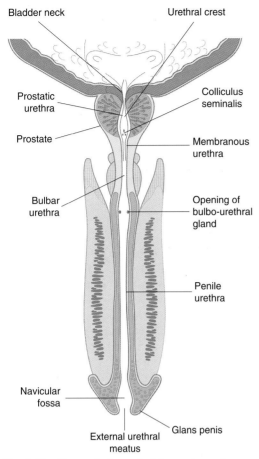

Bladder neck

Urethral crest

Prostatic urethra

Colliculus seminalis

Prostate

Membranous urethra

Bulbar urethra

Opening of bulbo-urethral gland

Penile urethra

Navicular fossa

External urethral meatus

Glans penis

Fig. 4.15n *The posterior wall of the male urethra.*

surrounded by the external sphincter of the urethra.

The commencement of the penile urethra in the bulb of the penis is relatively fixed, whereas its continuation in the corpus spongiosum of the penis is mobile. In the glans penis it widens as the navicular fossa. The external urethral meatus which is the narrowest part of the whole urethra appears as a sagittal slit at the tip of the penis. The narrowing helps to focus the urine as it comes through the dilatation of the navicular fossa.

The bulbourethral glands situated in the deep perineal pouch open into the bulbar part of the urethra. Besides this a number of mucous glands (of Littre) also open into the penile urethra with their orifices directed distally. These may get infected and also occasionally may cause confusion at the time of urethrography.

There are two sphincteric mechanisms for the bladder and urethra. The internal sphincter at the bladder neck is strong to maintain continence even if the external sphincter is destroyed. However its main role is to prevent retrograde ejaculation into the bladder. It closes the bladder neck during emission of semen into the prostatic urethra. The external sphincter surrounding the membranous urethra has an internal component, lissosphincter, of smooth muscle, and an external component, rhabdosphincter, made of striated muscle. The external sphincter is innervated by sensory and motor fibres from the pudendal nerve (somatic) as well as by the autonomic nerves.

FEMALE URETHRA (Fig. 4.15k)

The female urethra which is about 4 cm long lies on the anterior wall of the vagina and opens in the vestibule between the anterior ends of the labia minora and the clitoris (Fig 4.19b). The sphincter mechanism extends down the whole length of the urethra. Structurally the sphincter is similar to the external sphincter in the male with lissosphincter and rhabdosphincter components which are innervated by the pudendal and autonomic nerves. The sphincter is most well developed in the middle third of the urethra. Unlike in the male the female urethra does not have a well-defined sphincter at the bladder neck.

THE PELVIC WALL (Fig. 4.16a, b)

The pelvis contains the terminal parts of the alimentary and urinary systems and also parts of the reproductive system.

The bony pelvis is made up of three bones: the two hip bones and the sacrum. The hip bones articulate with each other in front at the pubic symphysis and with the sacrum at the back through the two sacroiliac joints. Each hip bone has three components, the ilium, the pubis and the ischium, the three fusing together in the acetabulum.

Three pairs of muscles are seen on the walls of the pelvis. The side wall has the obturator internus muscle covering the obturator foramen. Posteriorly, taking origin from the sacrum and passing through the greater sciatic foramen is the piriformis muscle. The two levator ani muscles fuse in the midline to form a gutter from the floor of the pelvis (Fig. 4.16 b, c).

The levator ani takes origin from a line extending from the back of the pubis to the ischial spine and is described as having three parts: the pubococcygeus, the iliococcygeus and the ischiococcygeus. The iliococcygeus does not arise from the ilium but instead

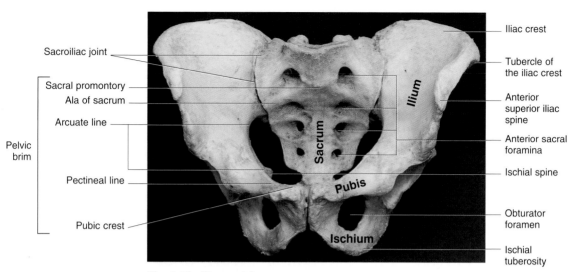

Iliac crest

Sacroiliac joint

Sacral promontory

Ala of sacrum

Arcuate line

Tubercle of
the iliac crest

Ilium

Sacrum

Anterior
superior iliac
spine

Anterior sacral
foramina

Ischial spine

Pelvic
brim

Pectineal line

Pubis

Obturator
foramen

Pubic crest

Ischium

Ischial
tuberosity

Fig. 4.16a *Bony pelvis.*

is attached to the fascia covering the obturator internus muscle.

The fibres of the levator ani run downwards medially and backwards. As they do so, the inner fibres of pubococcygeus are intimately related to the pelvic organs. The muscle is an important structure maintaining the normal positions of the pelvic organs. Fibres of the levator ani related to the prostate are known as the levator prostatae, those around the vagina form the sphincter vaginae. Behind these the

fibres are inserted into a tough fibromuscular nodule, the perineal body, in front of the anorectal junction. A number of perineal muscles are also inserted to the perineal body. The perineal body together with the muscles attached to it prevent the pelvic organs from prolapsing into the perineum.

Part of the levator ani around the anorectal junction is called the puborectalis muscle. The puborectalis fibres form a sling around the anorectal junction, i.e. fibres of one side become continuous with those of the

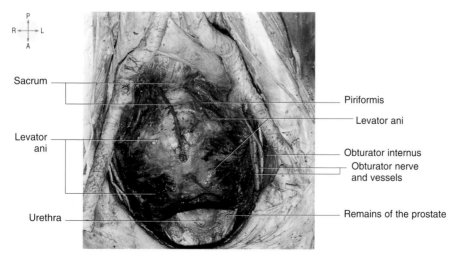

Sacrum

Levator
ani

Urethra

Piriformis

Levator ani

Obturator internus

Obturator nerve
and vessels

Remains of the prostate

Fig. 4.16b *The floor of the pelvis seen after removal of the pelvic organs.*

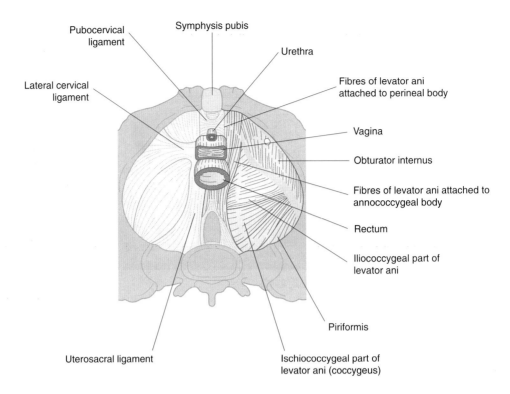

Fig. 4.16c *Floor of the pelvis and muscles and ligaments supporting the uterus and vagina — superior view. Ligaments are shown on the left side and muscles on the right.*

opposite side. This sling maintains the forward angulation of the anorectal junction. Fibres of the sling also fuse with the deep part of the external sphincter of the anal canal and contribute to the formation of the anorectal ring. This forms an important part of the sphincteric mechanism at the anorectal region.

More lateral fibres of the levator ani fuse in a fibrous raphe behind the anorectal junction, the anococcygeal raphe.

FEMALE INTERNAL GENITAL ORGANS
(Fig. 4.17a, b, c, d, e)

The ovary

The ovary is attached to the posterior leaf of the broad ligament by a double fold of peritoneum, the mesovarium. Continuation of the broad ligament from the ovary to the side wall of the pelvis is known as the suspensory ligament of the ovary. The ligament of the ovary, a thin fibrous cord, connects it to the uterus. This ligament then extends to the labium majus through the inguinal canal as the round ligament of

the uterus. The ovary lies on the side wall of the pelvis in the 'ovarian fossa' in the angle between the external and internal iliac vessels. The ureter lies close behind the ovary.

The ovary in its normal position may be just palpable by vaginal examination. It is laterally related to the obturator nerve. Inflammation of the ovary may cause pain along the distribution of the obturator nerve, along the medial aspect of the thigh.

The ovary is supplied by the ovarian artery given off just below the renal artery from the abdominal aorta. Veins form a plexus which eventually forms a single trunk. On the left side these drain into the renal vein and on the right side into the inferior vena cava. The lymphatics of the ovary drain into the para-aortic nodes. The blood supply of the ovaries and their lymphatic drainage is comparable to those of the testes.

The uterus (Fig. 4.17a, b, c, d, e)

Parts of the uterus are the fundus, body and the cervix (of the uterus). The lower part of the cervix is inside the vagina. The spaces around the cervix, inside the

Sigmoid colon

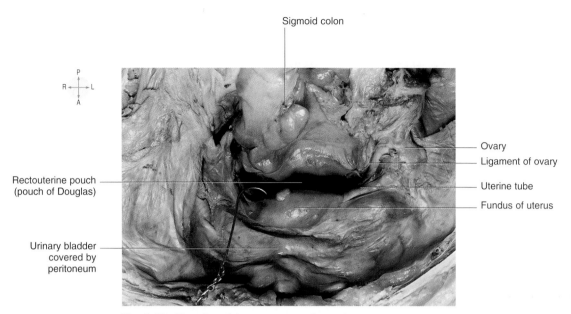

P
R ← → L
A

Rectouterine pouch
(pouch of Douglas)

Urinary bladder
covered by
peritoneum

Ovary

Ligament of ovary

Uterine tube

Fundus of uterus

Fig. 4.17a *Female pelvic organs seen from above.*

vagina, are the vaginal fornices. They are divided into anterior, posterior and lateral fornices according to their positions in relation to the vagina. The posterior fornix is deeper than the others. The opening of the cervix into the vagina is the external os.

In its normal position the uterus is angulated forward on the vagina (Fig. 4.5e). This is known as the anteverted position of the uterus and it is maintained by the levator ani (pelvic diaphragm) and the various ligaments connected to the uterus and vagina (Fig. 4.16c).

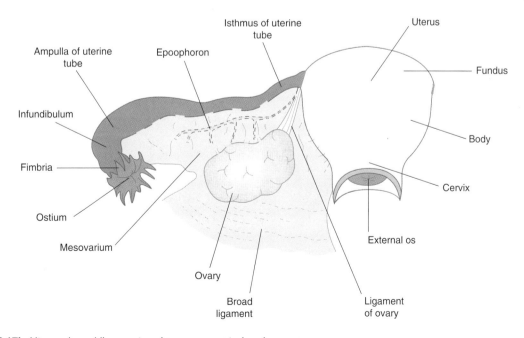

Isthmus of uterine
tube

Uterus

Ampulla of uterine
tube

Epoophoron

Fundus

Infundibulum

Body

Fimbria

Ostium

Cervix

Mesovarium

External os

Ovary

Broad
ligament

Ligament
of ovary

Fig. 4.17b *Uterus, broad ligament and ovary — posterior view.*

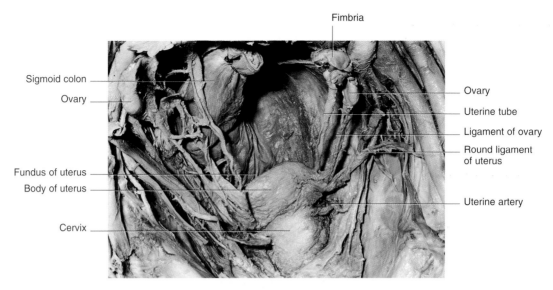

Fig. 4.17c *Female pelvic organs after removal of peritoneum. Uterus is lifted up to show the anterior surface of cervix. Part of the sigmoid colon and coils of intestines have been removed.*

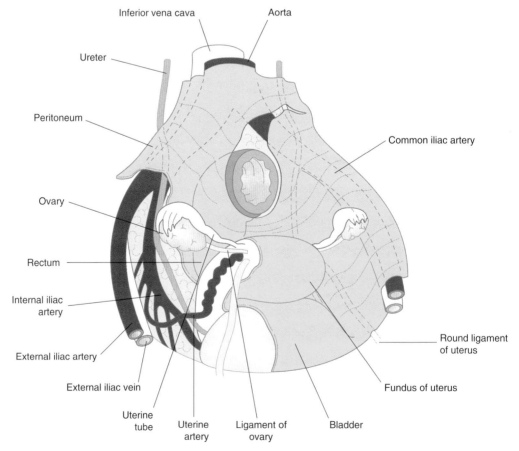

Fig. 4.17d *The female pelvic organs seen from above (diagrammatic). The peritoneum on the right side has been partially removed.*

Peritoneum covers the whole of the posterior surface and the upper third of the vagina and is reflected onto the rectum forming the rectouterine pouch (Fig. 4.5e).

Anteriorly, the supravaginal part of the cervix is not covered by peritoneum. This part enlarges during pregnancy and becomes the lower segment of the uterus and is the site of caesarean sections.

The uterine and the ovarian arteries supply the uterus. The uterine artery, a branch of the internal iliac artery, crosses above the ureter, adjacent to the lateral fornix, before ascending up in the broad ligament on the side of the uterus (see p.129). The ovarian artery runs along the uterine tube and anastomoses with the uterine artery (Fig. 4.17d, e).

Vagina

From the uterine end the vagina is directed downwards and forwards as it passes between the pubovaginalis part of the levator ani, the deep perineal pouch, to open in the vestibule which is the space between the two labia minora. It is highly stretchable having the benefit of being supplied by a number of arteries with a rich anastomosis on its wall (Fig. 4.17e).

A number of structures can be felt by vaginal examination which include cervix of the uterus and fornices of the vagina. Anteriorly the urethra, bladder and symphysis pubis and posteriorly the rectum as well as collection of fluid and malignant deposits in the pouch of Douglas can also be felt. The body of the uterus, ovaries and the uterine tubes may be felt with pressure applied to the lower abdominal wall.

The uterine tube

The uterine tube consists of from medial to lateral intramural part (in the uterine wall), isthmus, ampulla and the infundibulum or fimbriated end with a number of finger-like processes, the fimbriae, one of them applied to the ovary. It ends laterally near the ovary by opening into the peritoneal cavity. The opening is called the ostium. The tube lies inside the broad ligament (Fig. 4.17b).

The patency of the tube is essential for normal pregnancy. Infection of the tube (salpingitis) may result in scarring and closure of the tubes. In tubal sterilisation the uterine tubes are cut to prevent future pregnancies. In tubal ectopic pregnancies the fertilised ovum may implant in the uterine tube instead of passing into the uterus. The tube however cannot accommodate the growing fetus and the placenta and it will rupture into the peritoneal cavity resulting in bleeding and peritonitis.

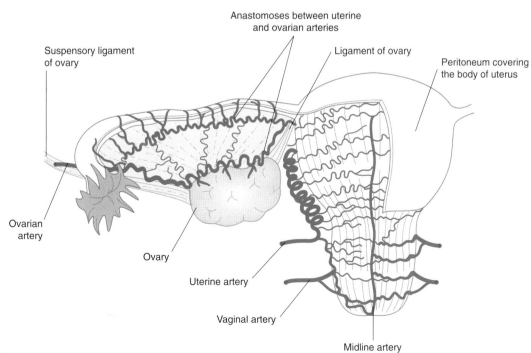

Fig. 4.17e *Arterial supply of the ovary, uterine tube, uterus and vagina.*

Anastomoses between uterine and ovarian arteries

Suspensory ligament of ovary

Ligament of ovary

Peritoneum covering the body of uterus

Ovarian artery

Ovary

Uterine artery

Vaginal artery

Midline artery

MALE INTERNAL GENITAL ORGANS
(Fig. 4.18)

The ductus deferens (vas deferens) starts at the inferior pole of the testis as a continuation of the epididymis. It passes through the inguinal canal and the deep inguinal ring before reaching the posterior surface of the bladder. The dilatation just before its termination is the ampulla of the vas deferens. The ductus terminates by joining the duct of the seminal vesicle to form the ejaculatory duct.

The seminal vesicles secrete the bulk of the seminal fluid. Rarely the seminal vesicle may become infected and the tenderness may be felt during rectal examination. Normal seminal vesicles are not palpable per rectum.

Prostate gland (Fig. 4.18a, b; Fig. 4.15l)

The prostate lies below the bladder. The urethra and the two ejaculatory ducts pass through the prostate. The ejaculatory ducts drain into the prostatic part of the urethra. The prostate has a base and an apex, the base which is the upper surface is fused with the bladder neck and the blunt apex is projecting downwards. The posterior surface of the prostate has a

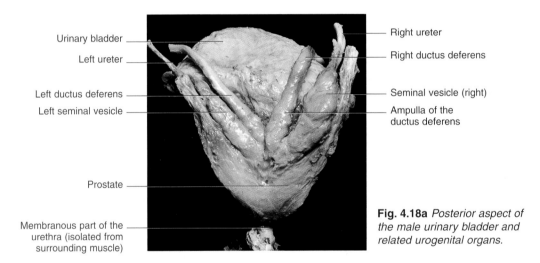

Urinary bladder

Left ureter

Left ductus deferens

Left seminal vesicle

Prostate

Membranous part of the urethra (isolated from surrounding muscle)

Right ureter

Right ductus deferens

Seminal vesicle (right)

Ampulla of the ductus deferens

Fig. 4.18a *Posterior aspect of the male urinary bladder and related urogenital organs.*

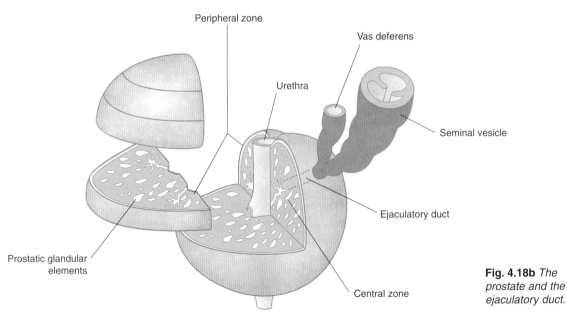

Peripheral zone

Vas deferens

Urethra

Seminal vesicle

Ejaculatory duct

Prostatic glandular elements

Central zone

Fig. 4.18b *The prostate and the ejaculatory duct.*

groove which is normally felt on rectal examination. When the prostate enlarges this groove disappears. Veins of the prostate drain into the prostatic venous plexus around the gland. This in turn is connected to the vertebral venous plexuses (Batson's veins). There are no valves in these connections. Malignant tumours of the prostate spread through these veins into the vertebral column.

The prostate contains fibromuscular tissues and glands which open into the urethra. The prostate has a central and a peripheral zone which respectively have approximately 25% and 75% of the glandular tissue each. The wedge-shaped central zone containing small glands which are not coiled forms the base of the gland. Its apex is at the verumontanum. The peripheral zone forming the lower part of the gland surrounds the central zone but does not reach the upper part of the gland. Glands of the peripheral zone are long and tortuous. The ducts of the central zone open on the verumontanum, whereas those of the peripheral zone open into the prostatic sinuses. Prostatic secretion added to the seminal fluid is important for the survival of spermatozoa.

Benign tumours of the prostate are extremely common in men above the age of 60. It is the central zone of the prostate which is usually affected by benign hypertrophy. The peripheral zone is almost exclusively the site of origin of carcinoma of the prostate.

PERINEUM (Fig. 4.19)

The space below the pelvic diaphragm is defined as the perineum. For descriptive purposes the perineum is divided by an imaginary line connecting the two ischial tuberosities into the anal triangle, which contains the anal canal, and the urogenital triangle, containing the urethra and the external genitalia.

Urogenital triangle

This part of the perineum has the superficial and the deep perineal pouches separated by the perineal membrane, a triangular sheet of fibrous tissue extending between the two ischiopubic rami.

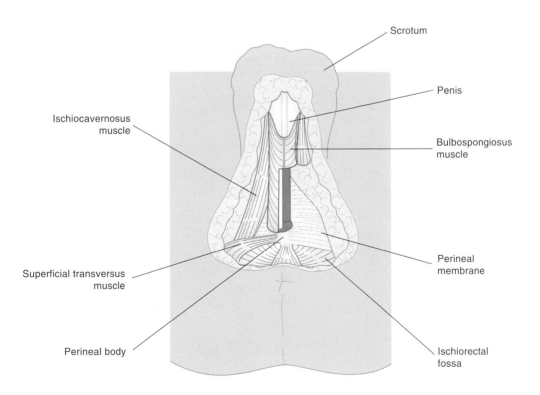

Fig. 4.19a *The superficial perineal pouch muscles of the male perineum and the perineal membrane — inferior view. The superficial muscles and part of the penis have been removed on the left side of the perineum to show the perineal membrane (scrotum and the penis are lifted up).*

The superficial perineal pouch

This space is superficial to the perineal membrane and is bounded externally by the membranous layer of the superficial fascia (Colle's fascia) which is an extension of the fascia from the anterior abdominal wall into the perineum. The superficial perineal pouch hence is continuous with the space under the membranous layer of the superficial fascia in the anterior abdominal wall.

In the male, the superficial perineal pouch contains the erectile tissues contributing to the formation of the penis and the thin muscles covering them. The urethra passes through the corpus spongiosum of the penis. If the urethra is ruptured urine will accumulate in the superficial pouch and spread upwards into the anterior abdominal wall into which the space extends.

In the female, as in the male, the superficial perineal pouch contains the erectile tissues These are the two crura forming the clitoris and a paired structure on either side of the vestibule, the bulb of the vestibule.

These erectile tissues also (as those in the male) are covered by thin muscles.

The perineum is supplied by the internal pudendal artery and the pudendal nerve. These leave the pelvis through the greater sciatic foramen and enter the perineum through the lesser sciatic foramen. The anterior part of the skin is supplied by the ilioinguinal nerve.

The deep perineal pouch

This space deep to the perineal membrane contains the deep transversus perineii muscle. The middle part of the muscle surrounds the urethra forming the external sphincter of the male urethra and exerts a prolonged tone on the urethra to keep it closed. This part of the urethra is called the membranous part of the urethra. In the female, the deep transversus perineii muscle is pierced by the urethra and the vagina. The external sphincter is similar to that in the male.

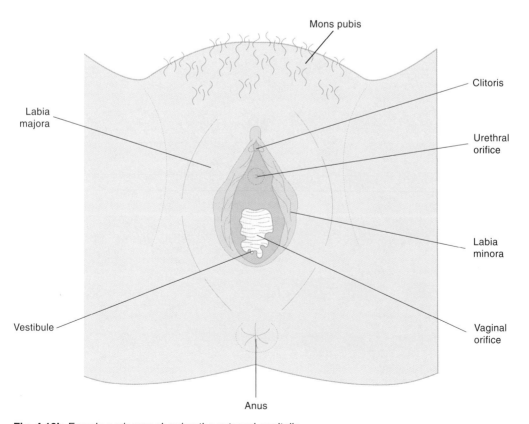

Fig. 4.19b *Female perineum showing the external genitalia.*

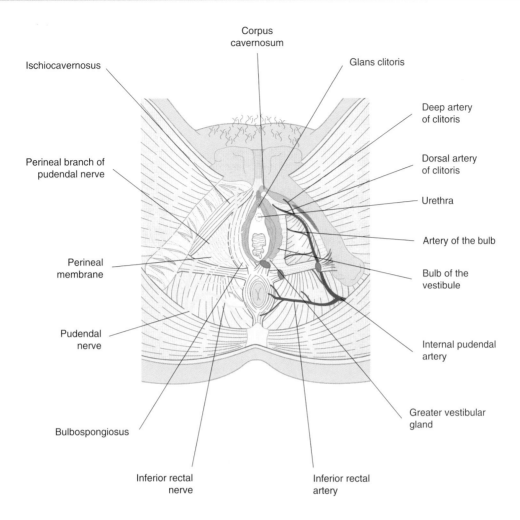

Corpus
cavernosum

Glans clitoris

Ischiocavernosus

Deep artery
of clitoris

Dorsal artery
of clitoris

Perineal branch of
pudendal nerve

Urethra

Artery of the bulb

Perineal
membrane

Bulb of the
vestibule

Pudendal
nerve

Internal pudendal
artery

Greater vestibular
gland

Bulbospongiosus

Inferior rectal
nerve

Inferior rectal
artery

Fig. 4.19c *Dissection of the female perineum. Arteries are shown on the left and nerves on the right. The superficial muscles have been removed on the left to show the bulb of the vestibule and the greater vestibular gland.*

THE PENIS (Fig. 4.20)

The attached parts of the penis known as the roots of the penis consist of a crus each on either side and the bulb in the midline, the former attached to the ischiopubic ramus and the perineal membrane and the latter to the perineal membrane. The crus continues forward as the corpus cavernosum and the bulb as the corpus spongiosum. The two corpora cavernosa are bound together on the dorsal aspect of the corpus spongiosum, all three contributing to the body or shaft of the penis. The corpus spongiosum extends beyond the anterior end of the corpora cavernosa and expands to become the glans penis. The penile urethra enters the bulb, traverses the whole length of corpus spongiosum to open at the external urethral meatus at the end of the glans penis. The skin of the penis is hairless and at the tip it folds on itself over the glans

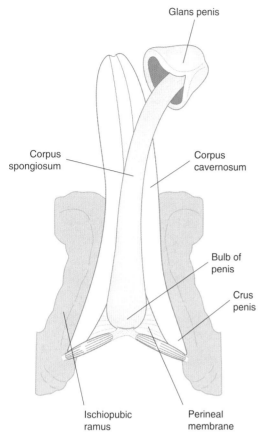

Glans penis

Corpus spongiosum

Corpus cavernosum

Bulb of penis

Crus penis

Ischiopubic ramus

Perineal membrane

Fig. 4.20a *Roots of the penis in the superficial perineal pouch.*

penis as the prepuce. The prepuce is attached to the neck of the glans. The frenulum, an extension of the skin from the prepuce to the undersurface of the glans, extends to the urethral orifice.

Blood supply

Three pairs of arteries, all branches of the internal pudendal artery, supply the penis. The artery to the bulb supplies the bulb, the corpus spongiosum and the glans. The deep artery of the penis supplies the corpus cavernosum. The dorsal artery of the penis supplies the skin, fascia and glans and anastomoses with the artery to the bulb. The venous drainage is partially through veins accompanying the arteries into the internal pudendal vein but mostly through the deep dorsal vein of the penis which pierces the suspensory ligament (connection of deep fascia to the pubic symphysis), and passing in the gap between the pubic symphysis and the perineal membrane enters the pelvis to join the vesicovenous plexus. The dorsal skin is drained by the superficial dorsal vein which joins the superficial external pudendal vein, a tributary of the long saphenous vein.

Nerve supply

The skin of the penis is supplied by the scrotal nerves and the dorsal nerves of the penis, all branches from the pudendal nerve. The dermatome involved mainly is S2, with a small area of supply by L1 via the ilio-inguinal nerve. The increased blood flow essential for erection is facilitated by parasympathetic stimulation whereas ejaculation is initiated by sympathetic stimulation.

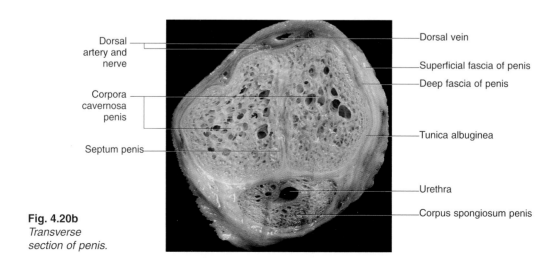

Dorsal artery and nerve

Corpora cavernosa penis

Septum penis

Dorsal vein

Superficial fascia of penis

Deep fascia of penis

Tunica albuginea

Urethra

Corpus spongiosum penis

Fig. 4.20b
Transverse section of penis.

VERTEBRAL COLUMN AND THE SPINAL CORD

VERTEBRAL COLUMN (Fig. 5.1a)

The vertebral column consists of: seven cervical vertebrae, 12 thoracic, five lumbar, the sacrum consisting of five fused vertebrae and the coccyx formed by the fusion of four or more rudimentary vertebrae. The vertebral column transmits the body weight on to the lower limbs through the sacroiliac joints. The spinal cord and its coverings and the spinal nerves are contained inside the vertebral canal.

Curvatures

The sinusoidal shape of the vertebral column is developed after birth. In the fetus the vertebral column is C shaped with the concavity facing anteriorly. After birth secondary curvatures with convexity develop in the cervical region when the child holds up its head and also in the lumbar region when the legs start weight bearing.

INDIVIDUAL VERTEBRAE (Fig. 5.1a, b, c, d)

Each individual vertebra consists of a body and a neural arch surrounding the vertebral foramen. The neural arch consists of a pedicle and a lamina on either side. The two laminae fuse to form the spinous process. The arch also has two transverse processes and a pair

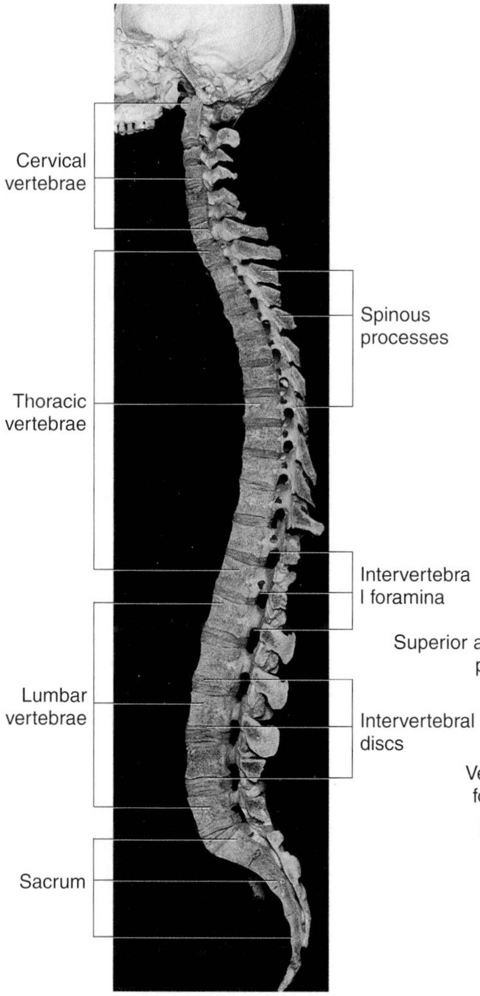

Fig. 5.1a *Sagittal section of the vertebral column viewed from the side.*

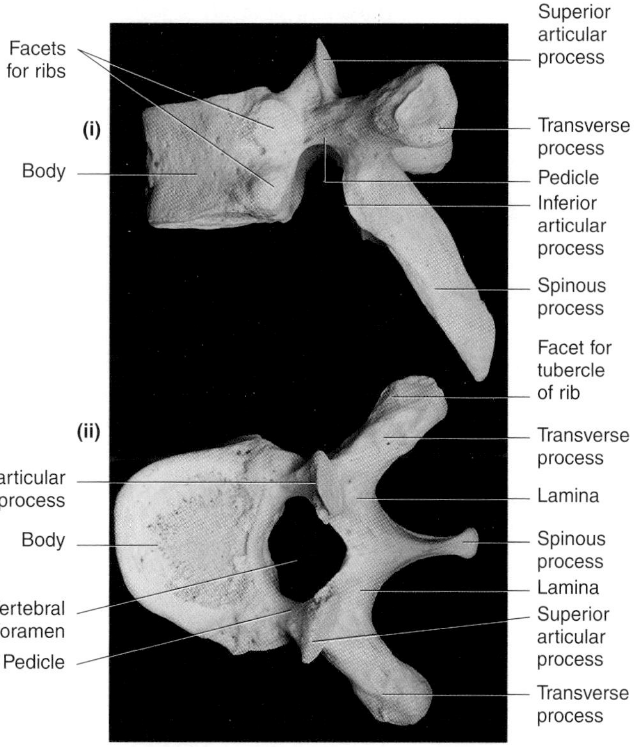

Fig. 5.1b *Thoracic vertebra:* **(i)** *lateral view;* **(ii)** *superior view.*

Spinous process

Superior articular processes

Transverse process

Pedicle

Lamina

Body

Vertebral foramen

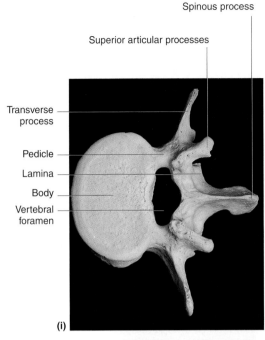

(i)

Superior articular facet

Lamina

Spinous process

Body

Vertebral foramen

Pedicle

Foramen transversarium

Transverse process

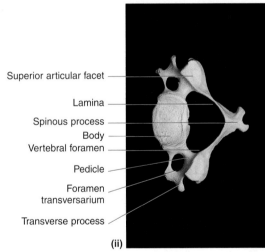

(ii)

Fig. 5.1c *Superior views:* **(i)** *lumbar vertebra;* **(ii)** *cervical vertebra.*

of superior and inferior articular processes for articulation with the adjacent vertebrae.

The cervical vertebrae can be distinguished from lumbar and thoracic vertebrae as they have small bodies, small and bifid spines (except C7) and the foramen transversarium in their transverse processes. The atlas (C1) has no body but has two lateral masses connected by the anterior and posterior arches. The atlas articulates above with the occipital bone and below with the axis (C2). Nodding and lateral flexion movements take place at the atlantooccipital joints. Projecting upwards from the body of axis is the odontoid process (dens) which articulates with the anterior arch of the atlas. Rotation of the head occurs in the atlantoaxial joints. An individual thoracic vertebra can be identified by noting the presence of articular facets on the body and on transverse processes (except T11 and T12). Lumbar vertebrae are massive to withstand body weight. The lumbar vertebrae and the intervening discs contribute 25% of the total length of the column.

Surface anatomy

The uppermost spinous process which is palpable is that of the seventh cervical vertebra known as the vertebra prominent as it has a long and non-bifid spine. The highest point of the iliac crest is in line with the interval between L3 and L4 spines.

JOINTS BETWEEN THE VERTEBRAE
(Fig. 5.1e, f, g)

The bodies of the adjoining vertebrae are joined by the intervertebral disc whereas the facet joints (zygopophyseal joints) which are synovial joints link the articular processes. The major longitudinal ligaments connecting the vertebrae are the anterior and posterior ligaments connecting the bodies of the vertebrae, ligamentum flavum in between the adjacent laminae and supraspinous and interspinous ligaments connecting the spines. These joints, ligaments, as well as the muscles of the back, stabilise the vertebral column. Movements of the vertebral column are forward flexion (40°), extension (15°), lateral flexion (30°) and rotation (40°). Rotation is maximum at the thoracic region whereas it is very limited in the lumbar spine. Flexion and extension on the other hand is limited in the thoracic region due to the presence of the rib cage.

The intervertebral discs are fibrocartilagenous

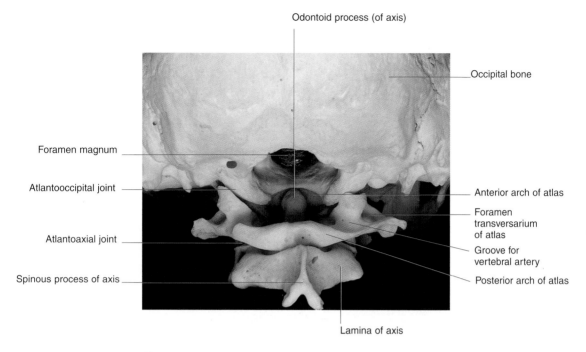

Odontoid process (of axis)

Occipital bone

Foramen magnum

Atlantooccipital joint

Anterior arch of atlas

Foramen transversarium of atlas

Atlantoaxial joint

Groove for vertebral artery

Spinous process of axis

Posterior arch of atlas

Lamina of axis

Fig. 5.1d *Atlas, axis and the occipital bone — viewed from behind.*

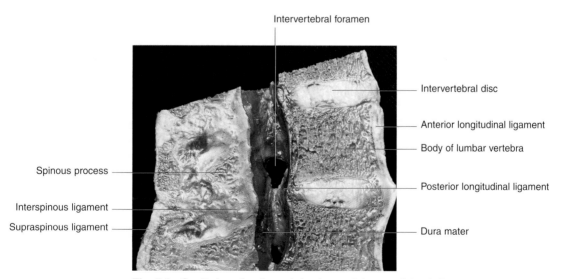

Intervertebral foramen

Intervertebral disc

Anterior longitudinal ligament

Body of lumbar vertebra

Spinous process

Posterior longitudinal ligament

Interspinous ligament

Supraspinous ligament

Dura mater

Fig. 5.1e *Sagittal section through lumbar vertebrae — lateral view.*

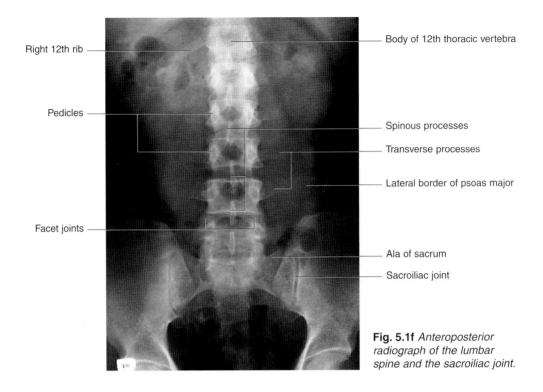

Right 12th rib

Pedicles

Facet joints

Body of 12th thoracic vertebra

Spinous processes

Transverse processes

Lateral border of psoas major

Ala of sacrum

Sacroiliac joint

Fig. 5.1f *Anteroposterior radiograph of the lumbar spine and the sacroiliac joint.*

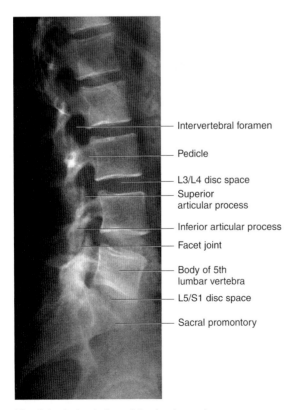

Intervertebral foramen

Pedicle

L3/L4 disc space

Superior articular process

Inferior articular process

Facet joint

Body of 5th lumbar vertebra

L5/S1 disc space

Sacral promontory

Fig. 5.1g *Lateral view of the lumbar spine.*

structures which are strong to withstand compression forces but are also flexible to allow movements between the vertebrae. Each disc has two parts, a nucleus pulposus surrounded by annulus fibrosus. The former is a well-hydrated gel having proteoglycan collagen and cartilage cells. The annulus fibrosus is made of 10–12 concentric layers of collagen whose obliquity alters in successive layers. Peripherally the annulus fibrosus is attached to the vertebral bodies as well as to the posterior longitudinal ligament. The annulus resists the expansion of the nucleus pulposus. However when the nucleus degenerates it can bulge through and even break through the annulus to produce nerve compression. As the nucleus is situated more towards the posterior aspect of the disc it herniates posterolaterally into the intervertebral foramen causing nerve compression. A straight posterior herniation is often prevented by the firm attachment of the disc to the posterior longitudinal ligament. More commonly this happens in the lumbar part of the vertebral column and can cause back pain or pain radiating to the leg (sciatica) by compression of the nerve roots.

The intervertebral foramina which transmit the spinal nerves and the accompanying radicular arteries (which supply the spinal cord) are on the lateral aspect of the vertebral column. Each foramen lying between the pedicles of the adjoining vertebrae are bounded anteriorly by the vertebral bodies and the disc and posteriorly by the facet joints. Herniation of the disc, arthritis of the facet joints as well as bony irregularities in the pedicle or vertebral body can narrow the intervertebral foramen and cause nerve root compression.

As there are eight cervical nerves and only seven cervical vertebrae the spinal nerves emerge through the intervertebral foramen in the following order. C1–C7 spinal nerves exit above their corresponding vertebrae. C8 nerve passes through the foramen between C7 and T1 vertebrae. All subsequent nerves emerge below their corresponding vertebrae.

THE SACROILIAC JOINT

The sacroiliac joint is a synovial joint through which the body weight is transmitted from the sacrum to the hip bone. The articular surface of the sacrum and the corresponding surface on the ilium are irregular and they fit together closely. The reciprocal irregularities of the joint surfaces and the strong ligaments of the joint make this a stable joint. However strain and arthritis of the joint causes back pain as one gets older.

SPINAL CORD AND MENINGES (Fig. 5.2)

The spinal cord extends from the lower end of the medulla oblongata at the level of the foramen magnum to the lower border of the first or the upper border of the second lumbar vertebra. The lower part of the cord is tapered to form the conus medullaris from which a prolongation of pia mater, the filum terminale, extends downwards to be attached to the coccyx. In the third

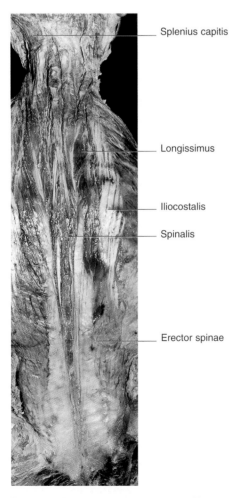

Splenius capitis

Longissimus

Iliocostalis

Spinalis

Erector spinae

Fig. 5.1h *Deep muscles of the back. Erector spinae and its three parts (spinalis longissimus and iliocostalis) exposed after removal of superficial muscles of the back.*

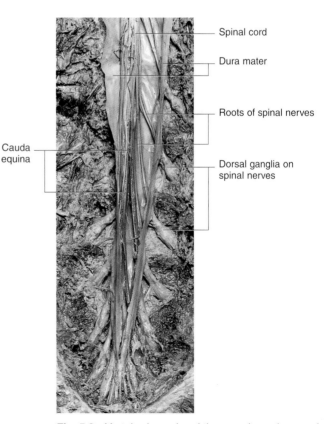

Spinal cord

Dura mater

Roots of spinal nerves

Dorsal ganglia on spinal nerves

Cauda equina

Fig. 5.2a *Vertebral canal and the sacral canal opened up from the back to show the cauda equina.*

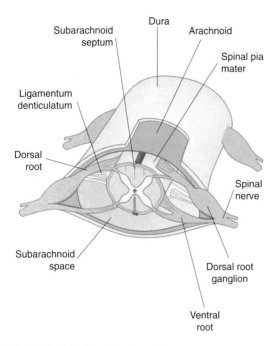

Fig. 5.2b *Spinal cord and meninges.*

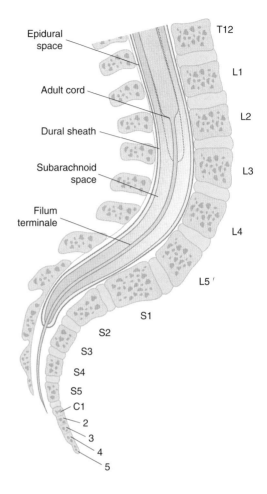

Fig. 5.2c *The termination of the spinal cord in the adult, showing its variation. This also shows the termination of the dural sheath.*

month of intrauterine life, the spinal cord fills the whole length of the vertebral canal but from then on the vertebral column grows more rapidly than the cord. At birth the cord extends as far as the third lumbar vertebra and eventually reaches its adult level gradually.

The three layers of the meninges envelop the spinal cord. The dura mater which is continuous with that of the brain extends up to the second sacral vertebra. The arachnoid mater lines the inner surface of the dura and pia mater is adherent to the surface of the cord. The subarachnoid space with the cerebrospinal fluid extends up to the level of the second sacral vertebra. The epidural space outside the dura contains fat and the components of the vertebral venous plexus.

The spinal cord is suspended in the dural sheath by the denticulate ligaments. This ligament which has a serrated lateral edge forms a shelf between the dorsal and ventral roots of the spinal nerves.

The cord has on its surface a deep anterior median fissure and a shallower posterior median sulcus. It also has, on either side, a posterolateral sulcus along which the dorsal roots of the spinal nerves are attached.

The area of the spinal cord from which a pair of spinal nerves are given off is defined as a spinal cord segment. The cord has 31 pairs of spinal nerves and hence 31 segments — eight cervical, 12 thoracic, five lumbar, five sacral and one coccygeal.

The dorsal root of the spinal nerve which carries sensory fibres has a dorsal root ganglion which has the cells of origin of the dorsal root fibres. The ventral (anterior) root which is motor emerges on the anterolateral aspect of the cord on either side. The anterior and posterior roots join together at the intervertebral foramen to form the spinal nerve, which on emerging from the foramen divides immediately into the anterior and posterior rami, each containing both motor and sensory fibres. The length of the nerve roots increases progressively from above downwards. The lumbar and sacral nerve roots below the termination of the cord form the cauda equina.

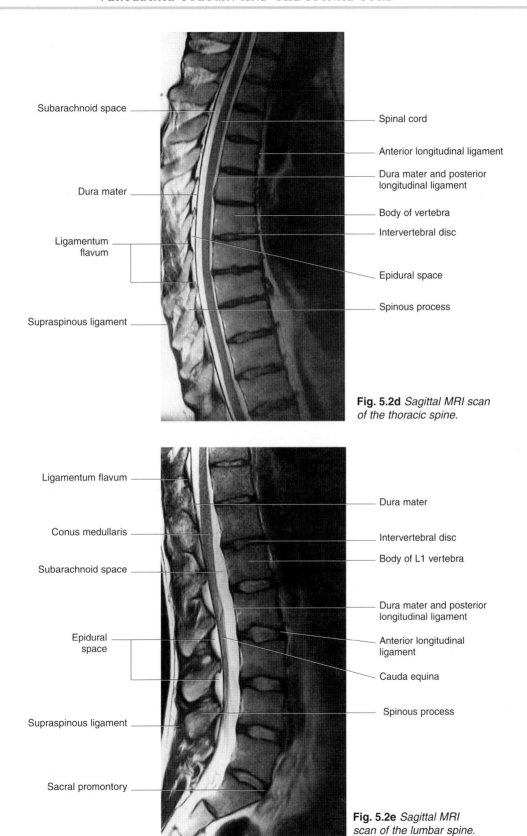

Subarachnoid space

Dura mater

Ligamentum flavum

Supraspinous ligament

Spinal cord

Anterior longitudinal ligament

Dura mater and posterior longitudinal ligament

Body of vertebra

Intervertebral disc

Epidural space

Spinous process

Fig. 5.2d *Sagittal MRI scan of the thoracic spine.*

Ligamentum flavum

Conus medullaris

Subarachnoid space

Epidural space

Supraspinous ligament

Sacral promontory

Dura mater

Intervertebral disc

Body of L1 vertebra

Dura mater and posterior longitudinal ligament

Anterior longitudinal ligament

Cauda equina

Spinous process

Fig. 5.2e *Sagittal MRI scan of the lumbar spine.*

Blood supply of the spinal cord

The blood supply of the spinal cord is derived from the anterior and posterior spinal arteries. The anterior spinal artery is a midline vessel lying in the anterior median fissure and is formed by the union of a branch from each vertebral artery. It supplies the whole of the cord in front of the posterior grey column. The posterior spinal arteries, usually one on either side posteriorly, are branches of the posterior inferior cerebellar arteries or arise directly from the vertebral arteries. They supply the posterior grey columns and the dorsal columns on either side.

The spinal arteries are reinforced at segmental levels by radicular arteries from the vertebral, ascending cervical, posterior intercostal, lumbar and sacral arteries. The radicular arteries enter the vertebral canal through the intervertebral foramina accompanying the spinal nerves and their ventral and dorsal roots. These arteries may be compromised in resection of segments of the aorta in surgery of aneurysms.

Internal structure of the spinal cord

The grey matter containing the sensory and motor nerve cells are surrounded by the white matter with the ascending and descending tracts.

In a transverse section the grey matter is seen as an H-shaped area containing in its middle the central canal. The central canal is continuous above with the fourth ventricle. The posterior (dorsal) horn of the grey matter has the termination of the sensory fibres of the posterior (dorsal) root. The larger anterior (ventral) horn contains motor cells which give rise to fibres of the anterior (ventral) roots. In the thoracic and upper lumbar regions there are lateral horns which have the cells of origin of the preganglionic sympathetic fibres.

The epidural space is the interval between the vertebrae and the dura mater of the spinal cord. It contains the small arteries which supply the spinal cord and the vertebral venous plexuses. Veins in these plexuses (Bateson's veins) contain no valves.

Metastases from malignant tumours in the breast and the prostate can reach the vertebrae through the vertebral venous plexuses which are connected to the veins draining these organs. Introduction of analgesic solutions into the epidural space in the lumbar region (epidural anaesthesia) is commonly performed to relieve pain during childbirth.

A sample of cerebrospinal fluid can be obtained by introducing a trochar and cannula into the subarachnoid space between the spinous processes of L3 and L4, which is at the level of the highest point of the iliac crest. As the spinal cord ends higher up this procedure will not damage the cord.

LOWER LIMB

INTRODUCTION (Fig. 6.1a, b, c)

The general plan of the lower limb is similar to that of the upper limb. It consists of the thigh, leg and foot which correspond to the arm, forearm and hand of the upper extremity. The gluteal region or the buttock lies behind the pelvis and hip above the back of the thigh. The boundary between the anterior abdominal wall and the thigh is the inguinal ligament which extends between the anterior superior iliac spine and the pubic tubercle. The femoral artery pulsation can be felt at the midinguinal point on palpation against the head of the femur. The structures in the thigh are arranged in three compartments—anterior or extensor, medial or adductor and posterior or flexor. The anterior or ventral position of the extensors and the posterior or dorsal position of the flexors are opposite to those seen in the upper limb. This is because the lower limb rotated medially during development unlike the lateral rotation which occurred in the upper limb. The leg also has three compartments—anterior or extensor, lateral or peroneal and posterior or flexor. The foot has dorsal and plantar aspects.

The function of the lower limb is to support the body weight and to propel it forward during locomotion. For this purpose it is constructed with large bones, massive muscles and stable joints.

The hip bone or the innominate bone connects the femur to the vertebral column at the sacrum. The thigh

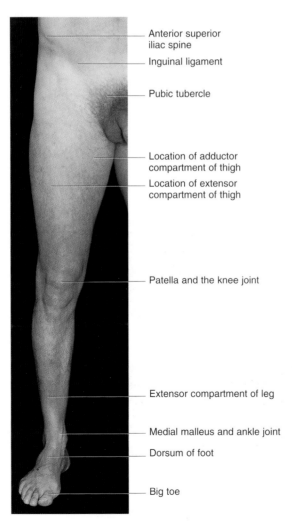

Fig. 6.1a *Parts of the lower limb viewed from the front.*

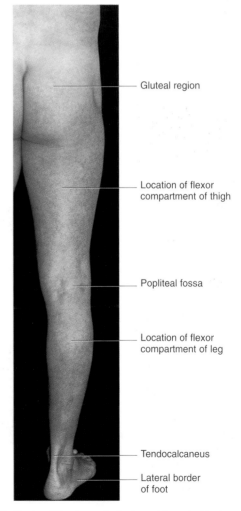

Fig. 6.1b *Parts of the lower limb viewed from behind.*

contains the femur which in turn connects the hip joint to the knee joint. The leg which extends from the knee to the ankle has the tibia and fibula. The foot contains the tarsal bones, the metatarsals and the phalanges.

The body weight in erect standing is transmitted from the vertebral column to the femur via the hip bone and from there through the tibia to the tarsal bones. The fibula, therefore, is a non-weight bearing bone.

The lower limb is innervated by nerves arising in the lumbar and sacral plexuses. The arterial supply is through the femoral artery and its continuation as the popliteal and anterior and posterior tibial arteries. As in the upper limb the venous drainage is via a superficial and deep set of veins. The lymph is drained into the inguinal group of lymph nodes.

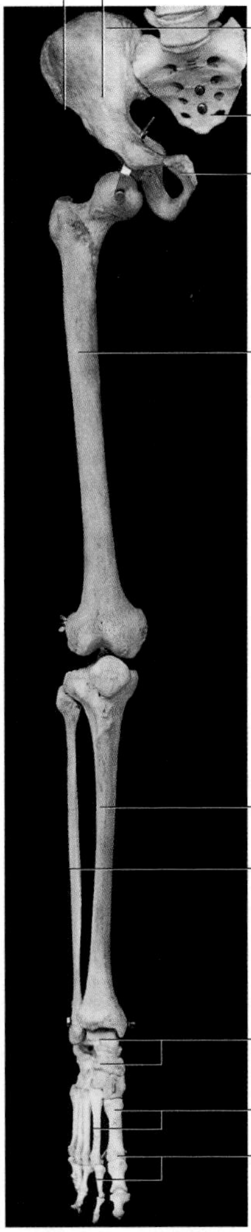

BONES OF HIP AND THIGH

Hip bone (Fig. 6.2)

The hip bone consists of a superior part, the ilium, a posteroinferior part, the ischium, and an anteromedial part, the pubis. All three contribute to the formation of the acetabulum where there is a triradiate cartilage separating the three components until 15–17 years of age. This fuses completely in the adult. The acetabulum articulates with the head of the femur. The iliac crest, posterior superior iliac spine, anterior superior iliac spine, pubic tubercle and the ischial tuberosity are palpable and are important landmarks in surface anatomy. The rest of the hip bone is covered by large muscles, and hence is not palpable.

Femur (Fig. 6.3)

The neck of the femur projects upwards and medially and also slightly forwards from the shaft forming an angle of 115–140° with the shaft. When the angle is

Anterior superior iliac spine

Hip bone

Iliac crest

Sacrum

Pubic tubercle

Femur

Tibia

Fibula

Tarsal bones

Metatarsals

Phalanges

Fig. 6.1c *The bones of the lower limb.*

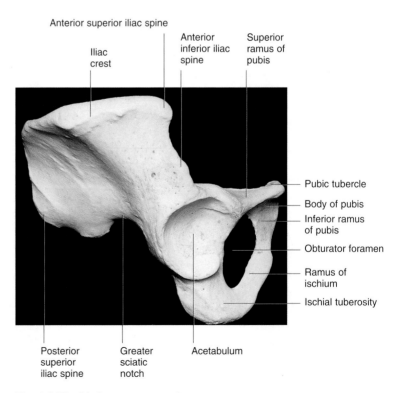

Anterior superior iliac spine

Iliac crest

Anterior inferior iliac spine

Superior ramus of pubis

Pubic tubercle

Body of pubis

Inferior ramus of pubis

Obturator foramen

Ramus of ischium

Ischial tuberosity

Posterior superior iliac spine

Greater sciatic notch

Acetabulum

Fig. 6.2 *The hip bone — external aspect.*

less than normal the condition is known as coxa vara and when more coxa valga. A fracture of the neck of femur, common in the elderly, can cause avascular necrosis of the head of the femur as the blood supply to the head reaches it through the neck. The greater trochanter is the only part which is palpable at the upper end of the femur. A number of major muscles are attached to the greater and lesser trochanters.

The shaft of the femur is related to a chain of arterial anastomoses. Severe haemorrhage occurs in a fracture of the shaft when these arteries are torn. A large number of muscles are attached to the linea aspera which is a sharp ridge at the posterior aspect of the femur.

FEMORAL TRIANGLE (FIG. 6.4)

The femoral triangle is in the upper part of the front of the thigh and it is bounded laterally by the medial border of sartorius and medially by the medial border of the adductor longus and above by the inguinal ligament. The muscles forming the floor from medial to lateral are the adductor longus, pectineus, the psoas major and the iliacus.

The femoral triangle contains from medial to lateral

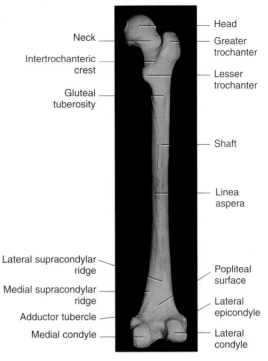

Fig. 6.3 *Femur — posterior aspect.*

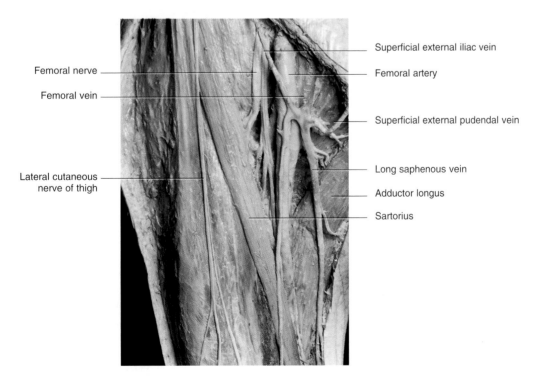

Fig. 6.4a *The femoral triangle. Contents of the femoral triangle — femoral artery, femoral vein and femoral nerve.*

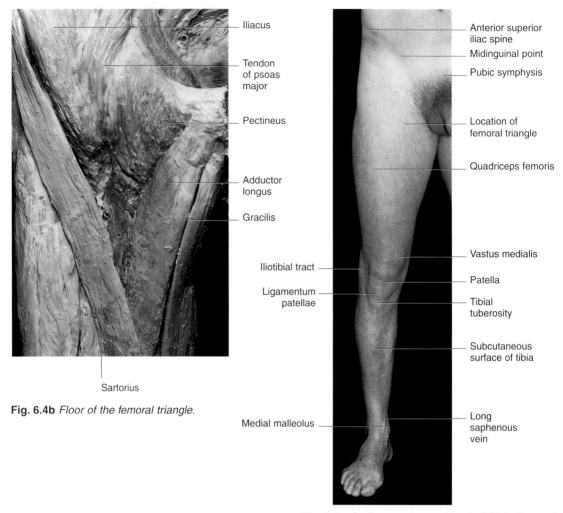

Fig. 6.4b *Floor of the femoral triangle.*

Labels for Fig. 6.4b:
- Iliacus
- Tendon of psoas major
- Pectineus
- Adductor longus
- Gracilis
- Sartorius

Fig. 6.4c *Surface anatomy of front of thigh, leg and foot. Location of femoral triangle and midinguinal point.*

Labels for Fig. 6.4c:
- Anterior superior iliac spine
- Midinguinal point
- Pubic symphysis
- Location of femoral triangle
- Quadriceps femoris
- Iliotibial tract
- Ligamentum patellae
- Vastus medialis
- Patella
- Tibial tuberosity
- Subcutaneous surface of tibia
- Medial malleolus
- Long saphenous vein

the femoral vein, the femoral artery and the femoral nerve.

The femoral artery, the continuation of the external iliac artery, and the femoral vein which continues into the abdomen as the external iliac vein are enclosed inside the femoral sheath, which has a potential space medial to the vein, the femoral canal. This communicates with the abdominal cavity through the femoral ring. A femoral hernia can pass through the femoral ring into the femoral canal.

The femoral artery enters the thigh at a point midway between the anterior superior iliac spine and the pubic symphysis (midinguinal point) where its pulsation can be felt easily. The artery is entered at this point for cannulation to place an arterial line.

The position of the vein in the living can be found by feeling the femoral artery pulsation which is immediately lateral to the vein just below the inguinal ligament. The long (great) saphenous vein receives a number of tributaries corresponding to the superficial branches of the femoral artery just before it joins the femoral vein. This is an identification point to distinguish it from the femoral vein at operation. The femoral vein here has only one tributary, the long saphenous vein.

The femoral nerve is lateral to the artery but is at a deeper plane compared to the artery and sometimes even posterior to the artery. It divides into its branches as soon as it enters the thigh. These anatomical variations make it a difficult nerve to block by injection of local anaesthetic agents. The nerve supplies the pectineus, the sartorius and the four parts of the quadriceps femoris, i.e. the rectus femoris, the vastus lateralis, the vastus intermedius and the vastus medialis. Its sensory branches are the medial and the intermediate cutaneous nerves of the thigh and the saphenous nerve.

Sartorius

The sartorius muscle extends from the anterior superior iliac spine to the medial condyle of the tibia. The sartorius is supplied by the femoral nerve. It is a flexor of the hip and knee and also, along with other long muscles connecting the hip bone to the leg, balances the hip bone on the femur.

The quadriceps femoris (Fig. 6.5a, b)

This major muscle consisting of the rectus femoris, the vastus lateralis, the vastus intermedius and the vastus medialis extends the knee joint. The rectus femoris, taking origin from the hip bone, is also a flexor of the hip joint. The other three components take origin from the femur and as such can act only on the knee.

To test the muscle the patient is asked to extend the knee against resistance. The muscle can be seen and felt as contracting. The four parts of the quadriceps are supplied by branches from the femoral nerve.

The three vasti and the rectus femoris are inserted into the patella through the quadriceps tendon (Fig. 6.5c). They then insert into the tibial tuberosity

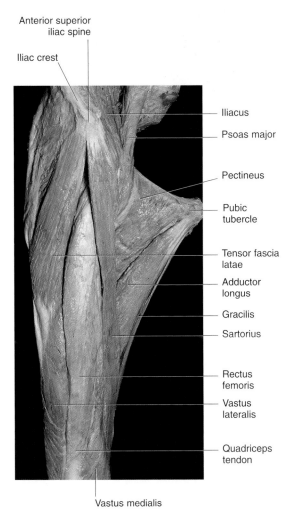

Fig. 6.5a *Muscles in the anterior and medial aspects of thigh. The quadriceps femoris.*

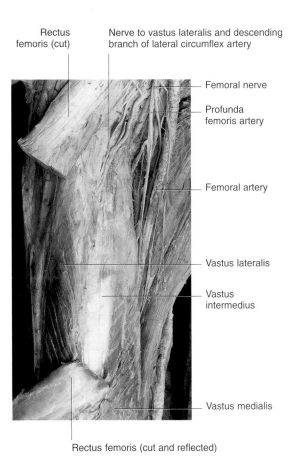

Fig. 6.5b *Vastus intermedius.*

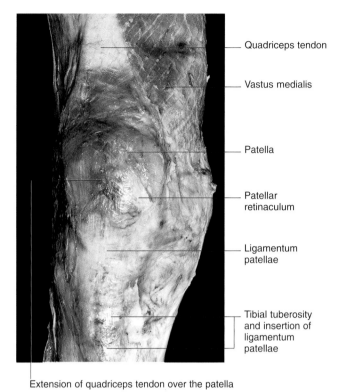

Quadriceps tendon

Vastus medialis

Patella

Patellar retinaculum

Ligamentum patellae

Tibial tuberosity and insertion of ligamentum patellae

Extension of quadriceps tendon over the patella

Fig. 6.5c *Quadriceps tendon, patella and ligamentum patellae.*

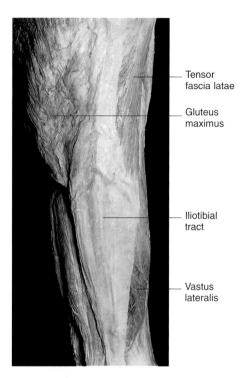

Tensor fascia latae

Gluteus maximus

Iliotibial tract

Vastus lateralis

Fig. 6.5d *Lateral aspect of thigh. Iliotibial tract and the insertion of gluteus maximus and tensor fascia latae (right side).*

through the patellar tendon or the ligamentum patellae. A thin sheet of the quadriceps tendon passes across the front of the patella into the ligamentum patellae and the retinacula. The patellar retinacula are expansions of the quadriceps tendon connecting the patella to the tibial condyles.

The vastus lateralis and vastus medialis mostly take origin from the linea aspera of the femur. The vastus intermedius arises from the anterior surface of the femur deep to the rectus femoris. Unlike the other members of the quadriceps, the vastus medialis is fleshy at its lower end and these fibres lie horizontally as they attach to the patella.

The long axis of the shaft of femur is not vertical but slants downwards and medially. Therefore when the quadriceps contracts its direction of pull is upwards and lateral causing the patella to move in the same direction. The patella thus has a tendency for

dislocating upwards and laterally. Pull of the lower horizontal fibres of the vastus medialis is an important factor preventing such dislocation.

Quadriceps contraction is an important factor in stabilising the knee joint. Without that the knee tends to flex when it is weight bearing. Persons with quadriceps paralysis tend to press the thigh to counteract the flexion of the knee whilst walking.

Iliotibial tract (Fig. 6.5d)

The deep fascia of the thigh, the fascia lata, has a thick lateral aspect. This is the iliotibial tract which extends from the iliac crest to the lateral condyle of the tibia. Along with the quadriceps muscle the iliotibial tract to which the gluteus maximus and the tensor fascia latae are attached is an important structure in stabilising the knee joint.

THE ADDUCTOR COMPARTMENT OR THE MEDIAL COMPARTMENT OF THE THIGH (Fig. 6.6)

The adductor compartment is separated from the anterior compartment by the medial intermuscular septum and contains: the adductors longus, brevis, magnus, gracilis and the obturator externus. All these muscles are supplied by the obturator nerve

The adductors are inserted into the linea aspera of the femur. The adductor longus has a tendinous origin from just below the pubic tubercle. Its tendon can be palpated in the living by adducting the thigh against resistance. The gracilis is a slender muscle connecting the pubic bone to the medial condyle of the tibia.

The adductor brevis lying deep to the adductor longus but anterior to the adductor magnus takes origin from the body of the pubis. It is inserted to the linea aspera behind the insertion of the adductor longus.

'Groin strain', a common sports injury among sprinters and footballers, usually results from abnormal stretching or tearing of the upper attachment of the adductor muscles.

Adductor magnus has adductor and hamstring components. The adductor component takes origin from the ramus of the pubis and its extensive insertion is into the linea aspera behind that of the adductor brevis. The hamstring part arises from the ischial tuberosity, and is inserted to the adductor tubercle of the femur and is supplied along with the rest of the hamstring muscles by the sciatic nerve. Its aponeurosis above the insertion has a hiatus through which the femoral vessels enter the popliteal fossa.

The obturator externus is a muscle covering the external aspect of the obturator foramen. It spirals posteriorly and laterally round the neck of the femur to its tendinous insertion to the trochanteric fossa of the femur.

Action of the adductors

As their names imply the three adductor muscles move the thigh towards the midline at the hip joint (as you settle down on a car seat). They are also important in balancing while standing, preventing abduction. The adductor longus and brevis can also act as medial rotators of the thigh (prevent lateral rotation while

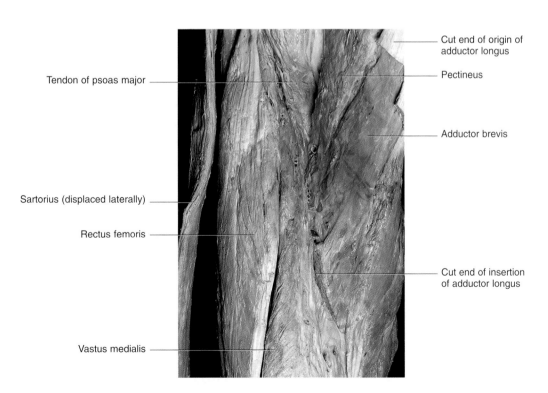

Cut end of origin of adductor longus

Tendon of psoas major

Pectineus

Adductor brevis

Sartorius (displaced laterally)

Rectus femoris

Cut end of insertion of adductor longus

Vastus medialis

Fig. 6.6a *The medial aspect of thigh. The adductor brevis seen after removal of adductor longus.*

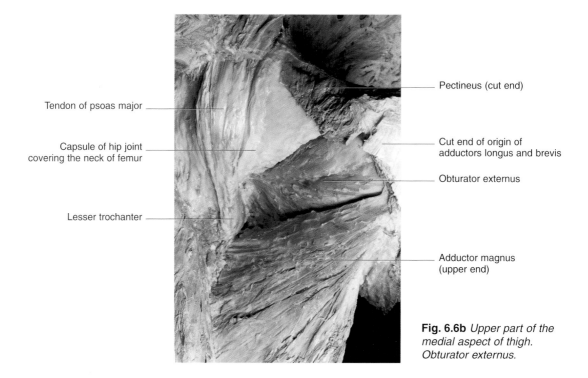

Pectineus (cut end)

Tendon of psoas major

Capsule of hip joint
covering the neck of femur

Cut end of origin of
adductors longus and brevis

Obturator externus

Lesser trochanter

Adductor magnus
(upper end)

Fig. 6.6b *Upper part of the medial aspect of thigh. Obturator externus.*

standing). The part of the adductor magnus originating from the ischial tuberosity, along with the other hamstring muscles, extend the hip joint. The obturator externus is one of the many lateral rotators of the hip joint.

Obturator nerve (Fig. 6.6c, d)

The obturator nerve supplies all the muscles in the medial compartment of the thigh. It enters the thigh by passing through the obturator foramen accompanied by the obturator artery. As it goes through the foramen it divides into anterior and posterior branches. The anterior division of the obturator nerve, lying deep to the adductor longus on the surface of the adductor brevis, gives branches to the adductor longus, adductor brevis and the gracilis and the skin of the medial part of the thigh. The posterior division of the obturator nerve emerges through the obturator externus after supplying it to lie on the adductor magnus. It supplies the adductor magnus and gives a branch which accompanies the femoral artery into the popliteal fossa to supply the capsule of the knee joint.

 Articular branches of the obturator nerve supply the hip and knee joints and hence pain produced in one joint can manifest as referred pain in the other.

Similarly pelvic inflammation involving the obturator nerve can produce referred pain along the medial aspect of the thigh.

Obturator artery

The obturator artery, a branch of the internal iliac artery, emerges through the obturator foramen and divides into branches which encircle the obturator foramen. Its branches anastomose with the medial circumflex artery. It gives a small articular branch to the hip joint.

Adductor canal (Fig. 6.7)

The subsartorial or the adductor canal which is also known as the Hunter's canal is the space containing the femoral artery and the vein below the femoral triangle. It is a gutter-shaped groove bounded laterally by the vastus medialis and medially by the adductor longus above and the adductor magnus below. Its contents are the femoral artery, the femoral vein, the nerve to vastus medialis and the saphenous nerve.

The femoral artery as it descends in the canal crosses from the lateral to the medial side of the femoral vein. The saphenous nerve crosses from the lateral side of

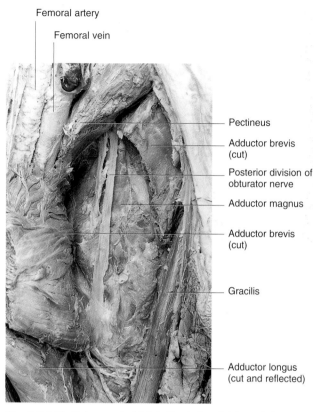

Femoral artery

Femoral vein

Pectineus

Adductor brevis (cut)

Posterior division of obturator nerve

Adductor magnus

Adductor brevis (cut)

Gracilis

Adductor longus (cut and reflected)

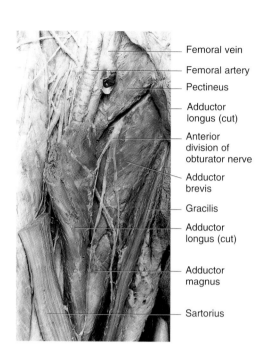

Femoral vein

Femoral artery

Pectineus

Adductor longus (cut)

Anterior division of obturator nerve

Adductor brevis

Gracilis

Adductor longus (cut)

Adductor magnus

Sartorius

Fig. 6.6c *Medial aspect of thigh. Obturator nerve — anterior division.*

Fig. 6.6d *Medial aspect of thigh. Posterior division of obturator nerve after reflection of adductor longus and adductor brevis.*

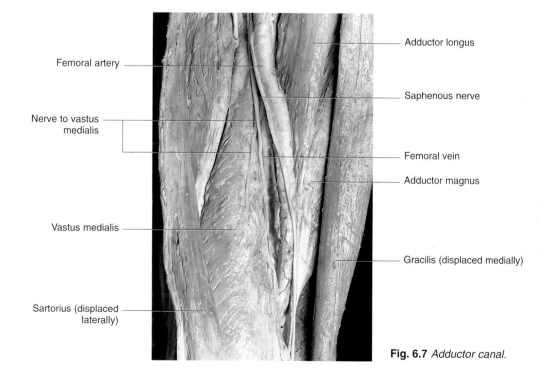

Femoral artery

Nerve to vastus medialis

Vastus medialis

Sartorius (displaced laterally)

Adductor longus

Saphenous nerve

Femoral vein

Adductor magnus

Gracilis (displaced medially)

Fig. 6.7 *Adductor canal.*

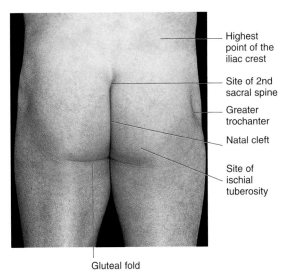

Highest point of the iliac crest

Site of 2nd sacral spine

Greater trochanter

Natal cleft

Site of ischial tuberosity

Gluteal fold

Fig. 6.8a *Surface anatomy of the gluteal region.*

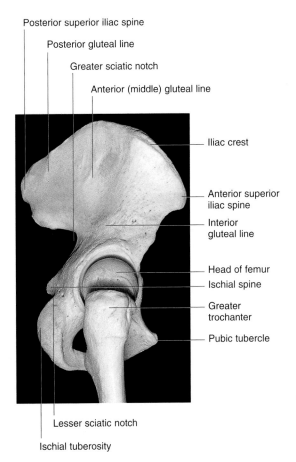

Posterior superior iliac spine

Posterior gluteal line

Greater sciatic notch

Anterior (middle) gluteal line

Iliac crest

Anterior superior iliac spine

Interior gluteal line

Head of femur

Ischial spine

Greater trochanter

Pubic tubercle

Lesser sciatic notch

Ischial tuberosity

Fig. 6.8b *The hip bone and the upper end of femur — lateral view.*

the artery to its medial side. The femoral artery and vein pass into the popliteal fossa from the adductor canal by passing through a hiatus in the adductor magnus. The saphenous nerve leaves the canal by passing along the posterior border of the sartorius and then accompanies the long saphenous vein as it descends in the leg.

GLUTEAL REGION (Fig. 6.8)

Surface anatomy and osteology

The gluteal region or the buttock lies above the hip joint on the posterior aspect of the pelvis and it extends from the iliac crest above to the gluteal fold below. The iliac crest is palpable throughout. The highest point of the iliac crest is at the level of the spinous process of the fourth lumbar vertebra, the level often used in examination of the vertebral column and for doing a lumbar puncture. The iliac crest terminates posteriorly as the posterior superior iliac spine. Its position is often indicated by a depression on the surface and it is at the level of the second segment of the sacrum. A hand's breadth below the middle of the iliac crest is the greater trochanter which can be seen and felt in front of the hollow on the side of the hip. It is the only part of the femur which is palpable at its upper end. The ischial tuberosity is palpated at the lower part of the buttock. It is covered by the gluteus maximus while standing whereas while sitting the muscle rises and uncovers the bone. Hence the ischial tuberosity which supports the body weight while sitting down is more easily felt in that position.

The prominence of the buttock is contributed by the gluteus maximus and the overlying fat. The natal cleft separates the buttocks. Its upper end corresponds to the third sacral spine. The gluteal region is a common site for intramuscular injections. These are given in the upper outer quadrant to avoid damage to the sciatic nerve

Gluteus maximus

Origin
From the ilium behind the posterior gluteal line, the sacrum and the sacrotuberous ligament, a thick ligament extending from the ischial tuberosity to the sacrum.

Insertion
Major part into the iliotibial tract (p. 156). The deeper portion into the gluteal tuberosity of the femur (p. 153).

Nerve supply
Inferior gluteal nerve
Action
Powerful extension of the hip joint as in running and climbing stairs. It acts as an antigravity muscle controlling flexion as in sitting down from the standing posture. It is also a lateral rotator of the hip. Through the iliotibial tract it can extend as well as stabilise the knee joint.

Gluteus medius

Origin
From the gluteal surface of the ilium between anterior and posterior gluteal lines.
Insertion
On the lateral surface of the greater trochanter.
Nerve supply
Superior gluteal nerve.

Gluteus minimus

Lies deep to the medius.
Origin
From the gluteal surface of the ilium between the anterior and inferior gluteal lines.

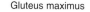
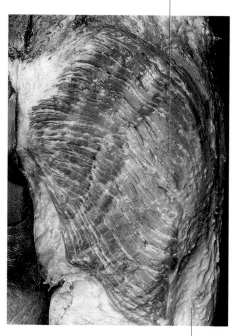

Fig. 6.8c *Gluteus maximus.*

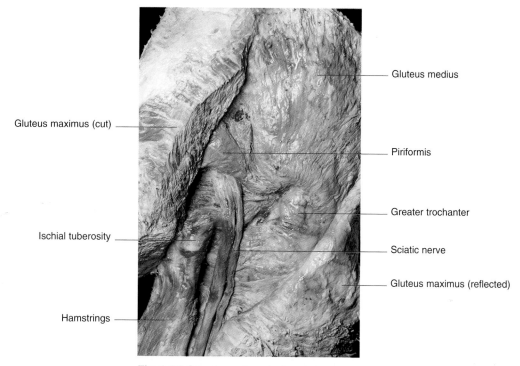

Fig. 6.8d *Structures deep to the gluteus maximus. The gluteus medius.*

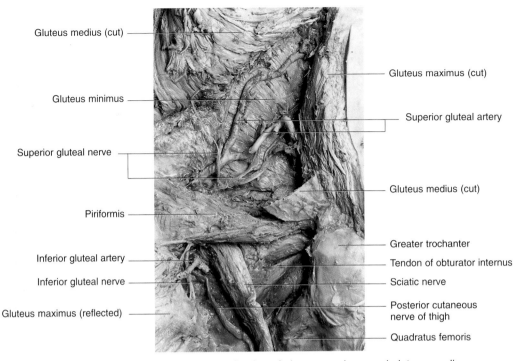

Gluteus medius (cut)

Gluteus minimus

Superior gluteal nerve

Piriformis

Inferior gluteal artery

Inferior gluteal nerve

Gluteus maximus (reflected)

Gluteus maximus (cut)

Superior gluteal artery

Gluteus medius (cut)

Greater trochanter

Tendon of obturator internus

Sciatic nerve

Posterior cutaneous nerve of thigh

Quadratus femoris

Fig. 6.8e *Structures of the gluteal region seen after reflection of gluteus maximus and gluteus medius.*

Insertion
On the anterior aspect of the greater trochanter.

Nerve supply
The superior gluteal nerve.

Action
The gluteus medius and minimus abduct the hip joint. When standing on one leg, gluteus medius and minimus of the supporting side prevent the hip from tilting to the unsupported side (it prevents adduction). When the muscles are paralysed, the tendency for tilting the pelvis to the unsupported side will be compensated by arching the trunk towards the supporting side.

The short lateral rotators of the hip
(Fig. 6.8e)

These consist of the piriformis, the obturator internus, the gemelli and the quadratus femoris. The obturator internus lies on the lateral wall of the pelvis. Its tendon emerges through the lesser sciatic foramen to be inserted on the greater trochanter. The two gemelli arise from the margin of the lesser sciatic notch and accompany the tendon of the obturator internus before inserting on the greater trochanter. The quadratus femoris takes origin from the ischial tuberosity and is

inserted to the greater trochanter. Besides laterally rotating the thigh these muscles help to do the fine adjustment and stabilise the hip joint.

Sciatic nerve

This, the largest nerve in the body, is formed in the sacral plexus (L4,L5,S1–3). It supplies the muscles of the posterior compartment of the thigh and those of the leg and foot. Its cutaneous branches supply the skin of the leg and foot except the skin along the medial border which is supplied by the saphenous nerve. The sciatic nerve in the lower third of the back of thigh divides into the common peroneal and the tibial nerves. However these two divisions of the nerve can remain separate almost throughout their course.

Posterior cutaneous nerve of the thigh
(**S2,S3**) (Fig. 6.8e)

This supplies the back of the thigh and upper half of the back of the leg. It is derived from the same nerve root as the pelvic splanchnic nerve which supplies the pelvic viscera (p. 131). Referred pain may sometimes be felt in pelvic inflammation along the back of the thigh and leg because of the common root value.

BACK OF THIGH (Fig. 6.9)

The hamstrings

Consist of the biceps, the semitendinosus, the semimembranosus and the hamstring part of adductor magnus.

Origin

Common origin from the ischial tuberosity. The short head of the biceps takes origin from the linea aspera of the femur.

Insertion

The biceps on the head of the fibula, the semitendinosus and the semimembranosus on to the medial condyle of the tibia, the adductor magnus into the adductor tubercle on the femur just above its medial condyle.

Nerve supply

The sciatic nerve.

Action

They are flexors of the knee joint. When the knee is straight they limit flexion of the hip. They also have an extensor action on the hip joint especially when the position of the hip is intermediate between full flexion and full extension. This extensor action is important in walking. The semitendinosus and the semimembranosus can medially rotate the flexed knee and the biceps can act as a lateral rotator.

'Pulled hamstrings' is a common injury in athletes and footballers caused by tearing of the attachments of the muscles to the ischial tuberosity.

Sciatic nerve

The sciatic nerve runs vertically down lying deep to the long head of the biceps. About a hand's breadth or more above the knee joint, at the apex of the popliteal fossa, the nerve divides into common peroneal and

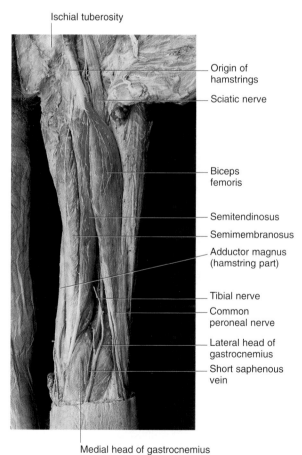

Ischial tuberosity

Origin of hamstrings

Sciatic nerve

Biceps femoris

Semitendinosus

Semimembranosus

Adductor magnus (hamstring part)

Tibial nerve

Common peroneal nerve

Lateral head of gastrocnemius

Short saphenous vein

Medial head of gastrocnemius

Fig. 6.9a *Posterior compartment of thigh and the popliteal fossa.*

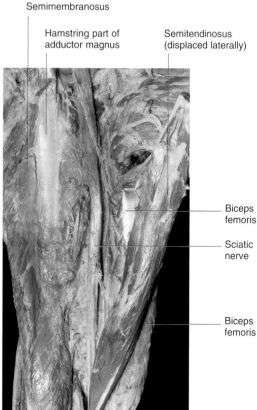

Semimembranosus

Hamstring part of adductor magnus

Semitendinosus (displaced laterally)

Biceps femoris

Sciatic nerve

Biceps femoris

Fig. 6.9b *Sciatic nerve in the posterior compartment of thigh.*

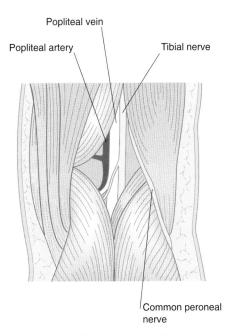

Popliteal vein

Popliteal artery

Tibial nerve

Common peroneal nerve

Fig. 6.10a *Popliteal artery, popliteal vein and the nerves in the popliteal fossa.*

tibial nerves. This division may occur at a higher level or the two components may emerge separate from the pelvis as they are formed separately in the sciatic plexus. The surface marking of the nerve is indicated by a line connecting the midpoint between the ischial tuberosity and the greater trochanter to the apex of the popliteal fossa.

THE POPLITEAL FOSSA (Fig. 6.10)

This space behind the knee joint is bounded above by the tendon of the biceps laterally, the semitendinosus and semimembranosus medially and below by the lateral and medial heads of the gastrocnemius. It contains the tibial and the common peroneal branches of the sciatic nerve, the popliteal artery and the popliteal vein.

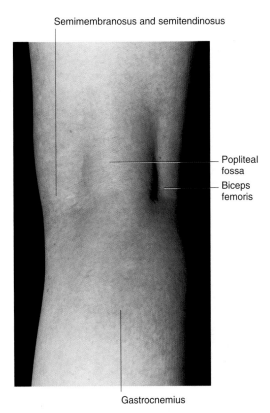

Semimembranosus and semitendinosus

Popliteal fossa

Biceps femoris

Gastrocnemius

Fig. 6.10b *Surface anatomy of the popliteal fossa.*

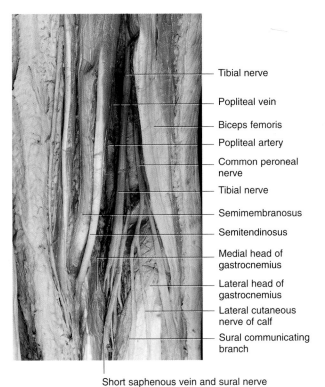

Tibial nerve

Popliteal vein

Biceps femoris

Popliteal artery

Common peroneal nerve

Tibial nerve

Semimembranosus

Semitendinosus

Medial head of gastrocnemius

Lateral head of gastrocnemius

Lateral cutaneous nerve of calf

Sural communicating branch

Short saphenous vein and sural nerve

Fig. 6.10c *The popliteal fossa, boundaries and contents.*

Common peroneal nerve

The common peroneal nerve lies along the posterior border of the tendon of the biceps and gives off a number of branches.

Sural (peroneal) communicating branch — joins the sural nerve in the leg to supply the lateral border of the foot. Lateral cutaneous nerve of the calf supplies the front and lateral aspect of the leg in its upper part. Superior and inferior lateral genicular branches accompany the corresponding arteries to supply the capsule and the lateral ligament of the knee joint.

The tibial nerve

Lies in the midline and disappears after passing deep to the two heads of the gastrocnemius. It supplies all the muscles which take origin in the popliteal fossa, i.e. two heads of the gastrocnemius, plantaris, soleus and popliteus. The sural nerve which accompanies the short saphenous vein supplies skin of the lateral border of the foot. The tibial nerve gives off three genicular branches.

The popliteal artery

The popliteal artery and vein lie at a deeper plane compared to the nerves. The vein, formed by the venae comitantes of the anterior and posterior tibial arteries, here is often joined by the short saphenous vein.

The popliteal artery is the continuation of the femoral artery after it has passed through the hiatus in the adductor magnus which is about a hand's breadth above the knee joint. It lies deep in the popliteal fossa and is separated from the tibial nerve by the popliteal vein. In the lower part of the popliteal fossa the artery bifurcates to form the anterior and posterior tibial arteries.

The popliteal artery pulsation can be felt on deep palpation after the knee is flexed to relax the muscles and the deep fascia.

The popliteal artery may be damaged in supracondylar fracture of the femur, especially if there is displacement of the lower fragment by the pull of the gastrocnemius.

The artery can be surgically exposed through posterior, medial or lateral approaches. The posterior

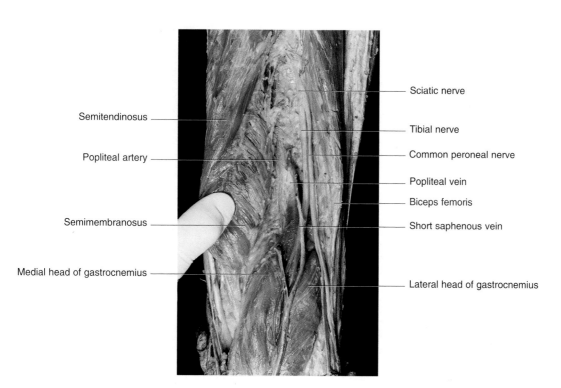

Fig. 6.10d *Structures in the popliteal fossa (tibial nerve displaced slightly laterally to show the popliteal vein and artery).*

approach is through the interval between the two heads of the gastrocnemius avoiding the nerves and the popliteal vein. In the medial approach the medial head of gastrocnemius is detached from its femoral attachment after retracting the semimembranosus and semitendinosus medially. In the lateral approach which passes behind the iliotibial tract and the lateral intermuscular septum the biceps is displaced backwards.

FRONT OF LEG AND DORSUM OF FOOT (Fig. 6.11)

The front of the leg has the subcutaneous medial surface of the tibia on the medial side and the extensor

compartment of the leg containing the dorsiflexors on the anterolateral side.

The extensor compartment

This compartment occupies the space between the tibia and fibula in front of the interosseous membrane. It contains the tibialis anterior, extensor hallucis longus, extensor digitorum longus and peroneus tertius muscles along with the deep peroneal nerve and the anterior tibial vessels. This is a tight space bounded by unyielding bones, deep fascia, intermuscular septae and the interosseous membrane and hence is a site where neurovascular structures can be compressed by haematoma or muscle oedema causing compartment syndrome.

The deep fascia in the lower part is thickened to form the superior and the inferior extensor retinacula which holds the tendons of the muscles against the ankle joint and prevents them from bowstringing.

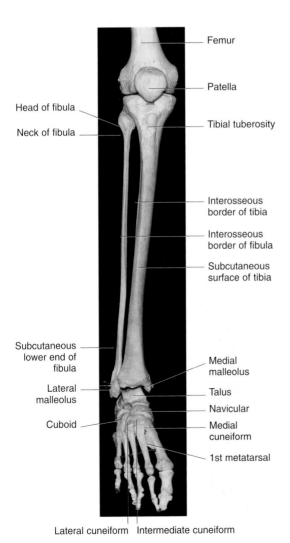

Femur

Patella

Head of fibula

Neck of fibula

Tibial tuberosity

Interosseous border of tibia

Interosseous border of fibula

Subcutaneous surface of tibia

Subcutaneous lower end of fibula

Medial malleolus

Lateral malleolus

Talus

Navicular

Cuboid

Medial cuneiform

1st metatarsal

Lateral cuneiform   Intermediate cuneiform

Fig. 6.11a *Bones of the leg and foot.*

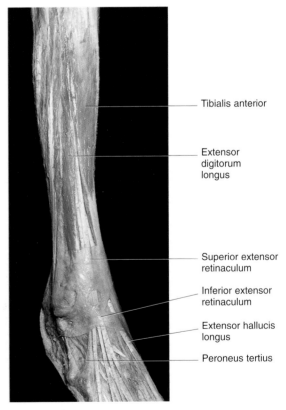

Tibialis anterior

Extensor digitorum longus

Superior extensor retinaculum

Inferior extensor retinaculum

Extensor hallucis longus

Peroneus tertius

Fig. 6.11b *Muscles of the extensor compartment of leg.*

Tibialis anterior

Origin
The anterolateral surface of the tibia and the interosseous membrane.
Insertion
The medial cuneiform and the adjoining first metatarsal bone.
Action
Dorsiflexes the ankle and inverts the foot.
Test
 By feeling the tendon at the ankle when the foot is dorsiflexed against resistance.

Extensor hallucis longus

Origin
From the fibula and the interosseous membrane.
Insertion
On the distal phalanx of the big toe.
Action
It is a dorsiflexor of the big toe and the ankle joint.
Test
By dorsiflexing the big toe against resistance.

Extensor digitorum longus

Origin
The extensor surface of the fibula, interosseous membrane as well as a small area on the lateral condyle of the tibia.
Insertion
It has four tendons which are inserted to the terminal phalanges of the lateral four toes. Their mode of insertion is similar to that of the extensor digitorum of the hand, as these tendons contribute to the dorsal extensor expansion over the proximal phalanges.
Action
The muscle dorsiflexes the lateral four toes and the tendons can be seen and felt as this is done against resistance.

Peroneus tertius

This arises from the lower third of the fibula and is inserted to the base of the fifth metatarsal bone with an extension of the insertion on its dorsal surface. It is an evertor of the foot.

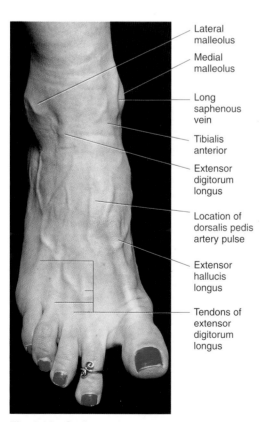

Fig. 6.11c *Surface anatomy of the dorsum of the foot.*

Lateral malleolus
Medial malleolus
Long saphenous vein
Tibialis anterior
Extensor digitorum longus
Location of dorsalis pedis artery pulse
Extensor hallucis longus
Tendons of extensor digitorum longus

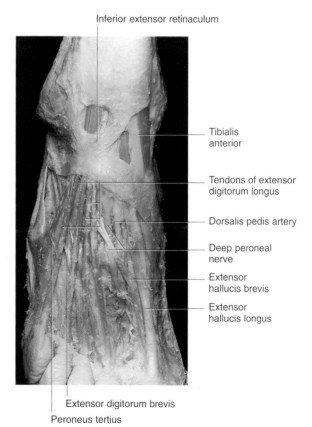

Inferior extensor retinaculum
Tibialis anterior
Tendons of extensor digitorum longus
Dorsalis pedis artery
Deep peroneal nerve
Extensor hallucis brevis
Extensor hallucis longus
Extensor digitorum brevis
Peroneus tertius

Fig. 6.11d *Structures on the dorsum of the foot.*

The deep peroneal nerve and the anterior tibial artery

All the muscles in the front of the leg are supplied by the deep peroneal nerve which accompanies the anterior tibial artery. These lie between the extensor hallucis longus and the tibialis anterior in front of the interosseous membrane. The nerve lies lateral to the artery and is one of the terminal branches of the common peroneal nerve. As it descends the nerve crosses over to the medial side of the artery but crosses back again to the lateral side in the lower part of the leg. The deep peroneal nerve emerges at the space between the big and second toes to supply the skin on its adjacent surfaces. Extensor digitorum brevis having tendons reaching the toes is a muscle arising from the dorsal surface of the calcaneum. The part going to the big toe separates off early from the main muscle mass and is known as the extensor hallucis brevis. Extensor digitorum brevis is also supplied by the deep peroneal nerve.

The anterior tibial artery enters the extensor compartment after it branches off from the popliteal artery by crossing over the interosseous membrane. The continuation of the artery on the dorsum of the foot is known as the dorsalis pedis artery.

The dorsalis pedis artery pulsation can be felt on the dorsum of the foot lateral to the tendon of the extensor

hallucis longus against the navicular and medial cuneiform bones. This artery may be replaced by a perforating branch of the peroneal artery, the pulsation of which may be palpable in front of the lateral malleolus.

LATERAL COMPARTMENT OF THE LEG (Fig. 6.12)

This muscular compartment which lies on the lateral aspect of the leg contains the peroneus longus and peroneus brevis muscles as well as the superficial peroneal nerve which supplies them. Peroneus longus takes origin from the upper two-thirds of the fibula and its tendon passes behind the lateral malleolus to enter the sole of the foot. It then crosses obliquely across to the medial aspect of the sole of the foot to be inserted to the medial cuneiform bone and the base of the first metatarsal. Peroneus brevis arises from the lower two-thirds of the lateral surface of the fibula and its tendon lying in front of that of the peroneus longus behind the lateral malleolus is inserted to the tubercle of the base of the fifth metatarsal bone. The peroneus longus and brevis are evertors of the foot. The two peronei tendons are bound down to the lateral malleolus by the superior and inferior peroneal retinacula. The superficial peroneal nerve begins in the substance of the peroneus

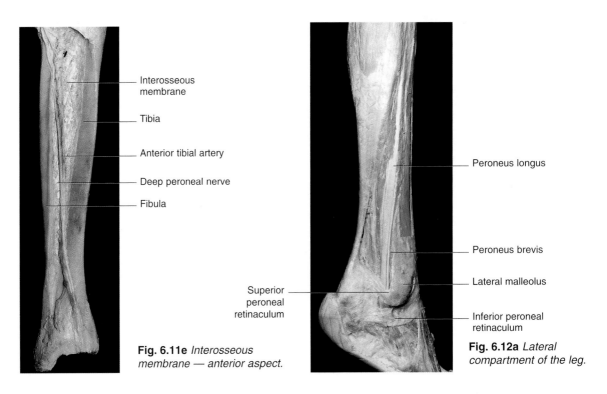

Interosseous membrane
Tibia
Anterior tibial artery
Deep peroneal nerve
Fibula
Superior peroneal retinaculum

Fig. 6.11e *Interosseous membrane — anterior aspect.*

Peroneus longus
Peroneus brevis
Lateral malleolus
Inferior peroneal retinaculum

Fig. 6.12a *Lateral compartment of the leg.*

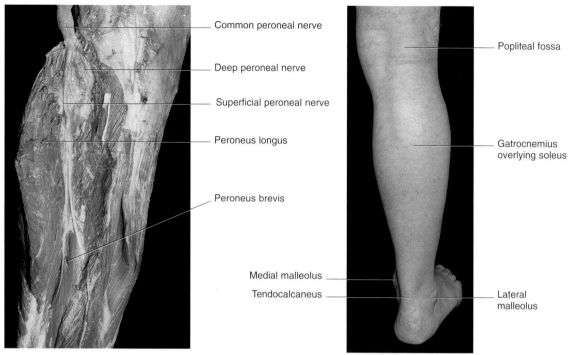

Common peroneal nerve

Deep peroneal nerve

Superficial peroneal nerve

Peroneus longus

Peroneus brevis

Popliteal fossa

Gatrocnemius overlying soleus

Medial malleolus

Tendocalcaneus

Lateral malleolus

Fig. 6.12b *Lateral compartment of the leg. Common peroneal nerve and its divisions.*

Fig. 6.13a *Surface anatomy of the back of the leg.*

longus at the division of the common peroneal nerve. It supplies the two peronei muscles as well as the skin of the lower part of the front of the leg and that of the dorsum of the foot.

The common peroneal nerve winds round the neck of the fibula and divides into superficial peroneal and deep peroneal nerves. It is very superficial as it lies on the neck of the fibula and can easily be damaged in injuries of this region causing a 'foot drop' as a result of paralysis of the dorsiflexors.

POSTERIOR COMPARTMENT OF THE LEG (Fig. 6.13)

Superficial structures

The small saphenous vein from the lateral aspect of the dorsal venous arch ascends behind the lateral malleolus to reach the back of the leg. It pierces the deep fascia anywhere between the middle of the calf and the roof of the popliteal fossa to drain into the popliteal vein. The vein which has several communications with the great saphenous vein is accompanied by the sural nerve.

The muscles of the calf which are the plantar flexors of the foot and of the toes are arranged in superficial

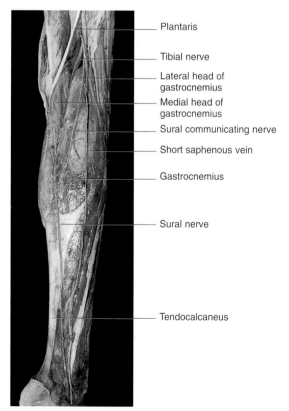

Plantaris

Tibial nerve

Lateral head of gastrocnemius

Medial head of gastrocnemius

Sural communicating nerve

Short saphenous vein

Gastrocnemius

Sural nerve

Tendocalcaneus

Fig. 6.13b *Superficial structures of the back of the leg.*

and deep compartments separated by the thick deep transverse fascia. The superficial muscles which are the main plantar flexors of the foot consist of the gastrocnemius, soleus and plantaris, the tendons of which converge to form the tendo calcaneus or Achilles' tendon. All the muscles in the posterior compartment are supplied by the tibial nerve. The artery of the posterior compartment is the posterior tibial artery, a terminal branch of the popliteal artery.

The gastrocnemius arises by two heads from the lateral and medial femoral condyles. The plantaris, with a small belly and a long slender tendon, originates from the lateral supracondylar ridge of the femur. Its tendon can be harvested for tendon grafting. However the muscle is absent in about 10% of subjects. The soleus takes origin from the upper third of the back of the fibula, the soleal line of the tibia and from a fibrous arch connecting these two origins. The muscle contains a venous plexus and the perforating veins connecting the superficial and deep groups of veins pass through it. Contraction of the soleus (soleal pump) aids venous

return and stagnation of venous blood here can produce deep vein thrombosis and pulmonary embolism.

Deep muscles

The deep group contains the flexor digitorum longus, flexor hallucis longus and the tibialis posterior. Flexor digitorum longus takes origin from the posterior surface of the tibia. The flexor hallucis longus, the bulkiest of the three deep flexor muscles, takes origin from the fibula and the interosseous membrane. It is fleshy until the heel and is known as the 'beef of the heel'. The tibialis posterior is the deepest muscle in the calf and its fibres arise from the back of the fibula and tibia and the interosseous membrane. The tendons of these three muscles pass deep to the flexor retinaculum to enter the sole of the foot. Their further course is described under 'The sole of the foot' below. The flexor retinaculum is a thickening of the deep fascia extending between the medial malleolus and the medial

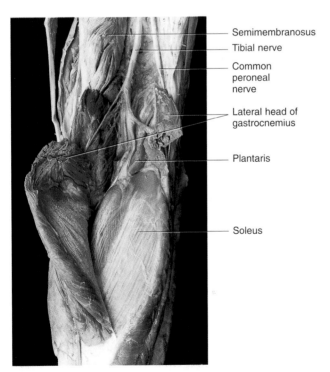

- Semimembranosus
- Tibial nerve
- Common peroneal nerve
- Lateral head of gastrocnemius
- Plantaris
- Soleus

Fig. 6.13c *Back of the leg. Structures under the gastrocnemius.*

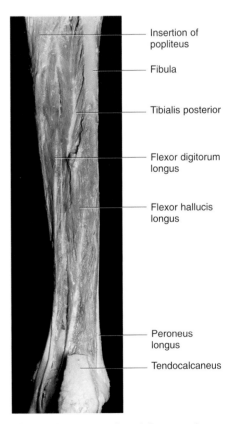

- Insertion of popliteus
- Fibula
- Tibialis posterior
- Flexor digitorum longus
- Flexor hallucis longus
- Peroneus longus
- Tendocalcaneus

Fig. 6.13d *Origin of deep muscles of the posterior compartment of the leg.*

tubercle of the calcaneus. This roofs the tarsal tunnel in which lies from anterior to posterior the tendons of tibialis posterior, flexor digitorum longus, posterior tibial artery, tibial nerve (which divides here to form the medial and lateral plantar nerves) and the tendon of flexor hallucis longus.

The tibial nerve

Supplies all the muscles in the posterior compartment. It lies deep to the soleus along with the posterior tibial artery. Its cutaneous branch, the sural nerve, often joined by the sural communicating branch from the common peroneal nerve supplies the lateral border of the foot. At the lower part of the leg the tibial nerve passes deep to the flexor retinaculum, where it divides into the lateral and medial plantar nerves, to supply the sole of the foot.

Posterior tibial artery

The posterior tibial artery commences at the lower border of the popliteus as one of the two terminal branches of the popliteal arteries, the other being the anterior tibial artery. It supplies the back of the leg and the sole of the foot. Near its commencement the artery

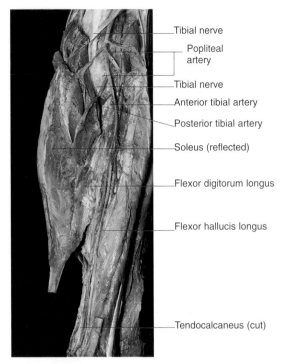

Tibial nerve

Popliteal artery

Tibial nerve

Anterior tibial artery

Posterior tibial artery

Soleus (reflected)

Flexor digitorum longus

Flexor hallucis longus

Tendocalcaneus (cut)

Fig. 6.13e *Deep structures of the back of the leg.*

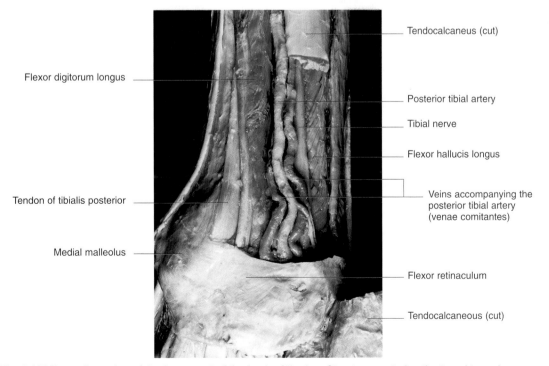

Tendocalcaneus (cut)

Posterior tibial artery

Tibial nerve

Flexor hallucis longus

Veins accompanying the posterior tibial artery (venae comitantes)

Flexor digitorum longus

Tendon of tibialis posterior

Medial malleolus

Flexor retinaculum

Tendocalcaneous (cut)

Fig. 6.13f *Deep dissection of the lower part of the back of the leg. Structures entering the tarsal tunnel. Right side — seen from the medial aspect.*

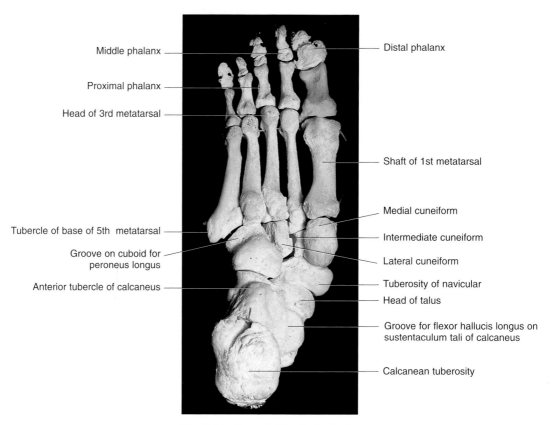

Middle phalanx

Proximal phalanx

Head of 3rd metatarsal

Distal phalanx

Shaft of 1st metatarsal

Medial cuneiform

Tubercle of base of 5th metatarsal

Intermediate cuneiform

Groove on cuboid for peroneus longus

Lateral cuneiform

Anterior tubercle of calcaneus

Tuberosity of navicular

Head of talus

Groove for flexor hallucis longus on sustentaculum tali of calcaneus

Calcanean tuberosity

Fig. 6.14a *Bones of the foot, plantar aspect.*

gives off the peroneal artery which supplies the deep muscles of the calf and the muscles in the lateral compartment and descends along the medial border of the fibula. The peroneal artery pierces the interosseous membrane to enter the extensor compartment and may replace or supplement the dorsalis pedis artery. The posterior tibial artery enters the sole of the foot by passing deep to the flexor retinaculum. Its pulsation can be felt midway between the medial malleolus and the medial border of the tendo calcaneus. The pulsation of the peroneal artery is felt in front of the lateral malleolus at its medial border.

THE SOLE OF THE FOOT (Fig. 6.14)

The muscles of the sole of the foot are arranged in four layers and they are covered by the plantar aponeurosis which is a thickening of the deep fascia. The plantar aponeurosis and the muscles of the sole of the foot, extending from the proximal part of the foot to its distal part, act like tie beams or bowstrings, to maintain the longitudinal arches of the foot.

Plantar aponeurosis

This is the thickened middle portion of the deep fascia which is attached proximally to the medial process of the calcanean tuberosity. Distally it divides into five slips, one to be attached to the fibrous flexor sheath on each toe as well as to the deep transverse metatarsal ligaments which connect the heads of the metatarsal bones.

Deep transverse metatarsal ligament

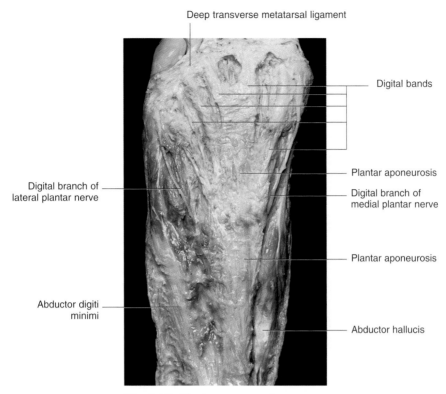

Digital bands

Plantar aponeurosis

Digital branch of
lateral plantar nerve

Digital branch of
medial plantar nerve

Plantar aponeurosis

Abductor digiti
minimi

Abductor hallucis

Fig. 6.14b *Plantar aponeurosis.*

Muscles of the first layer

ABDUCTOR HALLUCIS
Origin
Medial process of calcanean tuberosity, flexor
retinaculum.
Insertion
Medial side of base of proximal phalanx of big toe.

FLEXOR DIGITORUM BREVIS
Origin
Medial process of calcanean tuberosity, plantar
aponeurosis. Gives off four tendons, one for each toe.
Insertion
Middle phalanges of lateral four toes. Tendon splits for
passage of tendons of flexor digitorum longus.

ABDUCTOR DIGIT MINIMI
Origin
Medial and lateral processes of calcanean tuberosity.
Insertion
Lateral side of the base of the proximal phalanx of the
little toe along with the flexor digiti minimi brevis.

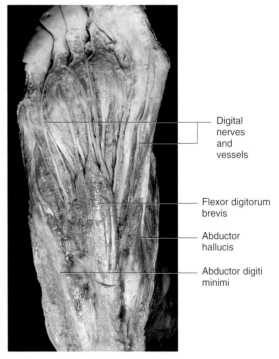

Digital
nerves
and
vessels

Flexor digitorum
brevis

Abductor
hallucis

Abductor digiti
minimi

Fig. 6.14c *Sole of the foot, first layer.*

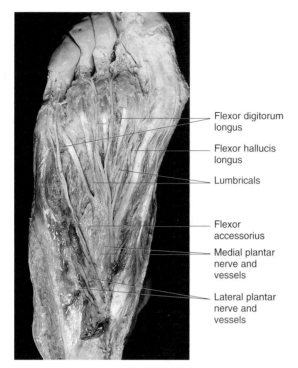

Flexor digitorum longus

Flexor hallucis longus

Lumbricals

Flexor accessorius

Medial plantar nerve and vessels

Lateral plantar nerve and vessels

Fig. 6.14d *Sole of the foot, second layer. Medial and lateral plantar nerves and vessels.*

The second layer

TENDON OF FLEXOR HALLUCIS LONGUS
Lies along the medial border of the foot like a bowstring maintaining the medial longitudinal arch and is crossed inferiorly by the tendon of the flexor digitorum longus. The tendon lies between the two sesamoid bones at the base of the big toe and is finally inserted to the base of the distal phalanx of the big toe.

TENDON OF THE FLEXOR DIGITORUM LONGUS
Proximally in the sole of the foot it divides into four tendons for the lateral four toes as it crosses the tendon of the hallucis longus. The four lumbricals take origin from these. The flexor accessorius is inserted to the digitorum longus tendon. The four tendons for the digits lie deep to those of the digitorum brevis until they reach the plantar surface of the toes where they pierce the brevis tendons to be inserted to the base of the distal phalanges. The arrangement of the lumbricals are similar to those in the palm of the hand.

THE LATERAL AND MEDIAL PLANTAR NERVES AND ARTERIES.
The medial plantar nerve supplies the abductor hallucis, flexor hallucis brevis, flexor digitorum brevis and the first lumbrical. All the remaining intrinsic

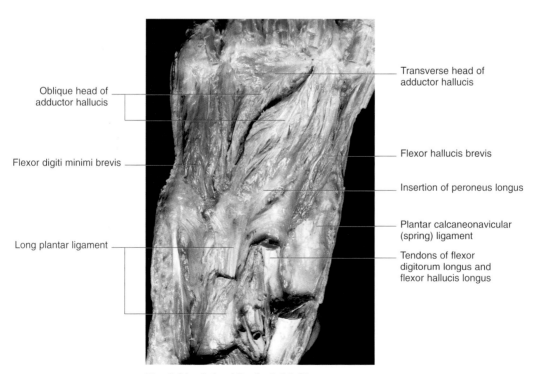

Oblique head of adductor hallucis

Flexor digiti minimi brevis

Long plantar ligament

Transverse head of adductor hallucis

Flexor hallucis brevis

Insertion of peroneus longus

Plantar calcaneonavicular (spring) ligament

Tendons of flexor digitorum longus and flexor hallucis longus

Fig. 6.14e *Sole of the foot, third layer.*

muscles including the adductor hallucis are supplied by the lateral plantar nerve. The cutaneous branches of the lateral plantar nerve supply the lateral third of the skin of the sole and the lateral one and a half digits. The sensory supply of the remaining skin is by the medial plantar nerve. Thus, the distribution of the two plantar nerves in the sole of the foot resembles the distribution of the median and the ulnar nerves in the palm of the hand: the lateral plantar is similar to the ulnar nerve and the medial plantar to the median.

The third layer

FLEXOR HALLUCIS BREVIS
Origin
Cuboid, tendon of tibialis posterior.
Insertion
Splits into two parts to be inserted to the lateral and medial sides of the proximal phalanx of the big toe along with abductor hallucis and adductor hallucis respectively. Small sesamoid bone in each tendon.

ADDUCTOR HALLUCIS
Origin
Oblique head from tendon of peroneus longus and metatarsals 2–4. Transverse head deep transverse

ligament and capsules of four metatarsophalangeal joints.
Insertion
Lateral aspect of proximal phalanx of big toe along with lateral part of flexor hallucis brevis.

FLEXOR DIGITI MINIMI BREVIS:
Origin
Base of fifth metatarsal.
Insertion
Lateral side of base of proximal phalanx of little toe.

The fourth layer

The peroneus longus tendon lies in the groove of the cuboid bone before reaching its insertion to the medial cuneiform and the first metatarsal bone. The tibialis posterior tendon is inserted into the tuberosity of the navicular bone and also into all the tarsal bones except the talus. There are two sets of interossei in this layer, three plantar and four dorsal. Toes 3–5 receive plantar interossei. They are arranged in such a way that they produce adduction of the toes by moving them towards the second toe. The dorsal interossei are abductors of the toes, i.e. moving the toes away from the axis of the movement going through the middle of the second toe. The second toe thus has two dorsal interossei, one on

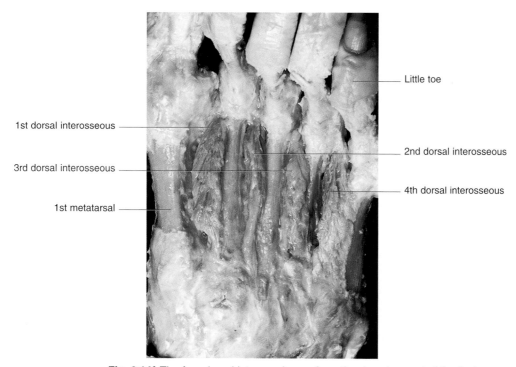

Fig. 6.14f *The four dorsal interossei seen from the dorsal aspect of the foot.*

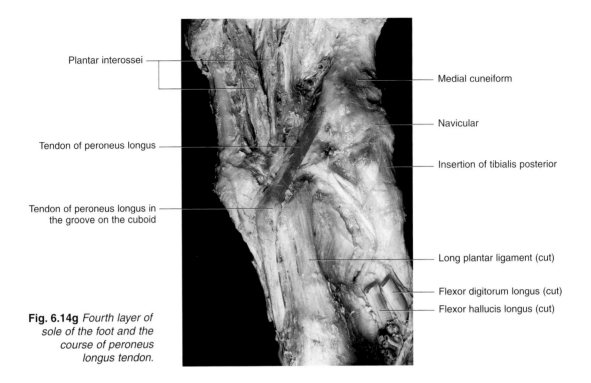

Plantar interossei

Tendon of peroneus longus

Tendon of peroneus longus in the groove on the cuboid

Medial cuneiform

Navicular

Insertion of tibialis posterior

Long plantar ligament (cut)

Flexor digitorum longus (cut)

Flexor hallucis longus (cut)

Fig. 6.14g *Fourth layer of sole of the foot and the course of peroneus longus tendon.*

either side. The other two are for toes 3 and 4. The arrangement of the interossei is comparable to those in the palm of the hand.

The long plantar ligament covers the undersurface of the calcaneus and distally is attached to the cuboid and the central three metatarsal bones. It converts the groove on the cuboid into a tunnel in which the tendon of the peroneus longus lies.

Plantar calcaneonavicular (spring) ligament

The spring ligament extends from the sustentaculum tali to the navicular bone. The head of the talus rests on its upper surface which forms part of the capsule of the subtalar joint.

THE HIP JOINT (Fig. 6.15)

The hip joint is a ball and socket type of synovial joint between the head of the femur and the acetabulum of the hip bone (innominate bone). As the joint supports the body weight in standing and also propels the trunk forward in locomotion it has to be stable and very mobile. Stability is achieved by a number of factors including its thick capsule and strong ligaments. The

mobility is due to the long femoral neck which joins the shaft at an angle.

Bony components

The acetabulum has a C-shaped articular surface, the lunate surface, which is lined by hyaline cartilage. The rim of the acetabulum is lined with a fibrocartilagenous acetabular labrum, part of which bridges across the acetabular notch as the transverse acetabular ligament. The deeper part of the acetabulum is non-articular and is occupied by the Haversian pad of fat. The head of the femur is mostly covered by articular cartilage (hyaline). The head has a pit (fovea) which is non-articular and receives the attachment of the ligament of the head of femur which extends to it from the transverse acetabular ligament.

Capsule

The fibrous capsule is strong, having its acetabular attachment around its margin just beyond the labrum and transverse ligament. The femoral attachment is on the intertrochanteric line anteriorly and about halfway down the neck posteriorly. The distal half of the posterior aspect of the neck is therefore extracapsular. From its attachment to the femoral neck, fibres of the

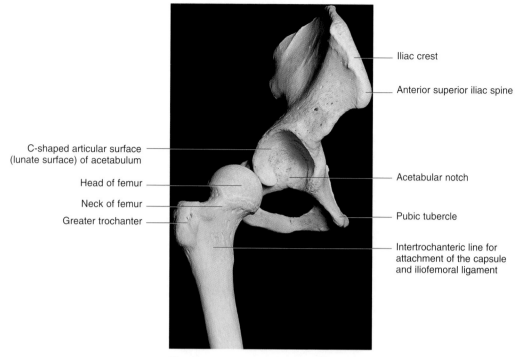

Iliac crest

Anterior superior iliac spine

C-shaped articular surface
(lunate surface) of acetabulum

Head of femur

Neck of femur

Greater trochanter

Acetabular notch

Pubic tubercle

Intertrochanteric line for
attachment of the capsule
and iliofemoral ligament

Fig. 6.15a *Hip bone and the upper end of femur.*

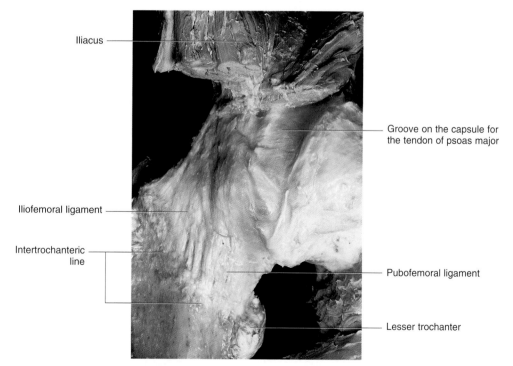

Iliacus

Groove on the capsule for
the tendon of psoas major

Iliofemoral ligament

Intertrochanteric
line

Pubofemoral ligament

Lesser trochanter

Fig. 6.15b *The capsule and ligaments of the hip joint — anterior aspect.*

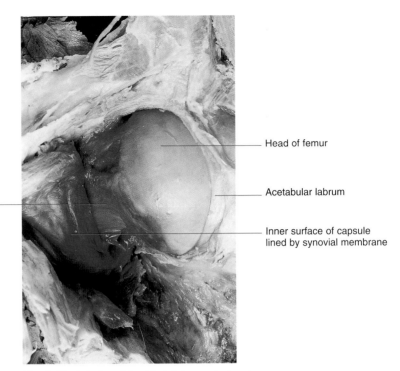

Head of femur

Acetabular labrum

Retinacula on neck of femur for transmission of blood vessels to the head of femur

Inner surface of capsule lined by synovial membrane

Fig. 6.15c *Interior of the hip joint — anterior view.*

capsule are reflected back along the neck as retinacular fibres. The blood vessels supplying the femoral head lie deep to these. Intracapsular fracture of the neck of femur, which is a common injury in the elderly, can result in avascular necrosis of the head of the femur due to rupture of the retinacular fibres and the blood vessels underneath.

Ligaments

The fibrous capsule is reinforced by three strong extracapsular ligaments. The iliofemoral ligament (ligament of Bigelow) reinforces the anterior aspect of the capsule. The ligament limits extension of the hip joint. The pubofemoral ligament blends with the capsule and the medial part of the iliofemoral ligament. The ischiofemoral ligament spirals on the femoral neck posteriorly.

Synovial membrane

The synovial membrane lines the capsule and all intracapsular structures except the articular cartilage in the acetabulum and on the femoral head. The synovial cavity often communicates with the iliac bursa through a gap in the capsule.

Relations

From medial to lateral the joint is covered anteriorly by the pectineus, tendon of psoas and the iliacus. The obturator externus spirals downwards and laterally on the inferior aspect of the joint. The pectineus separates the joint from the femoral vein and the psoas tendon separates it from the femoral artery. The iliac bursa lies between the iliacus and the joint capsule. The piriformis, the obturator internus tendon, the two gemelli and the sciatic nerve are the immediate posterior relations. The joint is laterally related to the iliotibial tract and medially to the structures in the pelvic cavity. As the acetabular fossa forms the lateral wall of the pelvis, the ovary in the female is separated from the joint only by obturator internus and the lining parietal peritoneum.

Movements

In flexion, the head of the femur rotates about a transverse axis up to about 120° when the knee is flexed. It is more limited when the knee is extended due to tension in the hamstrings. Flexion is achieved by the psoas major and the iliacus assisted by the sartorius, the rectus femoris and the pectineus. The movement is limited by the tension of the hamstrings. Extension, the

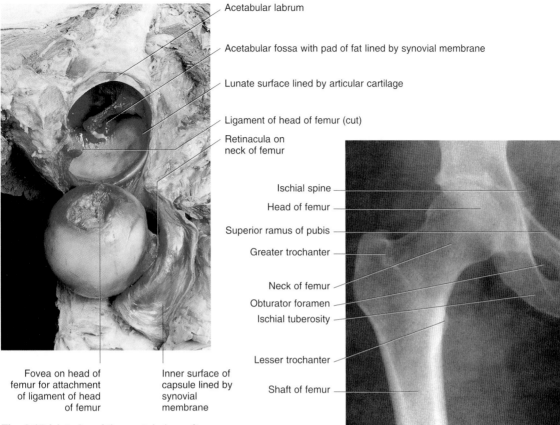

Acetabular labrum

Acetabular fossa with pad of fat lined by synovial membrane

Lunate surface lined by articular cartilage

Ligament of head of femur (cut)

Retinacula on neck of femur

Fovea on head of femur for attachment of ligament of head of femur

Inner surface of capsule lined by synovial membrane

Fig. 6.15d *Interior of the acetabulum after dislocation of head of femur.*

Ischial spine

Head of femur

Superior ramus of pubis

Greater trochanter

Neck of femur

Obturator foramen

Ischial tuberosity

Lesser trochanter

Shaft of femur

Fig. 6.15e *Radiograph of the anteroposterior view of the hip joint.*

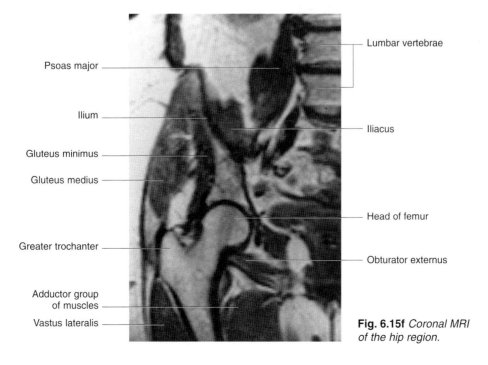

Psoas major

Ilium

Gluteus minimus

Gluteus medius

Greater trochanter

Adductor group of muscles

Vastus lateralis

Lumbar vertebrae

Iliacus

Head of femur

Obturator externus

Fig. 6.15f *Coronal MRI of the hip region.*

reverse of flexion, is possible to a range of about 20°
produced by gluteus maximus at the extremes of
movements and hamstrings in the intermediate ranges.
Tension of the iliofemoral ligament limits extension.
During abduction the head of femur rotates about an
anteroposterior axis up to about 60°. The movement is
produced by gluteus medius and minimus assisted by
tensor faciae latae and sartorius. Tension of the
adductors and the pubofemoral ligament limits
abduction. Adduction, the opposite of abduction, is by
adductors longus, brevis and magnus aided by the
pectineus and the gracilis. In lateral rotation the
femoral head rotates about a vertical axis passing
through the centre of head to the medial condyle. The
femoral neck swings backward about this axis. Due to
the angle between the neck and the shaft this axis of
rotation does not pass though the shaft of the femur.
The piriformis, the obturator internus, the superior and
inferior gemelli, the quadratus femoris, the obturator
externus, assisted by gluteus maximus and sartorius
are lateral rotators. Anterior fibres of the gluteus
medius and minimus assisted by tensor fasciae latae act
as medial rotators.

Contraction of the abductors is essential in one-leg
standing, in walking and running, to prevent

adduction of the hip. When the neck of the femur is
fractured rotation takes place about an axis passing
through the shaft of the femur. The psoas and the
iliacus then laterally rotate the femur which is
characteristic of a fractured femoral neck.

The hip joint can be dislocated due to violent trauma
as in a road traffic accident. Posterior dislocation is
more common than anterior and central (where the
head of the femur breaks through the acetabulum into
the pelvis) dislocations. The sciatic nerve is prone to
injury in posterior dislocations.

THE KNEE JOINT (Fig. 6.16)

In this, the largest synovial joint in the body, the
condyles of the femur articulate with those of the tibia
and the patella articulates with the femur. It is a
modified hinge joint where besides flexion and
extension there is a certain amount of rotation possible
when the joint is flexed.

The knee joint has on its medial aspect the medial
(tibial) collateral ligament and on its lateral aspect the
lateral (fibular) collateral ligament, posteriorly the
oblique popliteal ligament and the popliteus muscle and

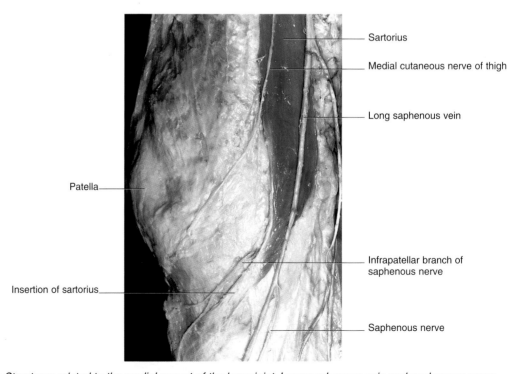

Fig. 6.16a *Structures related to the medial aspect of the knee joint. Long saphenous vein and saphenous nerve.*

anteriorly the tendon of the quadriceps, patella and the ligamentum patellae.

The quadriceps tendon, the patella and the ligamentum patella forming the anterior aspect of the joint have been described already (p. 155).

Tibial collateral ligament

This ligament is broad and it extends from the medial epicondyle of the femur to the medial surface of the tibia. It is crossed by the tendons of the sartorius, the gracilis and the semimembranosus with a bursa intervening. The ligment blends with the capsule of the knee joint and it is also posteriorly attached to the medial meniscus. Rupture of the ligament due to a blow on the lateral aspect of the joint can cause tearing of the medial meniscus. The medial inferior genicular vessels and nerves and an extension of the semimembranosus tendon insertion are deep to the distal part of the ligament.

Fibular collateral ligament

This is a cord-like ligament which is attached to the lateral epicondyle of the femur above and to the head of the fibula below. It is covered by the tendon of the biceps. Unlike the medial ligament it is not attached to the capsule of the joint or to the lateral meniscus.

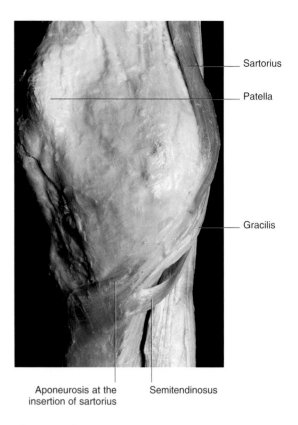

Fig. 6.16b *Structures related to the medial aspect of the knee joint. Sartorius, gracilis and semitendinosus.*

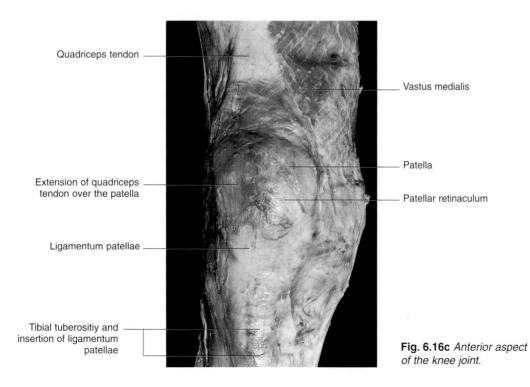

Fig. 6.16c *Anterior aspect of the knee joint.*

Oblique popliteal ligament

This ligament which blends with the posterior aspect of the capsule of the joint is an extension of the insertion of the semimembranosus from the posterior aspect of the medial tibial condyle upwards and laterally to the lateral condyle of the femur. The popliteal artery lies on it and the genicular nerves and vessels pierce it.

Cruciate ligaments

The two cruciate ligaments which lie within the capsule maintain the anteroposterior stability of the joint. They are named after their tibial attachments, the anterior cruciate ligament being attached to the anterior aspect of the intercondylar area of the tibia and the posterior cruciate ligament to the smooth impression on the posterior aspect. They are extrasynovial and when they cross the anterior cruciate is anterolateral to the posterior ligament.

The anterior cruciate ligament from its tibial attachment between the anterior horns of the medial and lateral menisci ascends posteromedially to be attached to the lateral femoral condyle at its posteromedial aspect.

The posterior cruciate ligament is the most posterior structure in the intercondylar area of the tibia and its attachment extends on to the posterior surface of the shaft. From there it ascends to its femoral attachment to the anterolateral aspect of the medial condyle. It is shorter and stronger than the anterior cruciate ligament.

The anterior cruciate ligament resists excessive forward glide of the tibia on the femur or backward glide of the femur on the tibia. The posterior cruciate ligament resists excessive posterior glide of the tibia on the femur or anterior glide of femur on tibia. They can be tested by bending the knee to 90° and rocking the tibia forward and backward (the drawer test).

The menisci are tough avascular fibrocartilages whose anterior and posterior ends are anchored to the intercondylar area of the tibia. They deepen the concavity of the tibial surface and also help to spread the synovial fluid. The medial meniscus is less mobile than the lateral meniscus and hence is more prone to injury. Its mobility is markedly restricted by its attachment to the tibial collateral ligament. The anterior horn of the meniscus is attached to the intercondylar area in front of the anterior cruciate ligament whilst its posterior horn is similarly attached

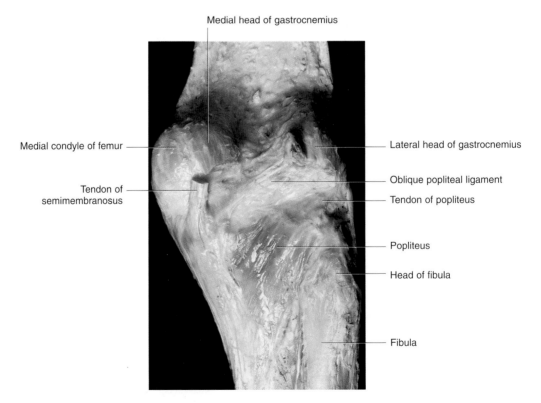

Fig. 6.16d *Posterior aspect of the knee joint. Oblique popliteal ligament.*

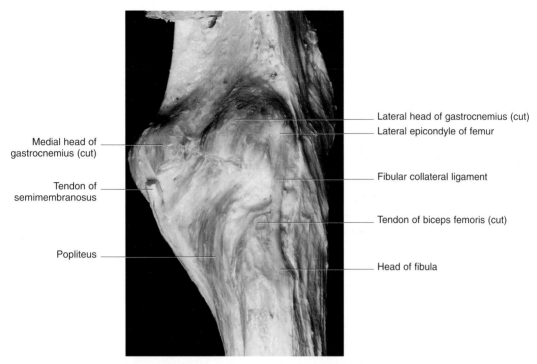

Lateral head of gastrocnemius (cut)

Lateral epicondyle of femur

Medial head of
gastrocnemius (cut)

Fibular collateral ligament

Tendon of
semimembranosus

Tendon of biceps femoris (cut)

Popliteus

Head of fibula

Fig. 6.16e *Posterolateral aspect of the knee joint. Fibular collateral ligament.*

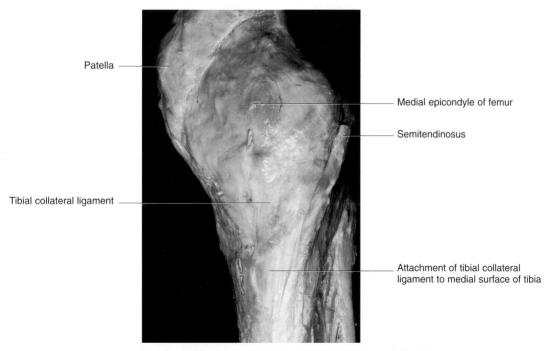

Patella

Medial epicondyle of femur

Semitendinosus

Tibial collateral ligament

Attachment of tibial collateral
ligament to medial surface of tibia

Fig. 6.16f *Medial aspect of the knee joint. Tibial collateral ligament.*

in front of the posterior cruciate ligament. The meniscus is broader posteriorly. The lateral meniscus is more circular and is attached to the popliteus which makes it more mobile and less prone to injury. Its anterior horn is attached behind the anterior cruciate ligament in front of the intercondylar tubercle of the tibia whilst the psoterior horn attachment is behind the tubercle but in front of the attachment of the posterior horn of the medial meniscus.

From the posterior aspect of the lateral meniscus the anterior and posterior meniscofemoral ligaments (of Humphry and Wrisberg) extend upwards and medially

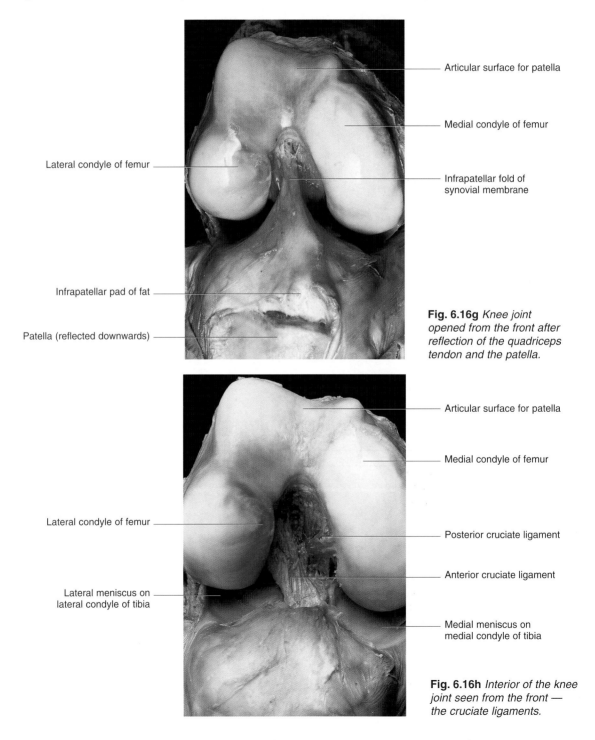

Lateral condyle of femur

Articular surface for patella

Medial condyle of femur

Infrapatellar fold of synovial membrane

Infrapatellar pad of fat

Patella (reflected downwards)

Fig. 6.16g *Knee joint opened from the front after reflection of the quadriceps tendon and the patella.*

Lateral condyle of femur

Articular surface for patella

Medial condyle of femur

Posterior cruciate ligament

Anterior cruciate ligament

Lateral meniscus on lateral condyle of tibia

Medial meniscus on medial condyle of tibia

Fig. 6.16h *Interior of the knee joint seen from the front — the cruciate ligaments.*

to the medial femoral condyle. The anterior meniscofemoral ligament lies in front of the posterior cruciate ligament and the posterior ligament behind.

The synovial membrane of the joint is extensive. The suprapatellar bursa, an extension of the synovial cavity, extends upwards under the quadriceps. The infrapatellar fold of synovial membrane extending from that covering the infrapatellar pad of fat is attached to the intercondylar area of the femur.

A number of bursae are associated with the knee joint besides the suprapatellar bursa. There are two subcutaneous bursae anteriorly, subcutaneous

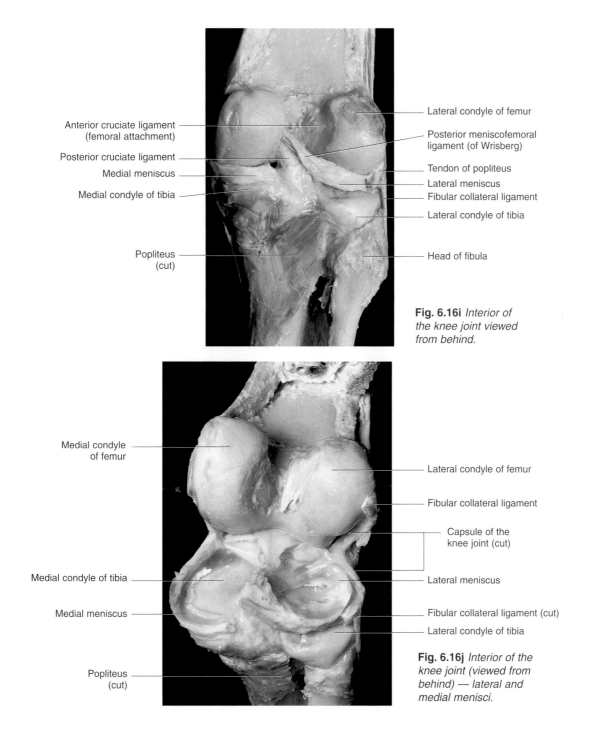

Anterior cruciate ligament (femoral attachment)

Posterior cruciate ligament

Medial meniscus

Medial condyle of tibia

Popliteus (cut)

Lateral condyle of femur

Posterior meniscofemoral ligament (of Wrisberg)

Tendon of popliteus

Lateral meniscus

Fibular collateral ligament

Lateral condyle of tibia

Head of fibula

Fig. 6.16i *Interior of the knee joint viewed from behind.*

Medial condyle of femur

Medial condyle of tibia

Medial meniscus

Popliteus (cut)

Lateral condyle of femur

Fibular collateral ligament

Capsule of the knee joint (cut)

Lateral meniscus

Fibular collateral ligament (cut)

Lateral condyle of tibia

Fig. 6.16j *Interior of the knee joint (viewed from behind) — lateral and medial menisci.*

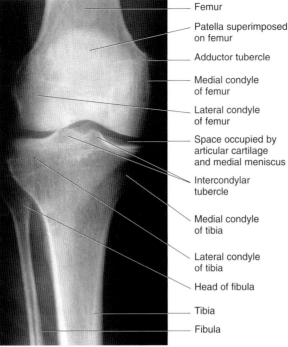

- Femur
- Patella superimposed on femur
- Adductor tubercle
- Medial condyle of femur
- Lateral condyle of femur
- Space occupied by articular cartilage and medial meniscus
- Intercondylar tubercle
- Medial condyle of tibia
- Lateral condyle of tibia
- Head of fibula
- Tibia
- Fibula

Fig. 6.16k *Anteroposterior radiograph of the knee joint.*

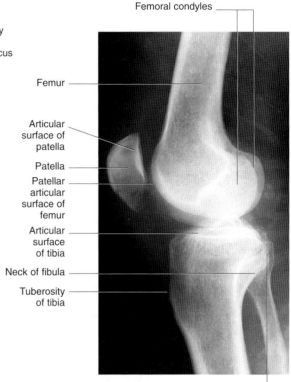

- Femoral condyles
- Femur
- Articular surface of patella
- Patella
- Patellar articular surface of femur
- Articular surface of tibia
- Neck of fibula
- Tuberosity of tibia
- Head of fibula

Fig. 6.16l *Lateral radiograph of the knee joint.*

infrapatellar bursa and the prepatellar bursa, in front of the tibial tubercle and the patella respectively. The deep infrapatellar bursa lies deep to the patellar ligament. Laterally there is a bursa between the fibular collateral ligament and the biceps femoris and another one deep to the fibular collateral ligament. Medially there is a bursa between the sartorius and the gracilis tendons and the tibial collateral ligament. The semimembranosus bursa is between that muscle and the medial head of gastrocnemius and may communicate with the joint cavity via a bursa which is deep to the gastrocnemius. Similarly the bursa under the popliteus also communicates with the joint cavity.

The popliteus which has a tendinous origin from the lateral condyle of the femur inside the joint is inserted to the upper part of the posterior surface of the tibia.

Movements

Flexion and extension are the main movements of the knee joint. When the knee is fully extended the posterior part of the capsule and all the ligaments except the posterior cruciate ligament are taut converting the leg and thigh into a rigid column—the knee is 'locked'. Flexion and extension of the tibia is

accompanied by rotation; medial rotation of the femur during extension and lateral rotation during flexion. During flexion the popliteus will rotate the femur laterally loosening the ligaments to 'unlock' the joint. Medial and lateral rotation can take place independently of flexion and extension in a flexed joint. The sartorius, the semitendinosus, the gracilis and the semimembranosus rotate the tibia medially and the biceps rotate it laterally.

The patella moves upwards during extension with a tendency for lateral displacement because of the pull of the quadriceps upwards and laterally parallel to the obliquity of the femur. Lateral dislocation of the patella is prevented by the prominence of the lateral condyle of the femur and by the horizontal fibres of the vastus medialis, which are inserted to the medial surface of the patella.

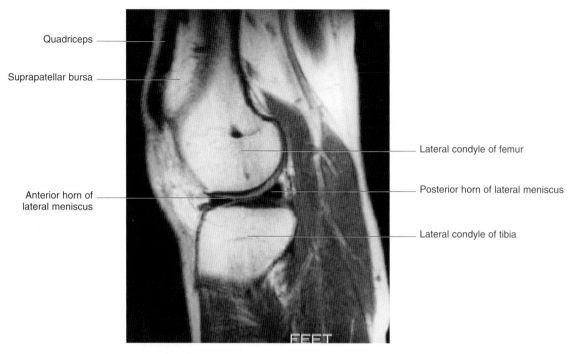

Quadriceps

Suprapatellar bursa

Anterior horn of
lateral meniscus

Lateral condyle of femur

Posterior horn of lateral meniscus

Lateral condyle of tibia

Fig. 6.16m *Sagittal MRI through the lateral part of right knee joint.*

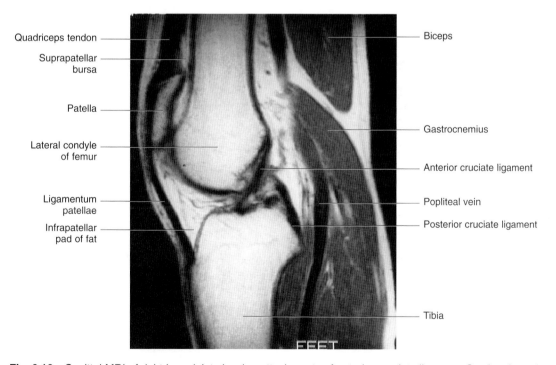

Quadriceps tendon

Suprapatellar
bursa

Patella

Lateral condyle
of femur

Ligamentum
patellae

Infrapatellar
pad of fat

Biceps

Gastrocnemius

Anterior cruciate ligament

Popliteal vein

Posterior cruciate ligament

Tibia

Fig. 6.16n *Sagittal MRI of right knee joint showing attachments of anterior cruciate ligament. Section through medial aspect of lateral femoral condyle.*

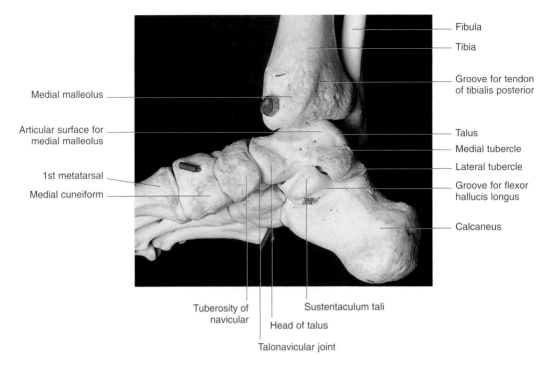

Fibula

Tibia

Groove for tendon of tibialis posterior

Medial malleolus

Articular surface for medial malleolus

Talus

Medial tubercle

Lateral tubercle

1st metatarsal

Medial cuneiform

Groove for flexor hallucis longus

Calcaneus

Tuberosity of navicular

Sustentaculum tali

Head of talus

Talonavicular joint

Fig. 6.17a *Tibia, fibula and the bones of the foot seen from the medial aspect.*

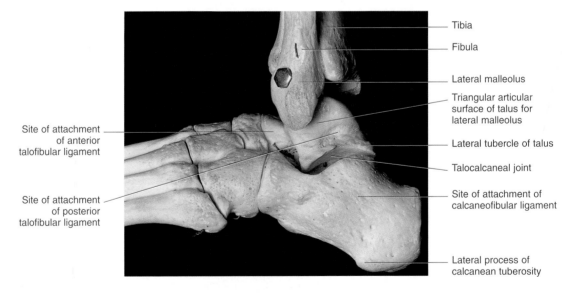

Tibia

Fibula

Lateral malleolus

Triangular articular surface of talus for lateral malleolus

Site of attachment of anterior talofibular ligament

Lateral tubercle of talus

Talocalcaneal joint

Site of attachment of posterior talofibular ligament

Site of attachment of calcaneofibular ligament

Lateral process of calcanean tuberosity

Fig. 6.17b *Tibia, fibula and bones of the foot seen from the lateral aspect.*

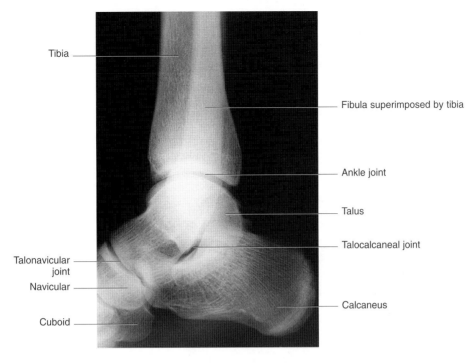

Tibia

Fibula superimposed by tibia

Ankle joint

Talus

Talocalcaneal joint

Talonavicular joint

Navicular

Cuboid

Calcaneus

Fig. 6.17c *Radiograph. Lateral view of the ankle joint.*

ANKLE JOINT (Fig. 6.17)

The tibia and fibula are connected to each other by the superior and the inferior tibiofibular joints as well as by the interosseous membrane.

The synovial joint between the lower ends of the tibia and fibula and the talus is the ankle joint. Plantar flexion and dorsiflexion of the foot are the main movements in this joint. The deep socket formed by the tibia and fibula with the medial and lateral malleoli gripping the sides of the talus along with the ligaments and the muscles crossing the joint stabilise the ankle joint.

Osteology

The medial surface of the lateral malleolus articulates with the lateral surface of the talus, the inferior surface of tibia with the superior articular surface (trochlear surface) of the talus and the lateral surface of the medial malleolus with the medial surface of the talus. The joint is most stable in dorsiflexion when the broad end of the trochlear surface fills the tibiofibular mortise.

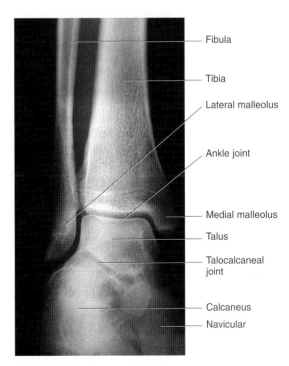

Fibula

Tibia

Lateral malleolus

Ankle joint

Medial malleolus

Talus

Talocalcaneal joint

Calcaneus

Navicular

Fig. 6.17d *Radiograph. Oblique — anteroposterior view of ankle.*

Capsule and ligaments

The fibrous capsule is thin in front and behind but is reinforced on either side by ligaments.

The deltoid ligament is a strong ligament on the medial aspect of the joint. Its narrow proximal part is attached to the medial malleolus, whereas distally it fans out to be attached to the calcaneus, talus and navicular.

On the lateral aspect there are three ligaments. The anterior talofibular ligament is a weak band connecting the lateral malleolus to the neck of the talus. The thick and horizontal posterior talofiblular ligament extends from the malleolar fossa to the lateral tubercle of the talus and the cord-like calcaneofibular ligament from the lateral malleolus extends from the tip of the malleolus to the lateral surface of the calcaneus.

Movements

Dorsiflexion and plantar flexion are the main movements. In the upright position with the foot at right angles to the leg the plantar flexion is about 20° and dorsiflexion about 10°. The range of passive movements is markedly more than these. The axis of movements is not horizontal but one which slopes from

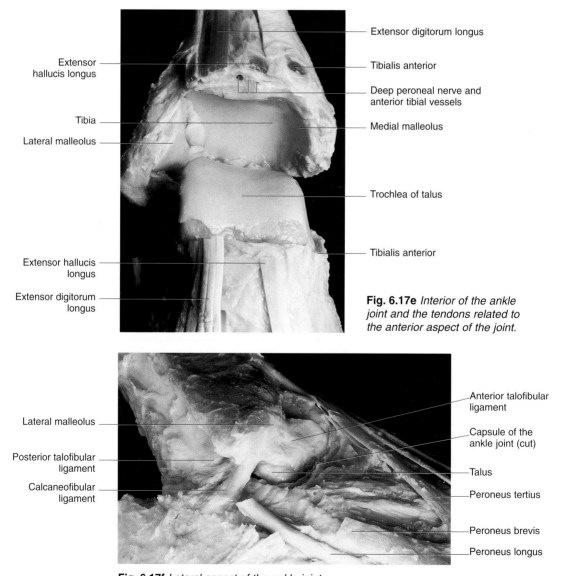

Fig. 6.17e *Interior of the ankle joint and the tendons related to the anterior aspect of the joint.*

Labels, Fig. 6.17e:
- Extensor hallucis longus
- Tibia
- Lateral malleolus
- Extensor hallucis longus
- Extensor digitorum longus
- Extensor digitorum longus
- Tibialis anterior
- Deep peroneal nerve and anterior tibial vessels
- Medial malleolus
- Trochlea of talus
- Tibialis anterior

Labels, Fig. 6.17f:
- Lateral malleolus
- Posterior talofibular ligament
- Calcaneofibular ligament
- Anterior talofibular ligament
- Capsule of the ankle joint (cut)
- Talus
- Peroneus tertius
- Peroneus brevis
- Peroneus longus

Fig. 6.17f *Lateral aspect of the ankle joint.*

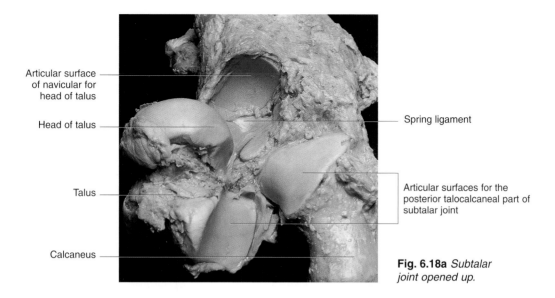

Articular surface of navicular for head of talus

Head of talus

Talus

Calcaneus

Spring ligament

Articular surfaces for the posterior talocalcaneal part of subtalar joint

Fig. 6.18a *Subtalar joint opened up.*

the lateral malleolus downwards and medially towards the medial malleolus contributing to slight eversion of the foot during dorsiflexion and inversion during plantar flexion.

Sprains and fractures

A sprained ankle is a common injury caused by an inversion twist of the foot. The weak anterior talofibular and or the calcaneofibular ligament is affected. Potts fracture, a much more serious injury, is caused by an eversion twist in which the strong deltoid ligament is torn often breaking the medial malleolus. The talus get displaced laterally fracturing the lateral malleolus or the lower end of the fibula. The posterior margin of the tibia may be sheared off by the talus as a result of the tibia getting displaced anteriorly.

JOINTS OF THE FOOT (Fig. 6.18)

Subtalar joint

There are two joints under the talus. Posteriorly the upper surface of the calcaneus articulates with the talus and anteriorly the head of the talus articulates with the the sustentaculum tali of calacaneus, the navicular and the intervening spring ligament. The subtalar joint and the midtarsal joint are involved in inversion and eversion of the foot. The anterior surface of the head of the talus articulating with the navicular bone along with the joint between the calcaneus and the cuboid (calcaneocuboid joint), form the midtarsal joint. The medial component of the midtarsal joint (the

talonavicular part) shares the same synovial cavity with the subtalar joint.

Inversion and eversion, which are twisting movements of the foot, enable one to walk on uneven

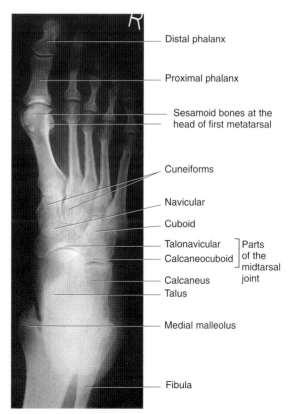

Distal phalanx

Proximal phalanx

Sesamoid bones at the head of first metatarsal

Cuneiforms

Navicular

Cuboid

Talonavicular ⎤ Parts
Calcaneocuboid ⎦ of the
                  midtarsal
Calcaneus   joint
Talus

Medial malleolus

Fibula

Fig. 6.18b *Radiograph of the foot. Dorsiplantar view. Parts of the midtarsal joint.*

ground. In eversion, the lateral border of the foot is slightly raised, making the sole of the foot face laterally. Inversion is the opposite movement, where the sole of the foot faces medially. The tibialis anterior and the tibialis posterior invert the foot. The peroneus longus and brevis are the main evertors. As the muscles involved are attached beyond the midtarsal joint, in the early part of inversion and eversion the midtarsal joint also moves. In inversion the midtarsal joint adducts and in eversion it abducts. When the foot is on the ground, adduction of the forefoot is masked by lateral rotation of the leg. Similarly, eversion of a fixed foot is accompanied by medial rotation of the leg.

The foot is one of the most dynamic parts of the body. It provides physical contact with the ground and supports the body weight. Yet the foot is flexible and resilient enabling it to absorb shocks transmitted to it. The foot also provides the spring and lift during walking, running and jumping. All these functions are achieved by the segmented but arched configuration of the foot. For descriptive purposes the arches of the foot are divided into the medial and lateral longitudinal arches and the transverse arch. Each arch consists of a number of bones and joints and is supported by muscles and ligaments. The arches are maintained by the shapes of the bones, the ligaments connecting them, the plantar aponeurosis as well as the muscles of the foot. The tendon of the flexor hallucis longus is the most important muscular structure supporting the medial longitudinal arch.

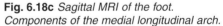

Tibia
Fibula

Talus
Calcaneus

Navicular
Medial cuneiform

1st metatarsal

Plantar muscles
Skin

Fig. 6.18c *Sagittal MRI of the foot. Components of the medial longitudinal arch.*

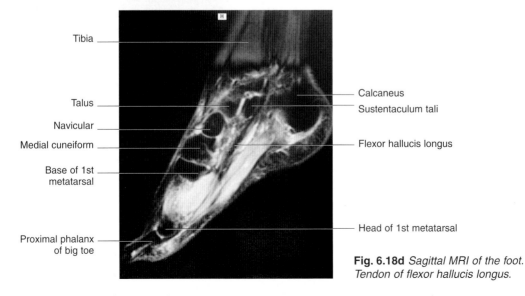

Tibia

Calcaneus
Sustentaculum tali

Talus

Navicular

Flexor hallucis longus

Medial cuneiform

Base of 1st metatarsal

Proximal phalanx of big toe

Head of 1st metatarsal

Fig. 6.18d *Sagittal MRI of the foot. Tendon of flexor hallucis longus.*

BLOOD SUPPLY OF THE LOWER LIMB
(Fig. 6.19)

Arterial supply of the lower limb

The femoral artery is the continuation of the external iliac artery beyond the midinguinal point. Its upper part is in the femoral triangle and the lower part in the adductor canal. After the first inch (2.5 cm) a major branch is given off, the profunda femoris. The main stem of the artery is also known as the common femoral, the profunda femoris as the deep femoral and the continuation of the main artery beyond the

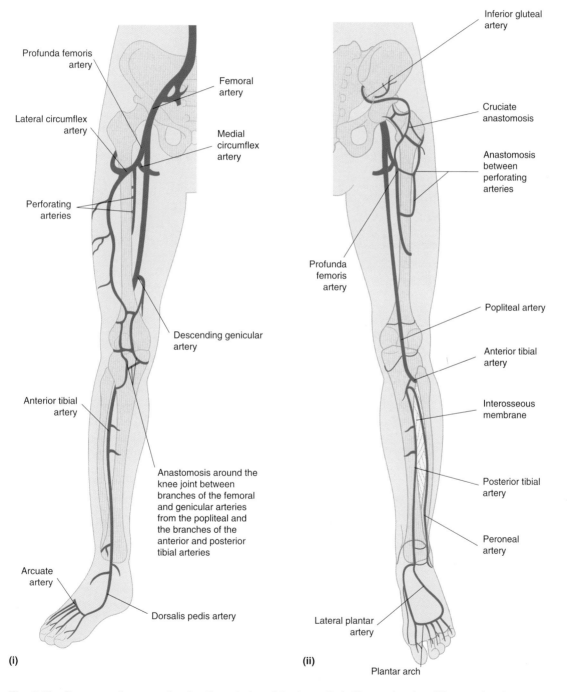

Fig. 6.19a *Summary diagrams showing the arteries of the lower limb:* **(i)** *anterior view;* **(ii)** *posterior view.*

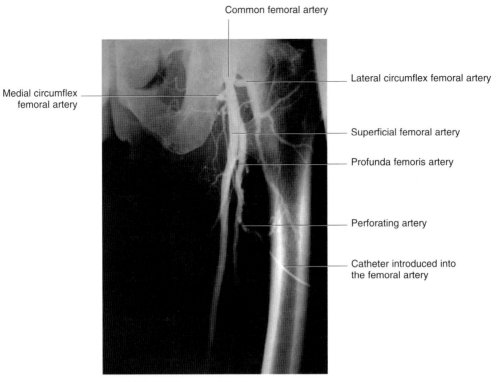

Common femoral artery

Lateral circumflex femoral artery

Medial circumflex femoral artery

Superficial femoral artery

Profunda femoris artery

Perforating artery

Catheter introduced into the femoral artery

Fig. 6.19b *Angiogram of the femoral artery.*

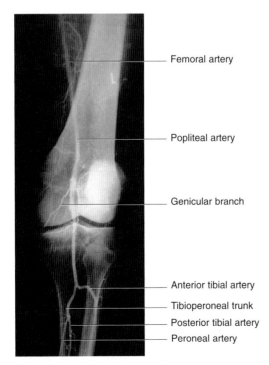

Femoral artery

Popliteal artery

Genicular branch

Anterior tibial artery

Tibioperoneal trunk

Posterior tibial artery

Peroneal artery

Fig. 6.19c *Popliteal artery and branches — angiogram.*

profunda the superficial femoral — the terms mostly used by radiologists and vascular surgeons. The pulsation of common femoral is easily palpable at the midinguinal point which is the midpoint of a line connecting the anterior superior iliac spine to the pubic symphysis (the joint between the two pubic bones). The artery can be easily catheterised in this part for the purpose of angiography and angioplasty. It is also a convenient site for taking samples to estimate blood gases.

There is a network of anastomoses between the branches of the profunda and those of the anterior and posterior tibial arteries (see below). When the superficial femoral is blocked these anastomoses will open up and act as a collateral channel.

The popliteal artery whose pulsation is palpable in the popliteal fossa (see p. 165) is the continuation of the femoral artery beyond the adductor hiatus. At the lower border of the popliteus muscle it divides into anterior and posterior tibial arteries. The former enters the anterior compartment by passing over the upper border of the interosseous membrane. The latter continues in the posterior compartment of the leg as the tibioperoneal trunk for about 2 cm and bifurcates into posterior tibial and peroneal arteries.

The anterior tibial artery from the anterior compartment of the leg continues on to the foot as the dorsalis pedis artery from which the arcuate artery and the dorsal metatarsal arteries arise (also see p. 168).

The posterior tibial artery descends in the posterior compartment of the leg and enters the sole of the foot by passing deep to the flexor retinaculum. The peroneal artery, though small, is important as it is usually not affected by atherosclerosis especially in diabetics (also see p. 171, 172).

The veins of the lower limb

A superficial and deep groups of veins drain the lower limb, the long saphenous and the short saphenous being the major ones in the former group.

The long (great) saphenous vein
This, the longest vein in the body, starts in the medial aspect of the dorsum of the foot. It crosses the ankle in front of the medial malleolus, a constant relationship

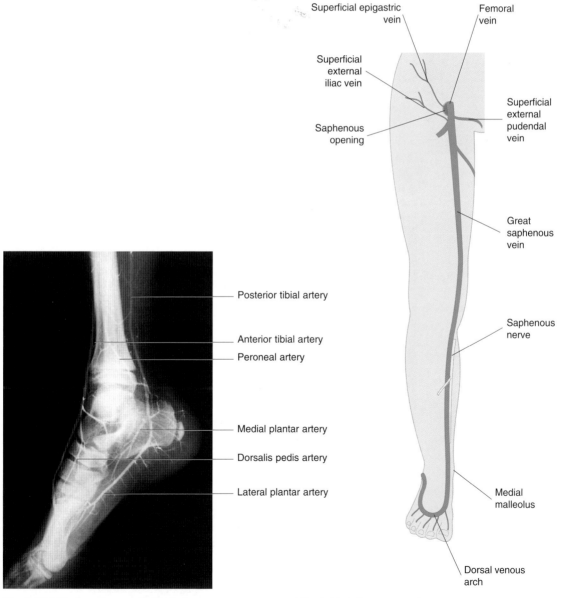

Fig. 6.19d *Foot angiogram. Lateral view.*

Fig. 6.19e *The great saphenous vein.*

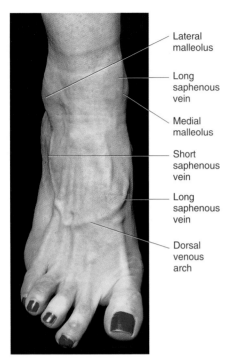

Fig. 6.19f *Surface anatomy of the veins on the dorsum of foot.*

- Lateral malleolus
- Long saphenous vein
- Medial malleolus
- Short saphenous vein
- Long saphenous vein
- Dorsal venous arch

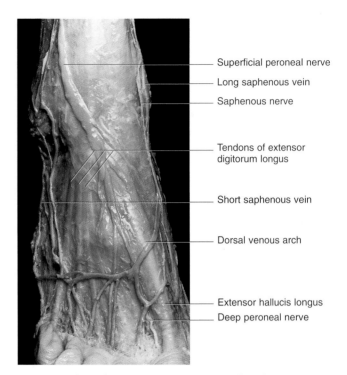

Fig. 6.19g *Superficial veins on the dorsum of the foot.*

- Superficial peroneal nerve
- Long saphenous vein
- Saphenous nerve
- Tendons of extensor digitorum longus
- Short saphenous vein
- Dorsal venous arch
- Extensor hallucis longus
- Deep peroneal nerve

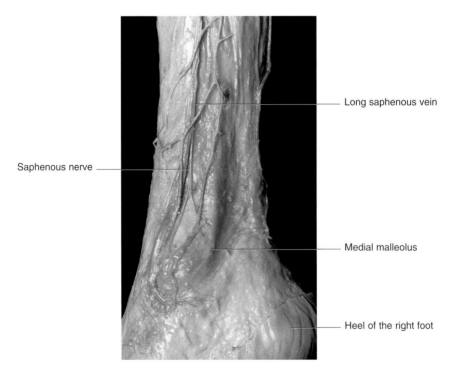

Fig. 6.19h *Long saphenous vein and the saphenous nerve in front of the medial malleolus.*

- Long saphenous vein
- Saphenous nerve
- Medial malleolus
- Heel of the right foot

which is useful in an emergency to do a cut-down for venous access. As it ascends it lies about a hand's breadth behind the medial border of the patella. About 3.5 cm below and lateral to the pubic tubercle, the vein goes through an opening in the deep fascia, the saphenous opening, to join the femoral vein. The vein is closely related to the saphenous nerve below the knee. Damage to the nerve while stripping the vein may cause numbness or paraesthesia along the medial border of leg and foot. In the treatment of varicose veins the long saphenous vein is usually stripped above the knee to avoid damage to the saphenous nerve (also see p. 154).

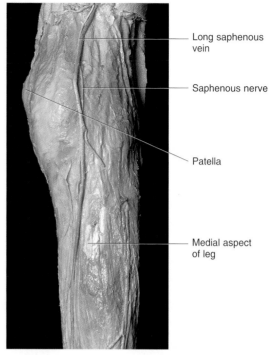

Long saphenous vein

Saphenous nerve

Patella

Medial aspect of leg

Fig. 6.19i *Medial aspect of leg and knee joint. Long saphenous vein and saphenous nerve behind the patella.*

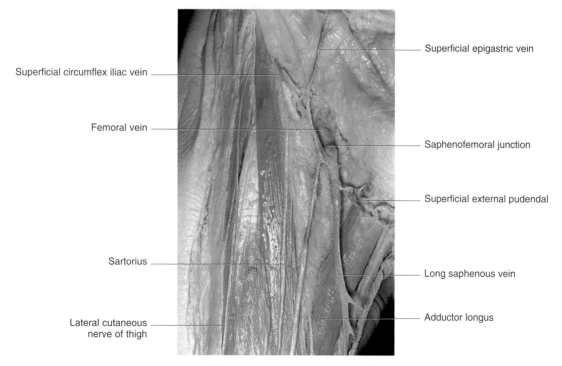

Superficial circumflex iliac vein

Femoral vein

Sartorius

Lateral cutaneous nerve of thigh

Superficial epigastric vein

Saphenofemoral junction

Superficial external pudendal

Long saphenous vein

Adductor longus

Fig. 6.19j *Long saphenous vein and the saphenofemoral junction.*

The short saphenous vein

Commencing from the lateral aspect of the dorsal venous arch the short saphenous vein ascends behind the lateral malleolus accompanied by the sural nerve. The nerve damage which may occur during stripping of the vein causes numbness or paraesthesia along the lateral border of the foot. The small saphenous vein perforates the deep fascia at a variable point between the middle of the calf and the roof of the popliteal fossa and usually ends in the popliteal vein.

Deep veins

These are named after the arteries they accompany and are present as venae comitantes in the lower part of the leg. Higher up the popliteal and femoral veins accompany the relevant arteries. The femoral vein continues into the pelvis as the external iliac vein.

Perforating veins

These connect the superficial veins to the deep veins and are seen at different levels. There is a valve close to where the perforating vein perforates the deep fascia. Common sites for the perforators are in the lower half of the medial aspect of calf, one just below the middle of the calf and another in the lower thigh. The lower perforators are joined by a longitudinal trunk, the posterior arch vein which usually joins the long saphenous vein below the knee. Blood flows from the

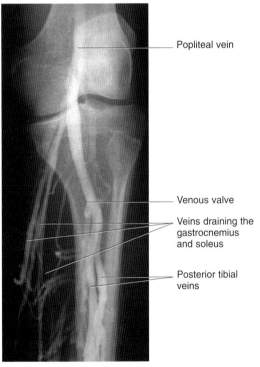

— Popliteal vein

— Venous valve

— Veins draining the gastrocnemius and soleus

— Posterior tibial veins

Fig. 6.19k *Deep veins of the leg — venogram.*

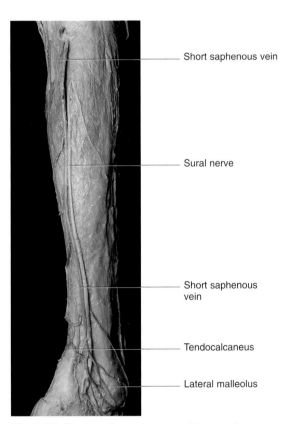

— Short saphenous vein

— Sural nerve

— Short saphenous vein

— Tendocalcaneus

— Lateral malleolus

Fig. 6.19l *Short saphenous vein and the sural nerve at the back of the leg.*

superficial to the deep veins through the perforating veins. Flow in the opposite direction is prevented by the valves, the incompetence of which causes varicose veins and venous ulcers.

SEGMENTAL AND CUTANEOUS INNERVATION (Fig. 6.20)

The dermatomes of the lower limb lie in a numerical sequence downwards at the front of the limb and upwards on its posterior aspect. The myotomes are: at the hip — L2,L3 flexors, L4,L5 extensors; knee — L3,L4, extensors, L5,S1 flexors; ankle — L4,L5 dorsiflexors, S1,S2 plantar flexors. Hence the segments tested by the knee jerk are L3,L4 and the ankle jerk S1,S2.

Cutaneous nerves

The ilioinguinal nerve (L1) emerges through the superficial inguinal ring to supply the root of the penis, anterior third of the scrotum and vulva, and an adjoining small area in the upper part of the thigh.

The genitofemoral nerve (L1,L2) divides into a genital and a femoral branch, the latter containing L1

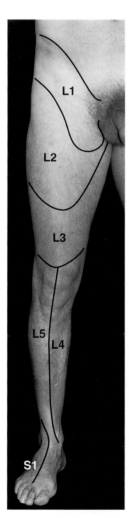

Fig. 6.20a *Dermatomes of the lower limb — anterior aspect.*

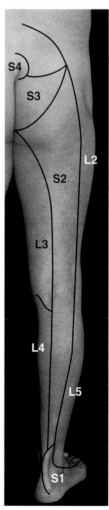

Fig. 6.20b *Dermatomes of the lower limb — posterior aspect.*

fibres enters the thigh accompanying the femoral artery and pierces the femoral sheath (see below) to supply the skin overlying the femoral triangle

The medial and intermediate femoral cutaneous nerves (L2,L3) are cutaneous branches of the femoral nerve, and they supply the medial and the anterior aspects of the thigh respectively. The saphenous nerve is the only branch of the femoral nerve to supply the leg and foot. It gives a cutaneous innervation to the medial surface of the leg and the medial border of the foot. In the leg it is closely related to the great saphenous vein and it can be rolled under the fingers

where it lies over the medial condyle of the tibia about a hand's breadth behind the medial border of the patella.

The lateral femoral cutaneous nerve (L2,L3) pierces the inguinal ligament a centimetre medial to the anterior superior iliac spine to supply the lateral aspect of the thigh. Compression of the lateral cutaneous nerve of the thigh at the point where it pierces the inguinal ligament or more proximally as it traverses the iliac fascia causes pain and a tingling sensation along the lateral aspect of the thigh, a condition known as meralgia paraesthetica.

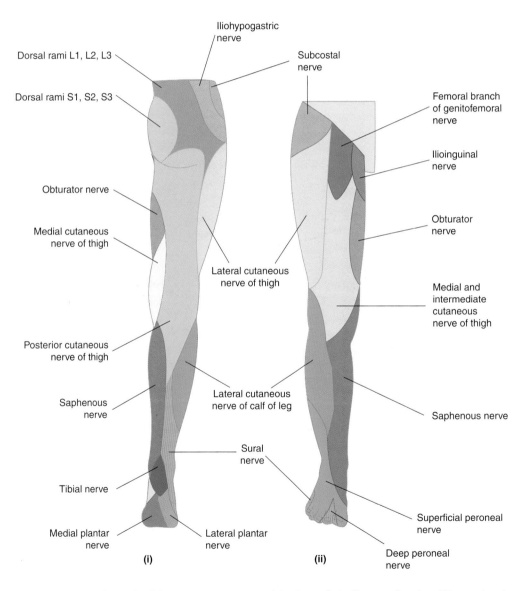

Fig. 6.20c *The territories of supply of the cutaneous nerves of the lower limb:* **(i)** *posterior view;* **(ii)** *anterior view.*

HEAD AND NECK

A thorough knowledge of anatomy is required to diagnose and treat a number of clinical conditions affecting the neck. The sternocleidomastoid muscle divides the neck into two large triangles, the anterior triangle between sternocleidomastoid and the midline and the posterior triangle between it and the trapezius.

THE FRONT OF THE NECK (Fig. 7.1)

The front of the neck, or the anterior triangle, has the thyroid gland, the carotid sheath and the infrahyoid muscles.

Surface anatomy

In the midline, from above downwards, the mandible, the hyoid bone, the thyroid cartilage, the cricoid cartilage, the tracheal rings and the suprasternal notch can be felt. The movement of the thyroid cartilage up and down with swallowing is easily visible. The two sternocleidomastoid muscles can be seen and felt by

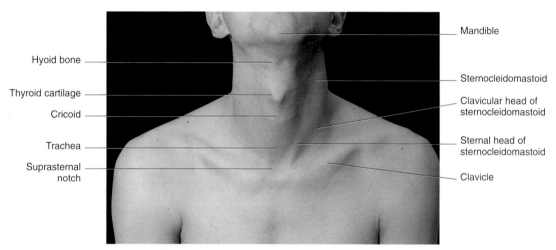

Hyoid bone —
Thyroid cartilage —
Cricoid —
Trachea —
Suprasternal notch —

— Mandible
— Sternocleidomastoid
— Clavicular head of sternocleidomastoid
— Sternal head of sternocleidomastoid
— Clavicle

Fig. 7.1a *Surface anatomy of the front of the neck.*

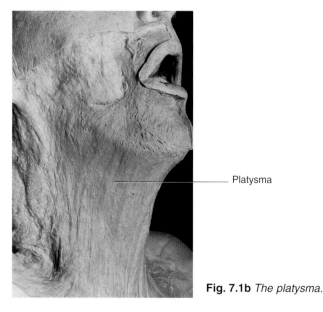

— Platysma

Fig. 7.1b *The platysma.*

turning the head against resistance to the opposite side. In the middle of the neck, at the anterior border of the sternocleidomastoid, the pulsation of the common carotid artery is palpable. The internal jugular vein lies lateral to the artery with the vagus nerve between the two vessels.

The lower border of the cricoid which is at the level of the sixth cervical vertebra is an important level in the neck and it corresponds to:

- the junction of the larynx with the trachea
- the junction of the pharynx with the oesophagus
- the site at which the carotid artery can be compressed against the carotid tubercle of the transverse process of the C6 vertebra.

SUPERFICIAL STRUCTURES

The superficial fascia contains the platysma, a striated muscle, which extends from the region of the clavicle, pectoralis major, and the deltoid to the mandible above.

To prevent retraction of the severed muscle contributing to a broad scar platysma is sutured with the skin when neck wounds are sutured. The muscle has good vascularity. Hence when skin flaps are raised platysma is included to maintain a good blood supply. The platysma is supplied by the cervical branch of the facial nerve.

INFRAHYOID MUSCLES

The sternohyoid, sternothyroid and thyrohyoid connect the sternum, hyoid bone and thyroid cartilage. The omohyoid extends between the hyoid and the scapula. These are known as the infrahyoid muscles or the strap muscles. They are supplied by the ansa cervicalis (C1,C2,C3) which is a nerve loop on the internal jugular vein. The branches to the muscles enter in their lower half. During exposure of a large goitre the strap muscles are cut in their upper half to preserve the nerve supply from the ansa cervicalis.

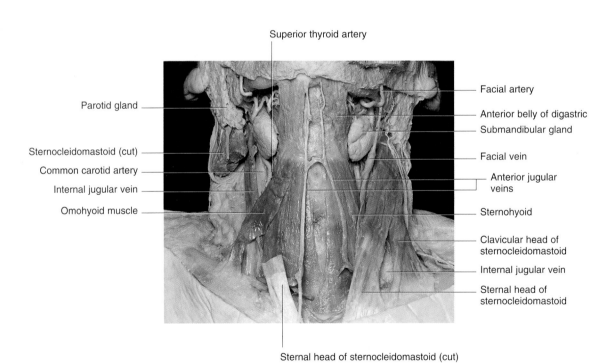

Fig. 7.1c *Superficial dissection of the anterior aspect of the neck.*

Fig. 7.1d (i) *Structures deep to the sternocleidomastoid on the left side. Left clavicle and sternocleidomastoid have been removed.* **(ii)** *Carotid arteries and internal jugular vein*

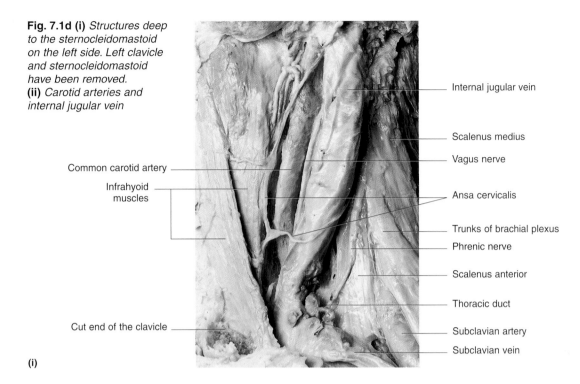

Internal jugular vein

Scalenus medius

Vagus nerve

Common carotid artery

Infrahyoid muscles

Ansa cervicalis

Trunks of brachial plexus

Phrenic nerve

Scalenus anterior

Thoracic duct

Cut end of the clavicle

Subclavian artery

Subclavian vein

(i)

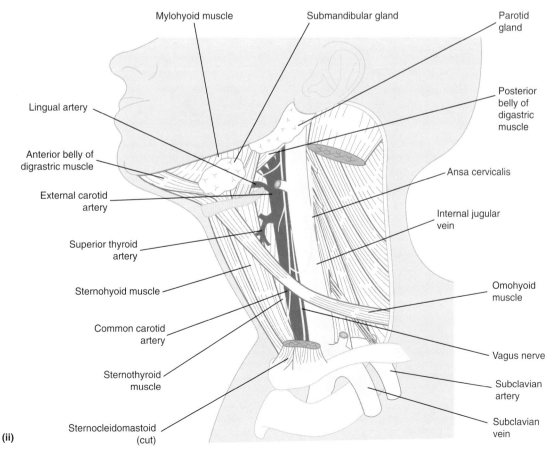

Mylohyoid muscle

Submandibular gland

Parotid gland

Lingual artery

Posterior belly of digastric muscle

Anterior belly of digastric muscle

Ansa cervicalis

External carotid artery

Internal jugular vein

Superior thyroid artery

Sternohyoid muscle

Omohyoid muscle

Common carotid artery

Sternothyroid muscle

Vagus nerve

Subclavian artery

Sternocleidomastoid (cut)

Subclavian vein

(ii)

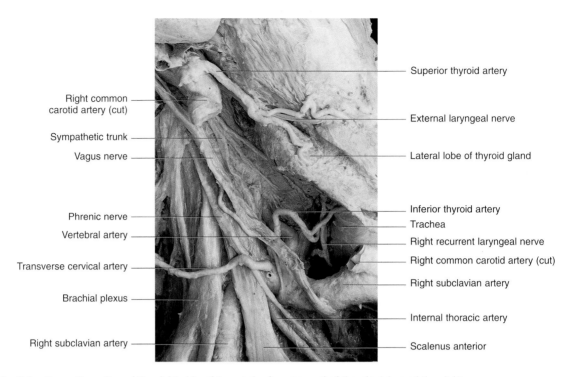

Right common carotid artery (cut)

Sympathetic trunk

Vagus nerve

Phrenic nerve

Vertebral artery

Transverse cervical artery

Brachial plexus

Right subclavian artery

Superior thyroid artery

External laryngeal nerve

Lateral lobe of thyroid gland

Inferior thyroid artery

Trachea

Right recurrent laryngeal nerve

Right common carotid artery (cut)

Right subclavian artery

Internal thoracic artery

Scalenus anterior

Fig. 7.1e *Deep dissection of the right side of the neck after removal of the clavicle and the right sternocleidomastoid showing branches of the subclavian artery and the structures related to the scalenus anterior.*

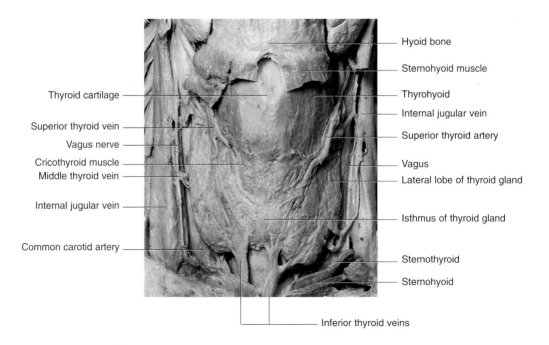

Thyroid cartilage

Superior thyroid vein

Vagus nerve

Cricothyroid muscle

Middle thyroid vein

Internal jugular vein

Common carotid artery

Hyoid bone

Sternohyoid muscle

Thyrohyoid

Internal jugular vein

Superior thyroid artery

Vagus

Lateral lobe of thyroid gland

Isthmus of thyroid gland

Sternothyroid

Sternohyoid

Inferior thyroid veins

Fig. 7.1f *Anterior view of the thyroid gland and its blood supply seen after removal of the sternocleidomastoid and the infrahyoid muscles.*

The common carotid artery

The right common carotid artery is a branch of the brachiocephalic trunk and the left is a direct branch from the arch of the aorta. At the upper border of the thyroid cartilage the common carotid artery divides into the external and the internal carotid arteries. The bifurcation can be at a higher level: a surgeon ligating the external carotid should be aware of this to avoid an inadvertent ligation of the common carotid. The common carotid and the internal carotid arteries are enclosed by the carotid sheath in which the internal jugular vein lies lateral to the arteries, with the vagus nerve in between the vein and the artery.

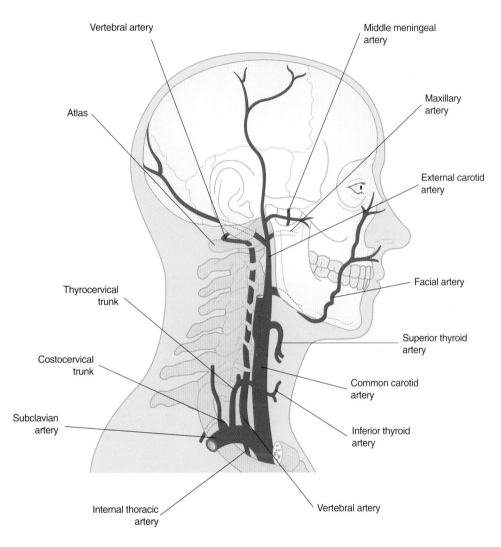

Fig. 7.1g *The subclavian and the carotid arteries.*

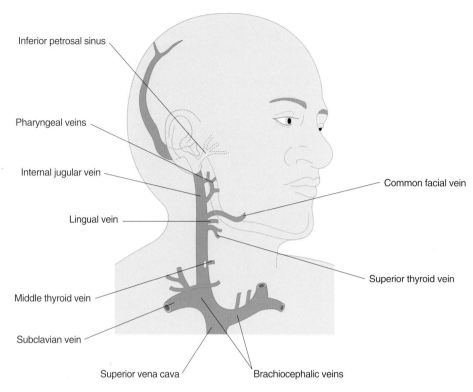

Inferior petrosal sinus

Pharyngeal veins

Internal jugular vein

Lingual vein

Common facial vein

Superior thyroid vein

Middle thyroid vein

Subclavian vein

Superior vena cava

Brachiocephalic veins

Fig. 7.1h *The internal jugular vein and its tributaries.*

The internal jugular vein (Fig. 7.1d, f, h)

This is the major vein in the neck draining the pharyngeal veins, the facial vein and the thyroid veins. It starts at the base of the skull as a continuation of the sigmoid venous sinus and terminates behind the sternoclavicular joint by joining the subclavian vein to form the brachiocephalic vein. Its tributaries are shown in Fig. 7.1h.

 Internal jugular vein cannulation is carried out at the middle of the anterior border of the sternocleidomastoid, immediately lateral to the carotid pulse or in a lower approach near the apex of the triangular gap between the sternal and the clavicular heads of the sternocleidomastoid (Fig. 7.1c).

The thyroid gland (Fig. 7.1f)

The thyroid gland has two lateral lobes connected by a midline isthmus. The gland is firmly bound to the larynx and trachea by the pre-tracheal fascia and hence moves with them during swallowing. The isthmus lies in front of the second, third and fourth tracheal rings. A pyramidal lobe, a remnant of the

thyroglossal duct, is sometimes seen as a midline extension of the isthmus upwards over the thyroid cartilage. The parathyroid glands are embedded in the posterior surface of the lateral lobes. The thyroid gland is covered anteriorly by the infrahyoid muscles.

The thyroid gland has a rich blood supply. The superior thyroid artery, a branch of the external carotid, enters the upper pole of the gland. The inferior thyroid artery (Fig. 7.1e, g), a branch of the thyro-cervical trunk of the subclavian, enters the middle of the posterior aspect. The inferior thyroid artery also supplies the parathyroid glands. Bilateral ligature of the inferior thyroid artery in thyroid surgery can cause ischaemia of the parathyroids. The venous drainage is extensive and variable. The superior thyroid vein accompanies the artery and drains into the internal jugular vein. The inferior thyroid veins are many and they drain into the subclavian or brachiocephalic veins. The middle thyroid veins are variable in number and may drain into the superior and inferior veins or by a short trunk into the internal jugular vein. Because the vein is short its careless handling may tear the internal jugular vein causing serious haemorrhage during thyroid surgery. The recurrent laryngeal nerve crosses the inferior thyroid artery very close to the thyroid gland. The nerve is usually deep to the artery but may be superficial to it or pass through its branches. It lies in the groove between the trachea and the oesophagus before reaching the inferior pole of the thyroid gland. The recurrent laryngeal nerves supply the muscles of the larynx. A malignant tumour of the thyroid gland may compress the recurrent laryngeal nerve affecting the movements of the vocal cords resulting in a change in the voice. The nerve is also prone to damage in thyroid surgery because of its close relation to the inferior thyroid artery. The external laryngeal branch of the superior laryngeal nerve is related to the superior thyroid vascular pedicle. Damage to the nerve paralyses the cricothyroid muscle causing a voice change.

The trachea lies in front of the oesophagus in the midline. Tracheostomy is an operation done to keep the airway patent. In this, a hole is made in the trachea at the level of the second or third tracheal ring and a tracheostomy tube is introduced. In a dire emergency an opening can be made through the cricothyroid ligament in the midline to maintain the airway.

At the lower part of the neck (root of the neck) the scalenus anterior muscle lies in between the subclavian artery and subclavian vein (Fig. 7.1d(i), f). The phrenic nerve lies on the scalenus anterior. As the right vagus crosses the subclavian artery to enter the thorax it gives off the right recurrent laryngeal nerve which winds round the artery to reach the groove between the trachea and the oesophagus. On the left side the thoracic duct arches laterally lying between the carotid sheath and the vertebral artery and enters the junction between the internal jugular and the subclavian veins. Inadvertant puncture or laceration of the thoracic duct will cause escape of lymph into the surrounding tissue and occasionally chylothorax.

The subclavian artery (Fig. 7.1d, e, g)

The right subclavian artery is a branch of the brachiocephalic trunk and the left arises directly from the arch of the aorta. It lies posterior to the insertion of the scalenus anterior on the first rib. The subclavian vein runs parallel to the artery but in front of the scalenus anterior slightly at a lower level. The roots and the trunks of the brachial plexus lie behind the subclavian artery on the first rib between the scalenus anterior and the scalenus medius muscles. The artery beyond the first rib continues into the axilla as the axillary artery.

The subclavian artery pulsations can be felt at the medial third of the clavicle near the lateral border of the SCM on deep palpatation against the first rib.

The branches of the subclavian artery are the vertebral artery, the internal mammary (thoracic) artery, the thyrocervical trunk and the costocervical trunk.

The vertebral artery is the first branch of the subclavian artery. It enters the foramen transversarium at the sixth cervical vertebra and ascends through the foramina transversaria of the sixth to the first cervical vertebrae and enters the cranial cavity and branches to supply the brain and spinal cord. The internal thoracic (mammary) artery passes vertically downwards a finger's breadth lateral to the sternum. In the sixth intercostal space it divides into the musculophrenic artery and the superior epigastric artery. The thyrocervical trunk is a branch of the subclavian artery medial to the scalenus anterior. It divides into the inferior thyroid artery, the transverse cervical and the suprascapular arteries. The inferior thyroid artery lies behind the carotid sheath and ascends in front of the scalenus anterior. At the level of the transverse process of the sixth cervical vertebra the artery arches medially and enters the posteromedial aspect of the capsule of the thyroid gland at its lower third. The recurrent laryngeal nerve is closely related to the artery and its branches near the lower pole of the thyroid gland.

The subclavian vein (Fig. 7.1d, h)

The subclavian vein follows the course of the subclavian artery in the neck, but lies in front of the scalenus anerior on the first rib. Veins accompanying the branches of the subclavian artery drain into the external jugular, the subclavian vein or its continuation, the brachiocephalic vein (formed by the union of the subclavian and the internal jugular veins). Sub-clavian venopuncture can be carried out by inserting the needle below the clavicle at the junction of its middle and medial thirds and advanced upwards and medially behind the clavicle towards the sterno-clavicular joint. There is the risk of pneumothorax and an inadvertent puncture of the subclavian artery in this procedure as the vein lies on the apex of the lung in front of the artery.

POSTERIOR TRIANGLE (Fig. 7.2)

The posterior triangle or the side of the neck contains the accessory nerve, external jugular vein, the cervical

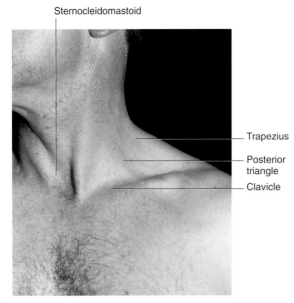

Fig. 7.2a *Surface anatomy of the posterior triangle.*

plexus and proximal parts of the brachial plexus of nerves supplying the upper limb.

Surface anatomy

The sternocleidomastoid and the trapezius muscles and the middle part of the clavicle form the boundaries of the posterior triangle. A line connecting the junction between the upper third and the lower two-thirds of the posterior border of the sternocleidomastoid to a point two fingers' breadths (5 cm) above the clavicle on the anterior border of the trapezius is the surface marking of the accessory nerve. The nerve can be identified as it enters the deep surface of the sternocleidomastoid about 4 cm below the mastoid. It is found just above Erb's point, where great auricular, transverse cervical and supraclavicular nerves (all branches of the cervical plexus) emerge from behind the sternocleidomastoid.

The external jugular vein drains the scalp and face. It lies in the superficial fascia, superficial to the sternomastoid, but in the lower part of the posterior triangle pierces the deep fascia and drains into the subclavian vein. The vein is prone to many variations and its size is inversely proportional to the size of other neck veins. The presence of a valve at its junction with the subclavian vein makes cannulation of the external jugular vein difficult. The vein is normally invisible but can be distended by straining or pressure at the root of

the neck. When the venous pressure rises as in heart failure the vein becomes prominent.

Sternocleidomastoid

Origin
By two heads from the manubrium of the sternum and the clavicle.
Insertion
The mastoid process and the superior nuchal line.
Nerve supply
The spinal accessory nerve.
Action
Turns the head to the opposite side.

The accessory nerve supplying the sternocleidomastoid and the trapezius can be easily damaged because of its superficial position in the posterior triangle. The trapezius muscle will be paralysed resulting in inability to lift the arm above the level of the shoulder.

Cervical plexus (Fig 7.2c, also see Fig. 7.3d)

Cutaneous branches of this plexus supply the skin of the neck, the shoulder and pectoral regions. They are: the great auricular nerve (C2,C3), the lesser occipital nerve (C2), the transverse cervical nerve (C2,C3) and the supraclavicular nerves (C3,C4).

The phrenic nerve (C3,C4,C5) supplying the diaphragm and the inferior root of the ansa cervicalis for the infrahyoid muscles are also branches of the cervical plexus.

THE FACE, THE FACIAL NERVE AND THE PAROTID GLAND (Fig. 7.3)

The superficial muscles of the face and the muscles of facial expression are attached to the skin. Contraction of the orbicularis oculi closes the eye. It has two parts: the palpebral part which arches across both the eyelids is used in blinking and the orbital part which circumscribes the orbital margin is used in shutting the eye more forcefully as in 'screwing up the eyes'. Orbicularis oculi facilitates drainage of the lacrimal secretion (tears). The blinking action enables the lacrimal fluid to spread medially towards the nose. A few fibres of the orbicularis oculi are attached to the lacrimal sac which dilates on contraction of the muscle thus sucking fluid into the sac. Elastic recoil of the sac empties the fluid into the nasal cavity through the nasolacrimal duct. The orbicularis oculi is supplied by

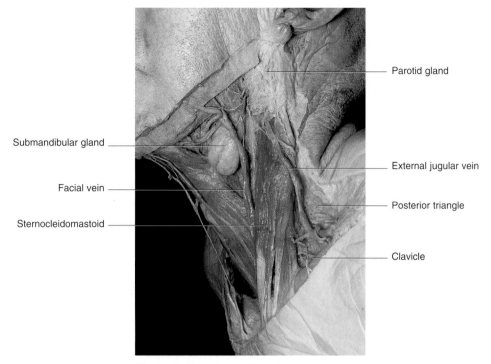

Parotid gland

Submandibular gland

External jugular vein

Facial vein

Posterior triangle

Sternocleidomastoid

Clavicle

Fig. 7.2b *External jugular vein.*

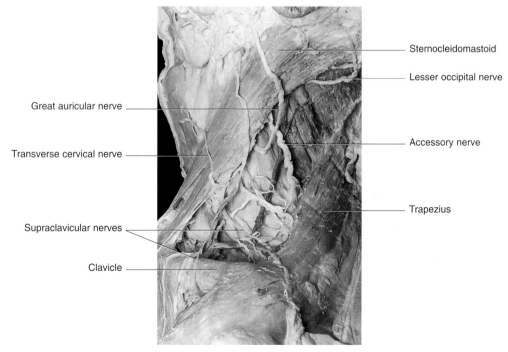

Sternocleidomastoid

Lesser occipital nerve

Great auricular nerve

Transverse cervical nerve

Accessory nerve

Trapezius

Supraclavicular nerves

Clavicle

Fig. 7.2c *Nerves of the posterior triangle (left side).*

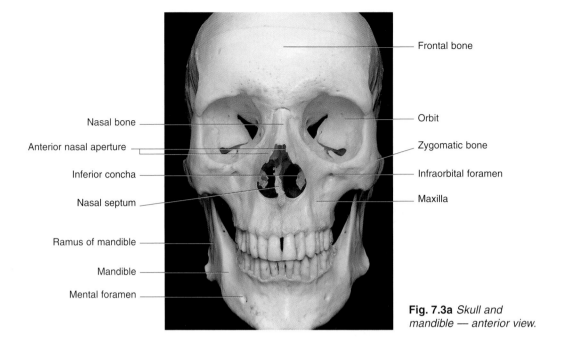

Fig. 7.3a *Skull and mandible — anterior view.*

- Frontal bone
- Orbit
- Zygomatic bone
- Infraorbital foramen
- Maxilla

- Nasal bone
- Anterior nasal aperture
- Inferior concha
- Nasal septum
- Ramus of mandible
- Mandible
- Mental foramen

the facial nerve. Paralysis of the orbicularis oculi, as may occur in facial nerve paralysis, will prevent the blinking action of the eyelid. This will fail to moisten the cornea and in turn lead to ulceration of the cornea.

The facial nerve (Fig. 7.3b, c)

The facial nerve (seventh cranial nerve) supplies the muscles of facial expression. It also conveys parasympathetic fibres to the lacrimal gland, glands in the nasal cavity, submandibular and sublingual glands

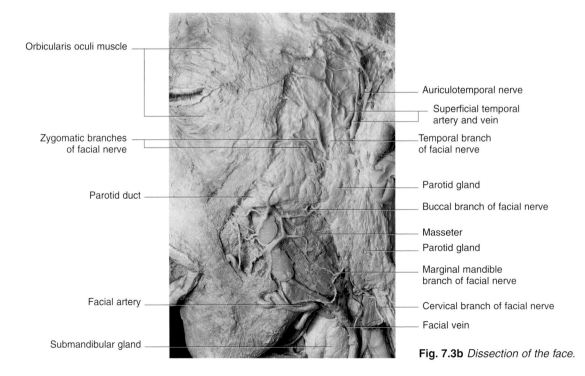

Fig. 7.3b *Dissection of the face.*

- Orbicularis oculi muscle
- Zygomatic branches of facial nerve
- Parotid duct
- Facial artery
- Submandibular gland

- Auriculotemporal nerve
- Superficial temporal artery and vein
- Temporal branch of facial nerve
- Parotid gland
- Buccal branch of facial nerve
- Masseter
- Parotid gland
- Marginal mandible branch of facial nerve
- Cervical branch of facial nerve
- Facial vein

and transmits taste fibres from the anterior two-thirds of the tongue.

The facial nerve originates from the pons and passes through the facial canal in the petrous temporal bone. It passes downwards on the posterior wall of the middle ear to emerge though the stylomastoid foramen at the base of the skull.

In the petrous temporal bone, the facial nerve gives off three branches:

- the greater petrossal nerve
- the nerve to stapedius
- the chorda tympani nerve.

The greater petrossal nerve transmits preganglionic parasympathetic fibres to the sphenopalatine ganglion, the postganglionic fibres from which supply the lacrimal gland and the glands in the nasal cavity. The chorda tympani nerve carries parasympathetic fibres to the submandibular and sublingual glands as well as taste fibres from the anterior two-thirds of the tongue.

After emerging from the stylomastoid foramen the nerve enters the parotid gland and divides into temporal, zygomatic, buccal, marginal mandibular and cervical branches. These supply the muscles of facial expression. Before entering the parotid gland the nerve supplies branches to the posterior belly of the digastric, stylohyoid and the muscles of the auricle.

The temporal branches of the facial nerve pass upwards to supply the frontalis muscle. The zygomatic branches cross the zygomatic arch and supply the orbicularis oculi. The buccal branches, passing anteriorly, supply the buccinator (buccinator is the

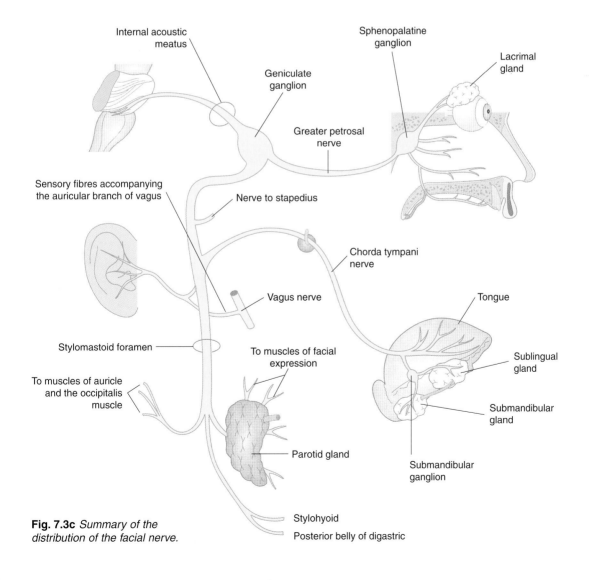

Fig. 7.3c *Summary of the distribution of the facial nerve.*

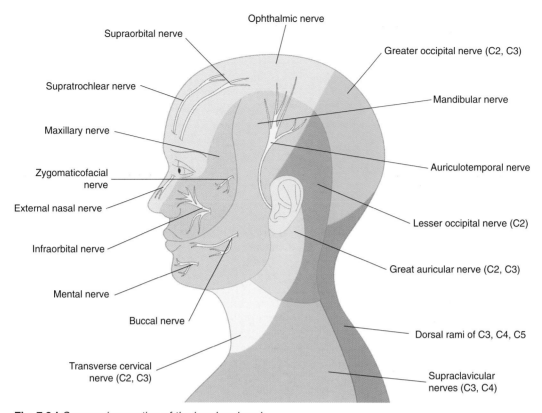

Fig. 7.3d *Sensory innervation of the head and neck.*

muscle of the cheek and functions to push the food medially from the space between the cheek and the teeth, i.e. the vestibule of the mouth). The marginal mandibular branch passes along the lower margin of the mandible to supply the muscles around the mouth including the orbicularis oris. The cervical branch passes downwards to supply the platysma.

The parotid gland (Fig. 7.3b)

The parotid gland is predominantly a serous salivary gland. It is situated below the external auditory meatus and extends on to the ramus of the mandible. It lies on the masseter, and the sternocleidomastoid. The deep part of the gland is irregular in shape and extends almost up to the side wall of the pharynx and the carotid sheath, from which it is separated by the styloid process and its attached structures. The parotid gland is traversed by the facial nerve, the retromandibular vein and the external carotid artery in that order from superficial to deep.

The parotid gland is enclosed inside a tough capsule derived from the investing layer of deep fascia of the

neck. Mumps, a virus infection of the gland, is painful because the gland swells within the thick fibrous capsule.

THE MUSCLES OF MASTICATION AND THE MANDIBULAR NERVE (Fig. 7.4)

The mandible, or the lower jaw, consists of a horizontal body bearing the alveolar process and the lower teeth, and a vertically orientated ramus. The junction between the body and the ramus is the angle of the mandible. The head articulates with the mandibular fossa at the base of the skull to form the temporomandibular joint.

On the medial aspect of the ramus is the mandibular foramen. This is guarded anteriorly by a projecting process called the lingula to which the sphenomandibular ligament is attached. The inferior alveolar (dental) nerve enters the mandibular foramen and transverses the body within the mandibular canal. It divides into the mental nerve and the incisive nerve. The incisive nerve which supplies the incisors and

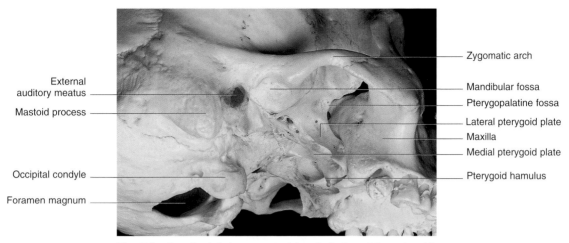

Fig. 7.4a *Anterior inferior aspect of the skull viewed from the side.*

External auditory meatus

Mastoid process

Occipital condyle

Foramen magnum

Zygomatic arch

Mandibular fossa

Pterygopalatine fossa

Lateral pterygoid plate

Maxilla

Medial pterygoid plate

Pterygoid hamulus

canine teeth continue beyond the mental foramen within the body in the incisive canal. The trunk of the inferior alveolar nerve supplies the premolars and the molars.

The mental nerve emerges through the mental foramen to supply the lower lip and the buccal and labial gingiva. A small groove runs inferiorly and forward from the mandibular foramen. This is the mylohyoid groove and is produced by the nerve to mylohyoid which supplies the mylohyoid and the anterior belly of the digastric muscles. Above the groove is a prominent ridge, the mylohyoid line, for the attachment of the mylohyoid muscle. The muscle extends from the level of the last molar tooth to the midline. The two mylohyoids which form the floor of the mouth separate the oral cavity from the neck. The lateral surface of the ramus gives attachment to the masseter which extends from the angle forward as far

as the external oblique line and the second molar tooth.

Fractures of the mandible happen more often than those of the upper facial skeleton. In many cases they are bilateral. The condyle of the mandible can fracture due to a blow to the chin and this may result in dislocation of the temporomandibular joint.

Fractures of the body of the mandible are most common in the canine region as the length of the root of the canine tooth weakens the bone in this position. Fractures of the body are always compound fractures lacerating the mucosa of the oral cavity.

The temporomandibular joint is a synovial joint where the head of the mandible articulates with the mandibular fossa (glenoid fossa) and the articular eminence of the temporal bone. The articular surfaces of this joint are covered by fibrocartilage (not hyaline) and there is also a fibrocartilaginous articular disc dividing the joint cavity into upper and lower

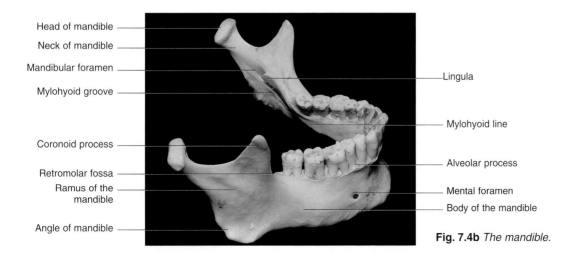

Head of mandible

Neck of mandible

Mandibular foramen

Mylohyoid groove

Coronoid process

Retromolar fossa

Ramus of the mandible

Angle of mandible

Lingula

Mylohyoid line

Alveolar process

Mental foramen

Body of the mandible

Fig. 7.4b *The mandible.*

compartments. The joints allow depression, elevation, protrusion, retraction, and side-to-side movements of the mandible.

Muscles of mastication (Fig. 7.4c, d, e)

There are four pairs of muscles in this group attaching the mandible to the base of the skull. The masseter extends from the zygomatic arch to the ramus of the mandible. It elevates the mandible. The temporalis takes origin from the temporal fossa and the temporal fascia covering the muscle and is inserted into the coronoid process. Its insertion extends into the retromolar fossa behind the last molar tooth. When lower dentures are fitted they should not extend into the retromolar fossa to avoid soreness of the mucosa due to contraction of the temporalis muscle. The temporalis elevates the mandible. Its posterior fibres retract the mandible after protrusion.

The pterygoid muscles lie medial to the ramus of the mandible. The lateral pterygoid which originates from the lateral surface of the lateral pterygoid plate and from the infratemporal surface of the skull is inserted into the capsule of the temporomandibular joint, the articular disc and also into the upper part of the neck of the mandible. Its contraction pulls the head of the mandible and the articular disc forward during protraction and during the act of opening the mouth. Unilateral contraction of the lateral pterygoid allows

the mandible to move to the opposite side. The forward movement of the disc may help to pack the space between the incongruent articular surfaces of the condyle and the articular eminence thus stabilising the joint.

The medial pterygoid extends from the medial surface of the lateral pterygoid plate to the medial surface of the ramus of the mandible. It is an elevator of the mandible. Unilateral contraction of the medial pterygoid is important in the side-to-side movement of the mandible as it deviates the jaw to the opposite side.

The four muscles of mastication are supplied by the mandibular division of the trigeminal nerve.

The mandibular nerve (Fig. 7.4d, e, f)

This branch of the trigeminal nerve having both motor and sensory fibres leaves the skull through the foramen ovale. The sensory fibres innervate the auricle and the external acoustic meatus, the skin over the mandible, the cheek, the lower lip, the tongue and the floor of the mouth, the lower teeth and the gums. The floor of the mouth and the inner gingiva of the lower jaw are supplied by the lingual nerve which is a branch of the mandibular nerve. The motor fibres supply the muscles of mastication — the temporalis, masseter, medial pterygoid and the lateral pterygoid. Branches from the mandibular division also innervate the tensor tympani and tensor palati as well as the anterior belly of the

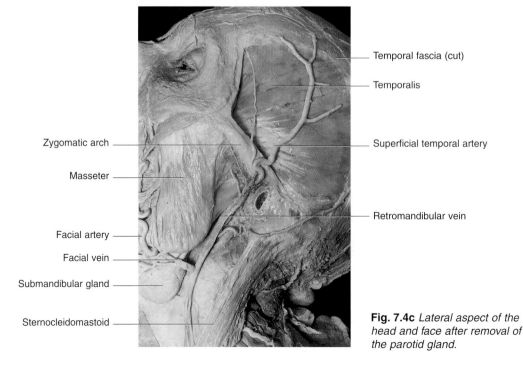

Temporal fascia (cut)

Temporalis

Superficial temporal artery

Zygomatic arch

Masseter

Retromandibular vein

Facial artery

Facial vein

Submandibular gland

Sternocleidomastoid

Fig. 7.4c *Lateral aspect of the head and face after removal of the parotid gland.*

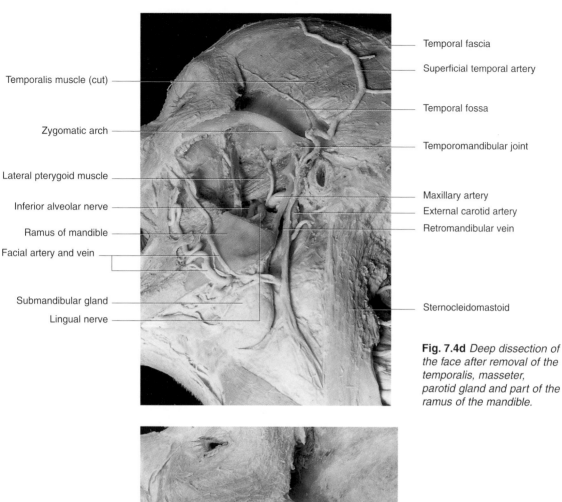

Temporalis muscle (cut)

Zygomatic arch

Lateral pterygoid muscle

Inferior alveolar nerve

Ramus of mandible

Facial artery and vein

Submandibular gland

Lingual nerve

Temporal fascia

Superficial temporal artery

Temporal fossa

Temporomandibular joint

Maxillary artery

External carotid artery

Retromandibular vein

Sternocleidomastoid

Fig. 7.4d *Deep dissection of the face after removal of the temporalis, masseter, parotid gland and part of the ramus of the mandible.*

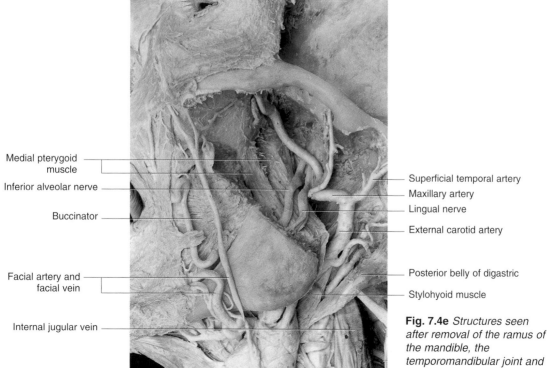

Medial pterygoid muscle

Inferior alveolar nerve

Buccinator

Facial artery and facial vein

Internal jugular vein

Superficial temporal artery

Maxillary artery

Lingual nerve

External carotid artery

Posterior belly of digastric

Stylohyoid muscle

Fig. 7.4e *Structures seen after removal of the ramus of the mandible, the temporomandibular joint and the lateral pterygoid muscle.*

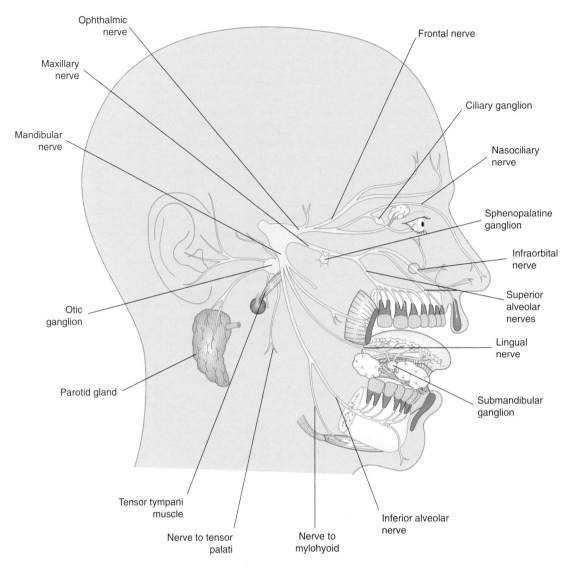

Fig. 7.4f *Summary of the distribution of the trigeminal nerve.*

digastric and the mylohyoid muscles (Fig. 7.4f). Proprioceptive fibres are contained in the branches innervating the muscles. The submandibular ganglion in which the parasympathetic nerve fibres to the submandibular and sublingual glands synapse is connected to the lingual nerve.

THE SUBMANDIBULAR REGION, THE SUBMANDIBULAR GLAND AND THE FLOOR OF THE MOUTH (Fig. 7.5)

The submandibular gland and the submandibular group of lymph nodes fill the submandibular triangle which is bounded by the anterior and posterior bellies of the digastric muscle and the lower border of the mandible. The superficial surface of the gland is crossed by the facial vein, the cervical branch of the facial nerve and also often by the marginal mandibular branch of the facial nerve. The marginal mandibular branch lies deep to the platysma and is one of the most important relations of the gland. Skin incisions in the

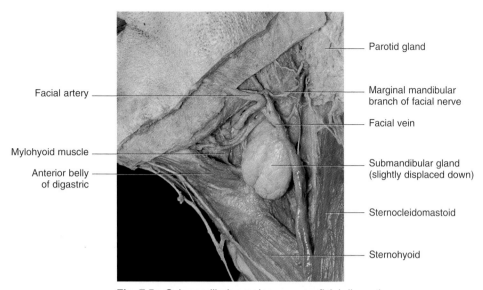

Facial artery

Mylohyoid muscle

Anterior belly of digastric

Parotid gland

Marginal mandibular branch of facial nerve

Facial vein

Submandibular gland (slightly displaced down)

Sternocleidomastoid

Sternohyoid

Fig. 7.5a *Submandibular region — superficial dissection.*

submandibular region are made about 4 cm below the mandible to avoid injury to the marginal mandibular branch.

Each submandibular gland has a larger, superficial part and a smaller deep part. The two are separated by the mylohyoid muscle. The two parts however are continuous with each other posteriorly and the concavity thus formed is occupied by the free posterior border of the mylohyoid muscle. The facial artery grooves the deep surface and emerges on to the face by passing between the gland and the mandible. Several submandibular lymph nodes lie on the superficial surface.

The deep part lies in the floor of the mouth, superior (deep) to the mylohyoid and is covered by the mucosa of the oral cavity. Medially it lies on the hyoglossus and is related to the lingual nerve, the submandibular ganglion and the hypoglossal nerve (Fig. 7.5c).

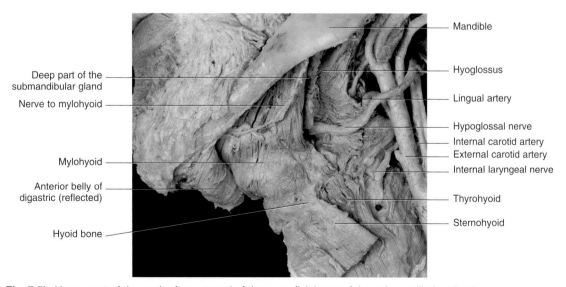

Deep part of the submandibular gland

Nerve to mylohyoid

Mylohyoid

Anterior belly of digastric (reflected)

Hyoid bone

Mandible

Hyoglossus

Lingual artery

Hypoglossal nerve

Internal carotid artery

External carotid artery

Internal laryngeal nerve

Thyrohyoid

Sternohyoid

Fig. 7.5b *Upper part of the neck after removal of the superficial part of the submandibular gland.*

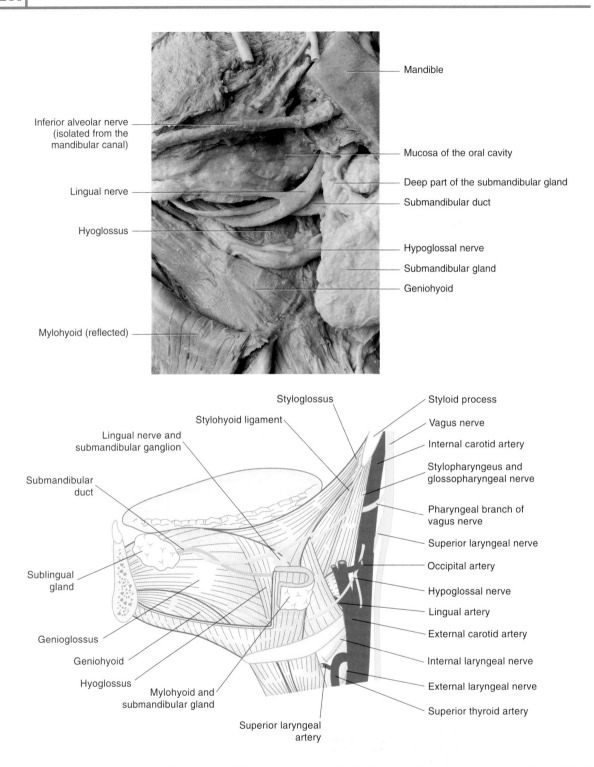

Fig. 7.5c *Deep structures in the submandibular region and the floor of the mouth seen after removal of the left half of the mandible and reflection of the left mylohyoid muscle — viewed from the left side. The lingual nerve, submandibular duct and the hypoglossal nerve are superficial to the hypoglossus whereas the glossopharyngeal nerve and the lingual artery pass deep to it.*

The submandibular duct (Fig. 7.5c)

The duct of the submandibular gland (Wharton's duct) starts in the superficial part, running posteriorly and superiorly to reach the deep part. Here it turns forward and medially and emerges on to the surface of the hyoglossus muscle. It runs forward deep to the mucosa of the floor of the mouth between the mucosa and the sublingual gland to open into the floor of the mouth on either side of the frenulum of the tongue (Fig. 7.6b). The duct, on the floor of the mouth, is closely related to the lingual nerve. As it goes forward it crosses medial to the nerve to lie above the nerve and then crosses back, this time lateral to it to reach a position once again below the nerve (Fig. 7.5c).

The floor of the mouth

The floor of the mouth separating the oral cavity from the neck is formed by the mylohyoid diaphragm formed by the fusion of the mylohyoid muscles of both sides along the midline raphe. Above the mylohyoid is the mouth and below is the neck. The mylohyoids are reinforced superiorly by the two geniohyoids. The anterior part of the tongue rests on the mucosa covering the floor of the mouth.

More posteriorly between the mylohyoid and the tongue lies the hyoglossus muscle which in fact is the side wall of the tongue. A number of important structures in the floor of the mouth lie on the hyoglossus. These from above downwards are the lingual nerve, the deep part of the submandibular gland and the submandibular duct and the hypoglossal nerve

The lingual nerve, a branch of the mandibular division of the trigeminal nerve, runs forward above the mylohyoid. It gives off a gingival branch which supplies the whole of the lingual gingiva and the mucous membrane of the floor of the mouth. The lingual nerve winds round the submandibular duct before getting distributed to the mucosa of the anterior two-thirds of the tongue. The submandibular ganglion is suspended from the lingual nerve as it lies on the hyoglossus. The preganglionic fibres in the chorda tympani synapse in this ganglion. Before reaching the floor of the mouth the lingual nerve lies against the periosteum of the alveolar process closely related to the third molar tooth. The nerve can be damaged here during dental extraction.

On the hyoglossus the hypoglossal nerve breaks up into branches to supply all the muscles (both extrinsic and intrinsic) of the tongue except the palatoglossus.

THE ORAL CAVITY (Fig. 7.6)

The tongue

The dorsum of the tongue is divided into an anterior two-thirds and a posterior third by a V-shaped groove, the sulcus terminalis, the apex of which has the foramen caecum from which the thyroglossal duct giving rise to the thyroid gland develops. The mucosa of the anterior two-thirds carries the filiform papillae, fungiform papillae and in front of the sulcus terminalis a row of vallate papillae, about 8–12 in number. The vallate papillae carry taste buds. The inferior surface of the tongue in the midline has the frenulum of the tongue. On either side of the frenulum the deep vein of the tongue can be seen and also the openings of the ducts of the submandibular glands.

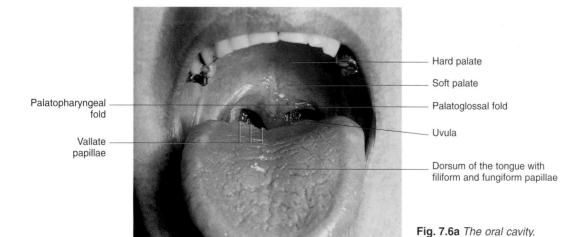

Palatopharyngeal fold

Vallate papillae

Hard palate

Soft palate

Palatoglossal fold

Uvula

Dorsum of the tongue with filiform and fungiform papillae

Fig. 7.6a *The oral cavity.*

Muscles (Fig. 7.5c; Fig. 7.7b)

A midline fibrous septum divides the tongue into right and left halves. Within these two compartments lie the intrinsic muscles which alter and control the shape of the tongue. The extrinsic muscles attach the tongue to the mandible (the genioglossus), hyoid bone (the hyoglossus), styloid process (the styloglossus) and the soft palate (the palatoglossus). They alter the position of the tongue.

Nerve supply (Fig. 7.6e)

This is based on the development. The lingual nerve which is a branch of the mandibular division of the trigeminal (nerve of the first branchial arch) carries common sensation from the anterior two-thirds. Taste is carried by the chorda tympani fibres within the lingual nerve. The sensory supply of the posterior third, including the vallate papillae, is by the glossopharyngeal nerve which is the nerve of the third branchial arch. The intrinsic and extrinsic muscles are supplied by the hypoglossal nerve. Paralysis of the hypoglossal nerve is manifested as fibrillation of the tongue as well as wasting of the muscles. The latter will show the mucosa loose on the paralysed side.

Blood supply

The tongue is supplied by the lingual artery, a branch of the external carotid artery. At the posterior third, branches from the tonsillar artery (branch of the facial) and ascending pharyngeal artery anastomose with those of the lingual artery. There is only a poor communication between the two lingual arteries across the median septum.

The venous drainage is by two main veins, the lingual vein accompanying the lingual artery and the deep lingual vein which is visible on the inferior surface.

Lymphatic drainage

Lymphatic spread in cancer of the tongue is by tumour emboli. The drainage is essentially to the deep cervical nodes along the internal jugular vein. In the anterior two-thirds there is only minimal communication of lymphatics across the midline septum so that meta-stases from this portion tend to be ipsilateral. Posterior third lymphatics form extrinsic networks and facilitate early bilateral metastases. Lymphatics from the tip of the tongue pass to the submental nodes and from there to the lower deep cervical nodes. From the midportion, lymphatics pass to the submandibular nodes and then

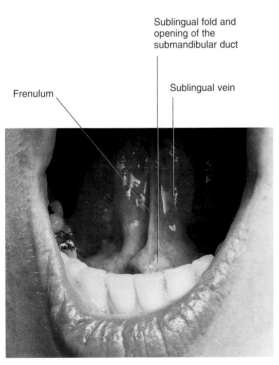

Fig. 7.6b *Inferior surface of the tongue and the floor of the mouth.*

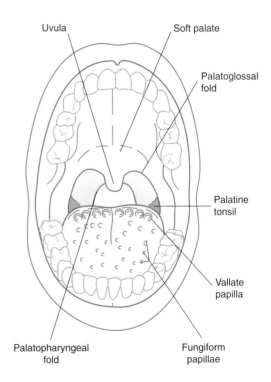

Fig. 7.6c *Oral cavity and oropharynx.*

to the deep cervical from the margin of the tongue ipsilaterally and the rest bilaterally. From the posterior third, the drainage is to the upper deep cervical of both sides.

The palate (Fig. 7.6a, c; Fig. 7.7a, b)

The roof of the mouth is the palate. The anterior two-thirds is bony, forming the hard palate and the posterior third, the soft palate, is muscular. The midline projection of the soft palate backwards is the uvula. If the subject says 'aah' the soft palate will move upwards. The palatine process of the maxilla and the horizontal plate of the palatine bones form the hard palate. The tensor palatini, the levator palatini, the musculus uvuli, the palatoglossus and the palato-pharyngeus form the muscular core of the soft palate. The tensor palatini winds round the pterygoid hamulus of the medial pterygoid plate to enter the cavity of the pharynx and its tendon spreads out to become the palatine aponeurosis to be attached to the posterior aspect of the hard palate. The levator palatini takes origin from the base of the skull inside the pharynx and is inserted to the palatine aponeurosis. The other palatine muscles merge with the aponeurosis. Both the tensor and the levator palatini in their upper part are attached to the cartilaginous part of the Eustachian (auditory) tube. Their contraction opens the tube to transmit air from the pharynx to the middle ear. Children with cleft palate may develop deafness as this mechanism is often affected.

The mucosa of the palate has stratified squamous epithelium on the oral surface and ciliated columnar epithelium on the surface facing the nasal cavity. The sensory nerve supply of the palate is by branches from the maxillary nerve and the motor supply is by the cranial part of the accessory nerve transmitted through the vagus as its pharyngeal branch.

THE PHARYNX AND RELATED STRUCTURES (Fig. 7.7)

External aspect of the pharynx

The pharynx is a muscular tube attached to the base of the skull. Below the level of the cricoid cartilage it opens into the oesophagus. For descriptive purposes the interior of the pharynx is divided into nasopharynx, oropharynx and hypopharynx or laryngeal part of the pharynx. The nasal cavity opens into the nasopharynx, the oropharynx is continuous with the oral cavity and the larynx opens into the hypopharynx.

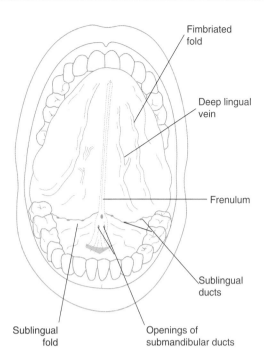

Fig. 7.6d *Inferior surface of the tongue and the floor of the mouth.*

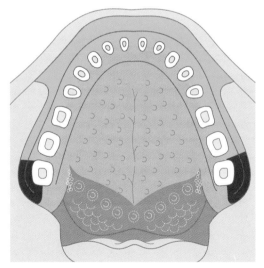

Mental nerve

Glossopharyngeal nerve

Inferior alveolar nerve

Lingual nerve

Buccal nerve

Fig. 7.6e *Sensory nerve supply of the tongue, lower lip and cheek.*

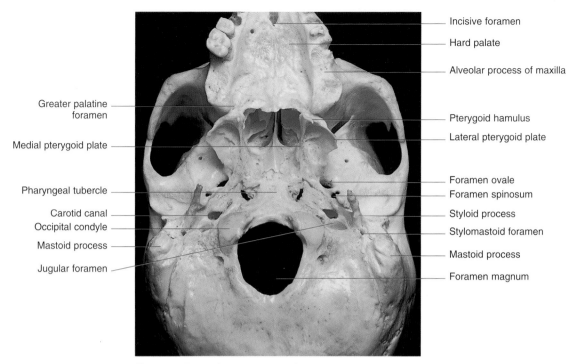

Incisive foramen

Hard palate

Alveolar process of maxilla

Pterygoid hamulus

Lateral pterygoid plate

Foramen ovale

Foramen spinosum

Styloid process

Stylomastoid foramen

Mastoid process

Foramen magnum

Greater palatine foramen

Medial pterygoid plate

Pharyngeal tubercle

Carotid canal

Occipital condyle

Mastoid process

Jugular foramen

Fig. 7.7a *Base of the skull seen from below.*

The origins of the constrictor muscles which form the wall of the pharynx are as follows. The superior constrictor takes origin from the pterygomandibular raphe which extends from the medial pterygoid plate to the mandible, the middle from the hyoid bone and the inferior constrictor from the thyroid cartilage (the thyropharyngeus) and the cricoid cartilage (the crico-pharyngeus). All the constrictors fuse together in a midline raphe on the posterior aspect. The pharyngeal raphe is attached to the pharyngeal tubercle on the base of the skull (Fig. 7.7a, c). The inner aspect of the constrictors is lined by the thick pharyngobasilar fascia which is attached to the pharyngeal tubercle, the auditory (Eustachian) tube and the medial pterygoid plate and this fascia bridges the gap between the superior constrictor and the base of the skull. The weakest part of the pharyngeal wall is in the midline at the back in the lower part of the pharynx. This lies between the diverging fibres of the cricopharyngeal and the thyropharyngeal part of the inferior constrictor. This area is known as the Killian's dehiscence and is the commonest site for a pharyngeal diverticulum (protrusion of the wall due to excessive pressure).

The stylopharyngeus takes origin from the styloid process and lies between the external and the internal

carotid arteries to reach the interval between the superior and the middle constrictor muscles. The glossopharyngeal nerve lies on the surface of the stylopharyngeus as it enters the pharynx. The glossopharyngeal nerve (IX cranial nerve) gives sensory innervation to the posterior third of the tongue and the oropharynx. Its tympanic branch supplies the middle ear and the auditory (Eustachian) tube. It also supplies the stylopharyngeus muscle.

The vagus nerve (X cranial nerve, Fig. 7.7g) has three major branches in the neck viz., the pharyngeal branch, the superior laryngeal nerve and the recurrent laryngeal nerve. The pharyngeal branch of the vagus gives motor innervation to the muscles of the pharynx and soft palate. Its fibres originate in the nucleus ambiguus in the brainstem and leave the brain as the cranial part of the accessory nerve. The superior laryngeal branch of the vagus lies deep to the external and the internal carotid arteries. It divides into the internal and the external laryngeal nerves. The external laryngeal nerve supplies the cricothyroid muscle as well as the cricopharyngeal part of the inferior constrictor. The internal laryngeal nerve is sensory and it supplies the hypopharynx and part of the larynx. The right recurrent laryngeal nerve

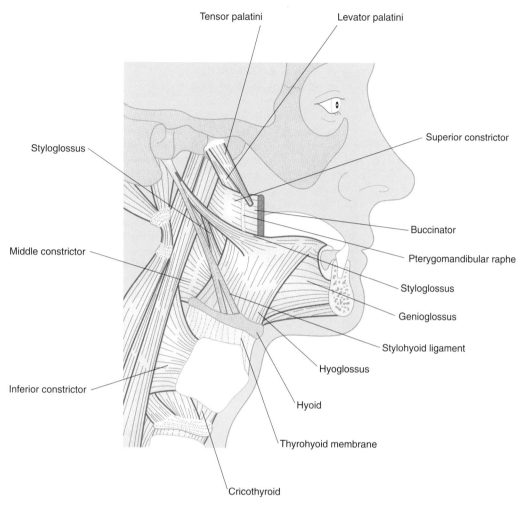

Fig. 7.7b *Muscles of the tongue and pharynx.*

branches off from the right vagus and winds round the subclavian artery. It lies in the groove between the trachea and the oesophagus and runs upwards until it disappears under the lower border of the inferior constrictor. The left recurrent laryngeal nerve lies in the groove between the trachea and the oesophagus on the left side. This nerve, unlike the one on the right, winds round the ligamentum arteriosum in the thorax. The two nerves are related to the thyroid gland.

In the posterior aspect of the pharynx the inferior thyroid artery arches to enter the back of the thyroid gland. The inferior thyroid artery crosses the recurrent laryngeal nerve at the lower pole of the thyroid gland.

The carotid sheath and the cervical part of the sympathetic trunk which lies on its posterior wall are also related to the pharynx. There are three cervical sympathetic ganglia in the neck, the superior, middle and inferior ganglia. The middle cervical ganglion may

be absent. The inferior ganglion often fuses with the first thoracic ganglion to form the stellate ganglion. The stellate ganglion is situated in front of the neck of the first rib and the transverse process of the seventh cervical vertebra. Paralysis of the sympathetic trunk at the root of the neck may occur as a result of compression from a tumour in the apex of the lung. This will produce Horner's syndrome characterised by absence of sweating, constriction of pupil and slight drooping of the eyelid (ptosis).

Interior of the pharynx

The nasopharynx is the part of the pharynx behind the nasal cavity. It has the opening of the Eustachian tube and, in a younger person, the nasopharyngeal tonsil or the adenoids. The opening of the Eustachian tube can be identified in the living by looking for the prominent

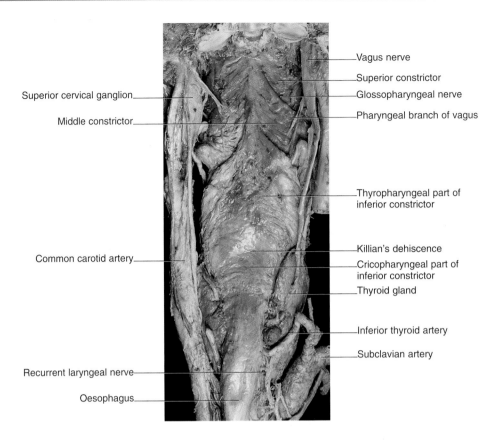

Superior cervical ganglion

Middle constrictor

Common carotid artery

Recurrent laryngeal nerve

Oesophagus

Vagus nerve

Superior constrictor

Glossopharyngeal nerve

Pharyngeal branch of vagus

Thyropharyngeal part of inferior constrictor

Killian's dehiscence

Cricopharyngeal part of inferior constrictor

Thyroid gland

Inferior thyroid artery

Subclavian artery

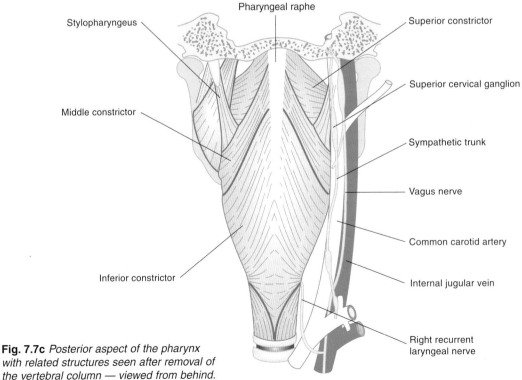

Stylopharyngeus

Middle constrictor

Inferior constrictor

Pharyngeal raphe

Superior constrictor

Superior cervical ganglion

Sympathetic trunk

Vagus nerve

Common carotid artery

Internal jugular vein

Right recurrent laryngeal nerve

Fig. 7.7c *Posterior aspect of the pharynx with related structures seen after removal of the vertebral column — viewed from behind.*

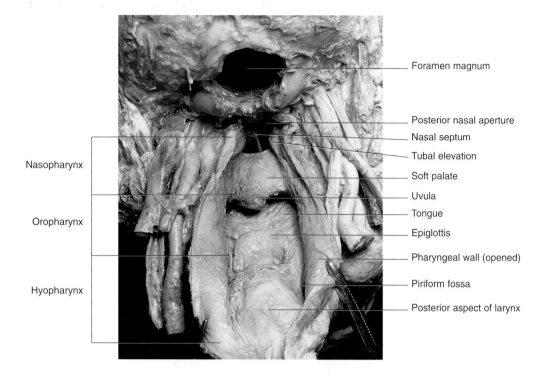

Foramen magnum

Posterior nasal aperture

Nasal septum

Tubal elevation

Soft palate

Uvula

Tongue

Epiglottis

Pharyngeal wall (opened)

Piriform fossa

Posterior aspect of larynx

Nasopharynx

Oropharynx

Hyopharynx

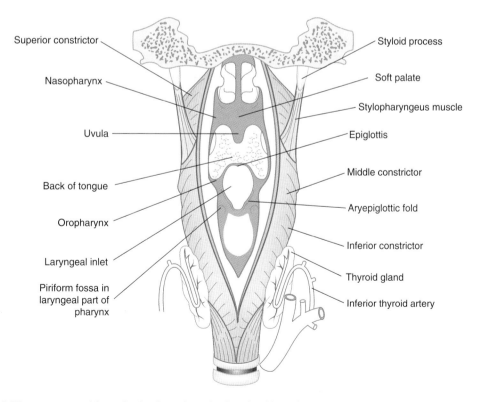

Superior constrictor

Nasopharynx

Uvula

Back of tongue

Oropharynx

Laryngeal inlet

Piriform fossa in laryngeal part of pharynx

Styloid process

Soft palate

Stylopharyngeus muscle

Epiglottis

Middle constrictor

Aryepiglottic fold

Inferior constrictor

Thyroid gland

Inferior thyroid artery

Fig. 7.7d *Pharynx opened from the back to show the interior. Nasopharynx, oropharynx and the laryngeal part of the pharynx are viewed from behind.*

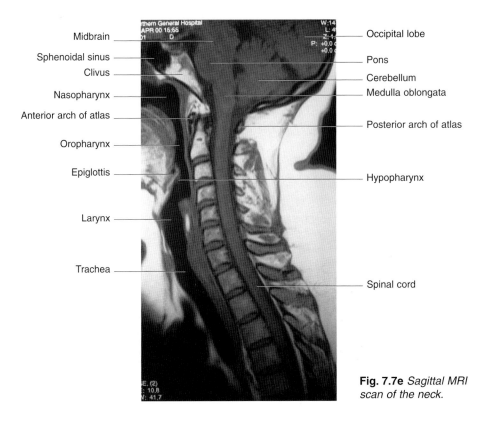

Midbrain

Sphenoidal sinus

Clivus

Nasopharynx

Anterior arch of atlas

Oropharynx

Epiglottis

Larynx

Trachea

Occipital lobe

Pons

Cerebellum

Medulla oblongata

Posterior arch of atlas

Hypopharynx

Spinal cord

Fig. 7.7e *Sagittal MRI scan of the neck.*

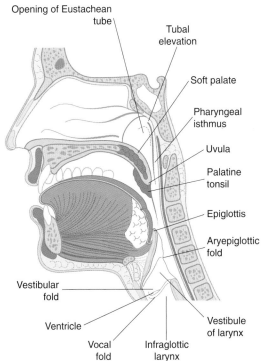

Opening of Eustachean tube

Tubal elevation

Soft palate

Pharyngeal isthmus

Uvula

Palatine tonsil

Epiglottis

Aryepiglottic fold

Vestibular fold

Ventricle

Vocal fold

Infraglottic larynx

Vestibule of larynx

Fig. 7.7f *Sagittal section of the head to show the larynx and pharynx.*

tubal elevation. The tubal opening is in front of the elevation. The salpingopharyngeal fold, produced by the muscle with the same name, extends downwards from the tubal elevation.

The Eustachian tube can be blocked by enlargement of the adenoids in throat infections. This condition is common in children. Infection from here can spread into the middle ear through the tube. An early sign of a malignant tumour in the nasopharynx may be deafness due to blockage of the auditory tube. The tumour can also spread through the pharyngeal wall into the branches of the trigeminal nerve which are lying just outside the nasopharynx. The sensory innervation of the nasopharynx is by the maxillary nerve via the pharyngeal branch of the sphenopalatine ganglion (Fig. 7.4f).

In the oropharynx the palatoglossal and the palatopharyngeal folds bound the tonsillar fossa. These are produced by the palatoglossal and palatopharyngeal muscles. The tonsillar bed is formed by the superior constrictor muscle. The main sensory innervation of the oropharynx is through the glossopharyngeal nerve.

The tonsil has a rich blood supply. The tonsillar

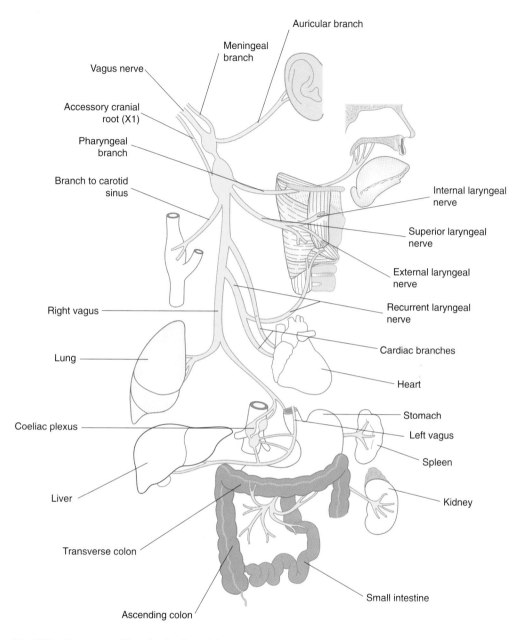

Fig. 7.7g *Summary of the distribution of the vagus nerve.*

branch of the facial artery enters it through the superior constrictor. The paratonsillar vein, lying deep to the tonsil, is a usual source of bleeding during tonsillectomy.

The hypopharynx (laryngeal part of the pharynx) has the laryngeal inlet. A forward extension of the hypopharynx forming a cul de sac by the side of the larynx is the piriform fossa. Malignant tumours arising in the piriform fossa may be 'silent' in the early stages. It may not produce difficulty in swallowing as the space is a recess extending from the main cavity of the pharynx. The sensory innervation of the hypopharynx is by the internal laryngeal nerve, a branch of the superior laryngeal branch of the vagus.

THE LARYNX (Fig. 7.8)

The larynx is held open by a series of cartilages on its wall. The cricoid cartilage has a narrow arch anteriorly and a broad lamina at the back. The cricotracheal ligament connects the cricoid to the first tracheal ring. The thyroid cartilage has two laminae meeting in the midline anteriorly and it articulates inferiorly with the cricoid at the cricothyroid joints. It is connected to the hyoid bone by the thyrohyoid ligament. The epiglottis is a leaf-shaped cartilage forming the anterior wall of the inlet of the larynx. The arytenoid cartilages, paired cartilages articulating with the lamina of the cricoid, have the vocal process projecting anteriorly and the muscular process laterally. The former receives attachment of the vocal ligament and the latter the abductors and adductors of the vocal cord.

There are two pairs of minor cartilages, corniculate cartilage articulating with the apex of the arytenoid and the cuneiform cartilage, a nodule in the aryepiglottic fold. Though small, these are essential for complete approximation of the inlet of the larynx.

The laryngeal inlet bounded by the epiglottis in front, the aryepiglottic folds on the side and the arytenoids and the corniculate cartilages at the back opens into the hypopharynx (laryngopharynx). The interior of the larynx is divided into different parts. The vestibule of the larynx extends from the inlet to the vestibular fold. The ventricle of the larynx is the short narrow space between the vestibular fold and the vocal fold. The space between the vocal cord, the rima glottidis, is the narrowest part of the upper airway.

The mucosa in the supraglottic region (above the vocal cords) is loosely bound to the underlying wall. In laryngeal oedema fluid accumulates in the submucous space and the mucosa swells up and obstructs the airway. The fluid cannot spread downwards, as at the vocal cord the mucosa is firmly adherent to the underlying structures without having a submucous space. The lack of a submucosal layer also makes the vocal cords relatively less vascular and hence it appears paler than the rest of the mucosa.

Muscles of the larynx

The extrinsic muscles are the suprahyoids and infrahyoids and are involved in the movements of the larynx during swallowing. Besides these there are intrinsic muscles. The paired posterior cricoarytenoid muscle abducts the cord. Their action is opposed by the lateral cricoarytenoids and the transverse arytenoid (interarytenoid) which act as adductors of the cords. The cricothyroid muscle arises from the oblique line on the lamina of the thyroid cartilage and is inserted to the anterior part of the arch of the cricoid. As it contracts it approximates the cricoid and the thyroid

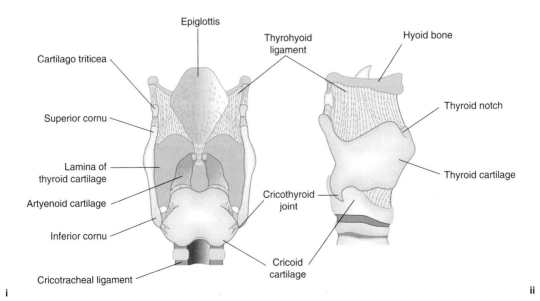

i

ii

Fig. 7.8a *The cartilages of the larynx and the hyoid bone:* **(i)** *posterior view;* **(ii)** *lateral view.*

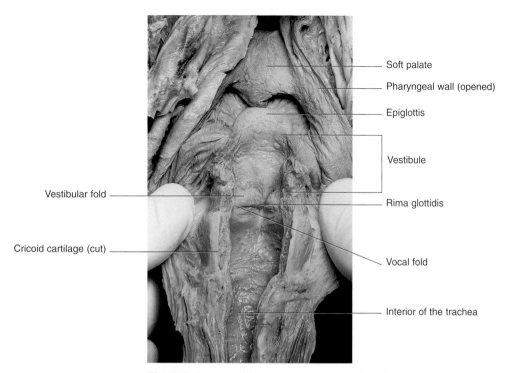

Soft palate

Pharyngeal wall (opened)

Epiglottis

Vestibule

Vestibular fold

Rima glottidis

Cricoid cartilage (cut)

Vocal fold

Interior of the trachea

Fig. 7.8b *Interior of the pharynx, larynx and trachea.*
Pharynx, larynx and the trachea opened from the back.

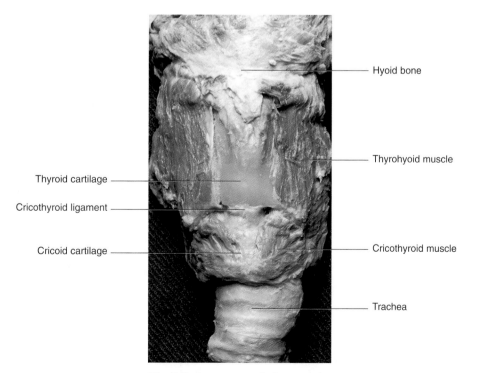

Hyoid bone

Thyrohyoid muscle

Thyroid cartilage

Cricothyroid ligament

Cricoid cartilage

Cricothyroid muscle

Trachea

Fig. 7.8c *Larynx — anterior aspect.*

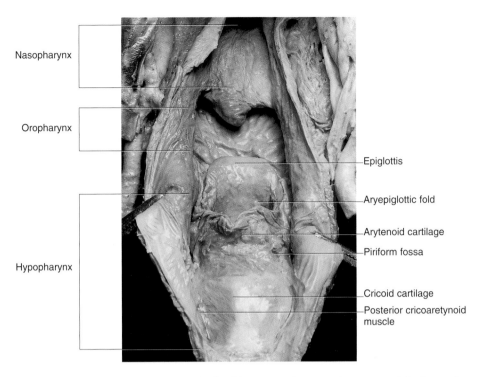

Nasopharynx

Oropharynx

Hypopharynx

Epiglottis

Aryepiglottic fold

Arytenoid cartilage

Piriform fossa

Cricoid cartilage

Posterior cricoaretynoid muscle

Fig. 7.8d *Interior of the pharynx and the laryngeal inlet. Mucosa on the posterior aspect of the larynx is removed to show the cricothyroid muscles.*

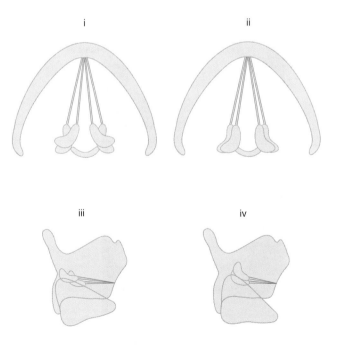

i   ii

iii   iv

Fig. 7.8e *Movements of the vocal cords.* **(i)** *Abduction by posterior cricoarytenoid.* **(ii)** *Adduction by transverse and oblique arytenoids.* **(iii)** *Tensing by cricothyroid.* **(iv)** *Relaxation by thyroarytenoid.*

cartilages anteriorly, increasing the distance between the attachments of the cords, and thus lengthens them. The thyroarytenoid muscle lying in the cord shortens the cord. A component of it, known as the vocalis, is said to be important in adjusting the tension of the cord.

The aryepiglottic muscle and the oblique arytenoid muscle are small muscles, but are important in reducing the size of the laryngeal inlet as in swallowing.

The recurrent laryngeal nerve innervates all the intrinsic muscles of the larynx except the cricothyroid. The cricothyroid is innervated by the external laryngeal branch of the superior laryngeal nerve. The recurrent laryngeal nerve also gives sensory innervation to the part of the larynx below the level of the vocal cord. The part above is supplied by the internal laryngeal nerve. The blood supply of the larynx is derived from the superior and inferior laryngeal arteries. The vocal cords have no lymphatic drainage and hence this region acts as a lymphatic watershed. The supraglottic part drains to the upper deep cervical nodes and the subglottic part drains to the prelaryngeal and pretracheal nodes and also to the inferior deep cervical nodes.

THE NASAL CAVITY AND THE PARANASAL SINUSES (Fig. 7.9)

Each nasal cavity has a roof, floor, a lateral wall and a medial wall formed by the nasal septum. It is pyramidal in shape with a narrow upper part and a slightly wider base. The roof is formed by the cribriform plate of the ethmoid and the body of the sphenoid. The hard palate forms the floor.

The nasal septum has a bony and a cartilaginous part. In the upper part it is formed by the perpendicular plate of the ethmoid bone and behind and below by the vomer, a single midline bone. The gap in front, between these two bones, is bridged by the septal cartilage. The septum may often be deflected to one side. This condition may cause nasal obstruction and headache.

The lateral wall is formed by the maxilla. Here the opening of the maxillary sinus is overlapped by the ethmoid, the lacrimal bone, the perpendicular plate of the palatine bone and the inferior concha. Projecting from the lateral wall are the superior, middle and inferior conchae dividing the nasal cavity into the superior, middle and inferior meatuses. Each meatus is seen below the respective concha. The inferior concha is the largest and is a separate bone. The other two are parts of the ethmoid bone.

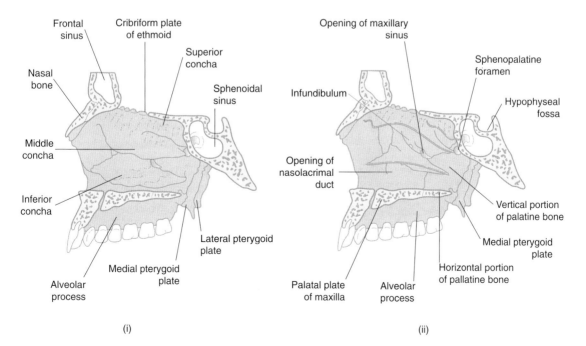

Fig. 7.9a *The bony lateral wall of the nasal cavity.* **(i)** *Bones complete.* **(ii)** *After partial removal of the conchae.*

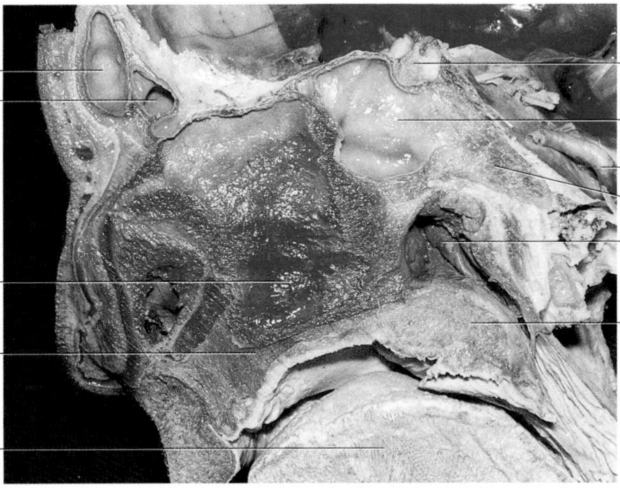

Frontal sinus

Nasal septum

Hard palate

Tongue

Pituitary gland

Sphenoidal sinus

Vertebral artery

Clivus

Tubal elevation

Soft palate

Fig. 7.9b *Sagittal section of the head.*

The inferior meatus is the widest part of the nasal cavity. Nasal intubations are done through this region. Hypertrophy of the inferior concha may produce difficulty in such intubation.

The space above and behind the superior meatus, the sphenoethmoidal recess, receives the opening of the sphenoidal sinus. The posterior ethmoidal sinus opens into the superior meatus and the sphenoidal sinus into the sphenoethmoidal recess. The pituitary fossa lies above the sphenoidal sinus which is also closely related to the cavernous sinus and the internal carotid artery. Surgical access to the pituitary gland is often through the nasal cavity and the sphenoidal sinus. The openings of the frontal, anterior ethmoidal and the maxillary sinuses are in the middle meatus. They all open in close proximity in the hiatus semilunaris and hence infection

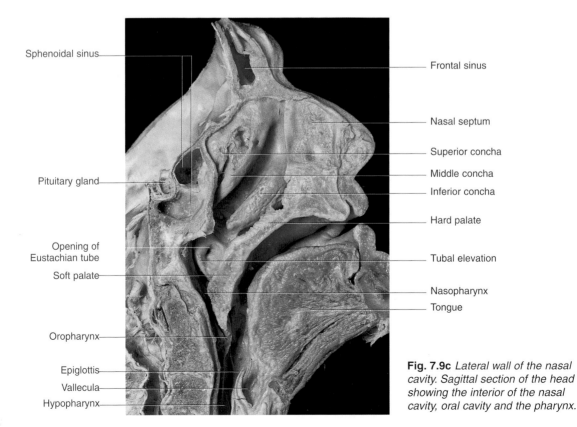

Sphenoidal sinus

Pituitary gland

Opening of Eustachian tube

Soft palate

Oropharynx

Epiglottis

Vallecula

Hypopharynx

Frontal sinus

Nasal septum

Superior concha

Middle concha

Inferior concha

Hard palate

Tubal elevation

Nasopharynx

Tongue

Fig. 7.9c *Lateral wall of the nasal cavity. Sagittal section of the head showing the interior of the nasal cavity, oral cavity and the pharynx.*

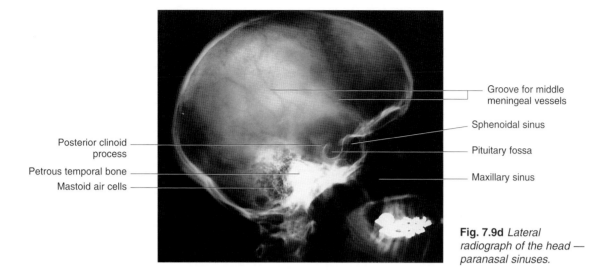

Groove for middle meningeal vessels

Sphenoidal sinus

Posterior clinoid process

Pituitary fossa

Petrous temporal bone

Maxillary sinus

Mastoid air cells

Fig. 7.9d *Lateral radiograph of the head — paranasal sinuses.*

from one sinus can easily spread to another. The nasolacrimal duct extends from the lacrimal sac to the inferior meatus. It drains the lacrimal fluid from the conjunctival sac.

Malignant tumours in the upper part of the nasal cavity, which are often silent in the early stages, can spread into the cranial cavity through the cribriform plate of the ethmoid. They can also spread into the orbit.

The innervation of the nasal cavity is by branches of the maxillary and the ophthalmic nerves. The arterial supply comes from the branches of the external and internal carotid arteries. Bleeding from the nasal cavity (epistaxis) is common. The commonest site is 'Little's area', in the anteroinferior part of the septum, where many vessels anastomose.

Paranasal sinuses

The maxillary sinus

This is the largest of the paranasal sinuses with a mean volume of about 10 ml. The medial wall or base is composed of thin and delicate bones on the lateral wall of the nasal cavity. The opening of the sinus into the hiatus semilunaris lies high on the medial wall, just below the floor of the orbit. As the ostium is high on the wall drainage depends on ciliary action and not gravity. The roof of the sinus is the floor of the orbit. The floor is the alveolar process of the maxilla overlying the second premolar and the first molar teeth. A tooth abscess may rupture into the sinus. The floor of the maxillary sinus is at a more inferior level than the floor of the nasal cavity.

Carcinoma of the maxillary sinus may invade the palate and cause dental problems. It may block the nasolacrimal duct causing epiphora. Spread of the tumour into the orbit causes proptosis. The maxillary division of the trigeminal nerve supplies the sinus through its infraorbital and superior dental nerves. The pain due to sinusitis may often manifest itself as toothache.

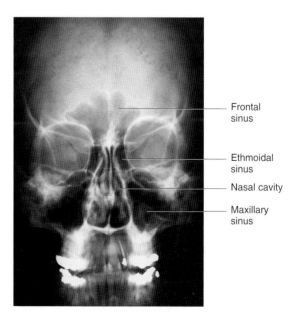

Frontal sinus

Ethmoidal sinus

Nasal cavity

Maxillary sinus

Fig. 7.9e *Radiograph of the paranasal sinuses.*

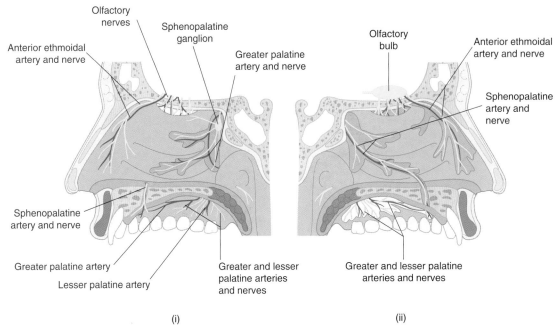

Fig. 7.9f *The arteries and nerves of the nasal cavity.* **(i)** *Lateral wall.* **(ii)** *Nasal septum.*

The ethmoidal air cells (ethmoidal air sinuses)

The ethmoidal air cells which are thin-walled cavities in the ethmoidal labyrinth vary in their size and number. Acute ethmoiditis in childhood and ethmoidal carcinoma may spread upwards causing meningitis and cerebrospinal fluid leakage or it may spread laterally into the orbit causing proptosis and diplopia.

The frontal sinus

The frontal sinuses are not present at birth but start to appear in the second year of life.

The frontal sinus drains by the infundibulum or the frontonasal duct into the hiatus semilunaris of the middle meatus. Infection of the frontal sinus is often associated with infection of the maxillary sinus as their openings are very close to each other.

Acute sinusitis can spread posteriorly into the anterior cranial fossa causing extradural and subdural abscesses or meningitis. The pus in the sinus can be drained by wash-out through the nose or by a small incision on its wall joint just below the medial end of the eyebrow.

The sphenoidal sinus

The sphenoidal sinus, like the maxillary sinus, is very small at birth. It occupies the body of the sphenoid but may extend into its greater and lesser wings. The sphenoidal sinus opens into the sphenoethmoidal recess of the nasal cavity.

The floor of the sinus is in the roof of the nasal cavity and the nasopharynx. The roof of the sinus is thin. The pituitary fossa bulges into the roof in its posterior half and anteriorly the roof separates the sinus from the optic chiasma and the optic nerves. The lateral wall is also thin and separates the sinus from the cavernous sinus and the internal carotid artery.

THE BRAIN AND THE CRANIAL CAVITY

The cranial fossae (Fig. 7.10)

The floor of the cranial cavity has three cranial fossae, the anterior, middle and the posterior cranial fossae, each progressively lower than the one in front. The anterior cranial fossa overlies the orbit and the nasal cavities. The frontal lobe of the brain lies in the anterior cranial fossa. The middle cranial fossa lies below and behind the anterior and contains the temporal lobes. Most posteriorly the posterior cranial fossa lies at the lowest level and contains the brainstem and the cerebellum.

In the anterior cranial fossa the falx cerebri is attached to the crista galli. The cribriform plate of the ethmoid forms the roof of the nasal cavity and transmits the olfactory nerves. Tumours from the upper part of the nasal cavity can spread into the anterior cranial fossa through the cribriform plate. Fractures of the anterior cranial fossa may produce bleeding and leakage of cerebrospinal fluid through the nasal cavity.

The optic canal connecting the middle cranial fossa to the orbit transmits the optic nerve and the ophthalmic artery. The optic nerve commences at the

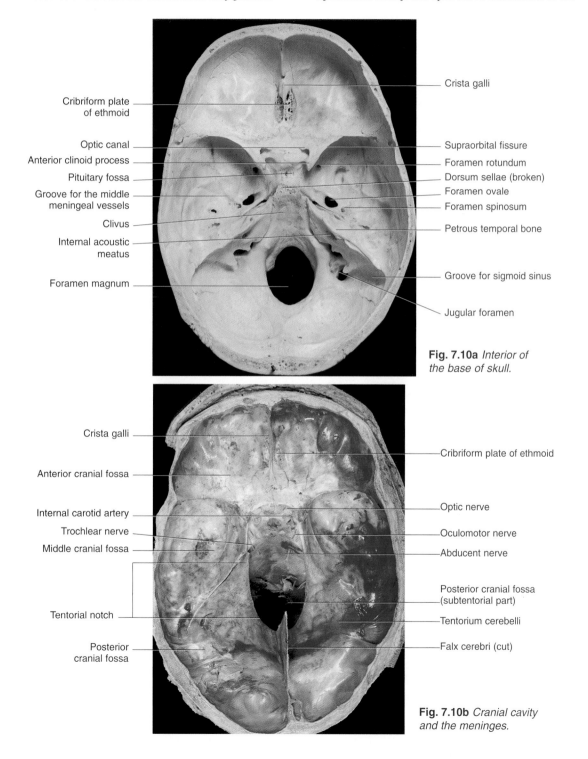

Crista galli

Cribriform plate of ethmoid

Optic canal
Anterior clinoid process
Pituitary fossa
Groove for the middle meningeal vessels
Clivus
Internal acoustic meatus
Foramen magnum

Supraorbital fissure
Foramen rotundum
Dorsum sellae (broken)
Foramen ovale
Foramen spinosum
Petrous temporal bone

Groove for sigmoid sinus

Jugular foramen

Fig. 7.10a *Interior of the base of skull.*

Crista galli
Anterior cranial fossa
Internal carotid artery
Trochlear nerve
Middle cranial fossa

Tentorial notch
Posterior cranial fossa

Cribriform plate of ethmoid

Optic nerve
Oculomotor nerve
Abducent nerve

Posterior cranial fossa (subtentorial part)
Tentorium cerebelli
Falx cerebri (cut)

Fig. 7.10b *Cranial cavity and the meninges.*

lamina cribosa, where the axons of the ganglion cells of the retina pierce the sclera of the eyeball. The nerve covered by the dura, arachnoid and pia runs posteromedially in the orbit to enter the optic canal. The ophthalmic artery gives off the central artery of the retina which sinks into the inferomedial aspect of the optic nerve. The nerve has a short course in the middle cranial fossa before uniting with the nerve of the opposite side at the optic chiasma. At the chiasma, nerve fibres from the temporal half of the retina lie laterally and those from the medial half lie in the middle. The middle fibres decussate. All the fibres that arise from the ganglion cells medial to a line passing through the fovea centralis cross from the optic nerve of that side to the optic tract of the opposite side. The left optic tract thus contains fibres from the temporal half of the left retina and nasal half of the right retina. As the temporal half of the retina perceives light from the nasal half of the visual field and the nasal half of the retina from the temporal half of the visual field, the left optic tract transmits data from the right half of the visual field (and the right tract from the left half of the visual field).

In the middle of the middle cranial fossa is the pituitary fossa or sella turcica (hypophyseal fossa)

containing the pituitary gland. It is roofed by a fold of dura mater, the diaphragma sellae, and this is pierced by the infundibulum. The diaphragma sellae is attached to the anterior and posterior clinoid processes which bound the fossa.

Lateral to the pituitary gland, the dura mater contains the cavernous sinus, one on either side. The oculomotor, trochlear, and the ophthalmic and maxillary divisions of the trigeminal, the abducent nerve and the internal carotid artery pass through the cavernous sinus. The S-shaped artery inside the sinus is known as the carotid syphon. Infection can reach the cavernous sinus from the face and the eye because of its venous connections.

The trigeminal nerve as it enters the middle cranial fossa takes a prolongation of the dura from the posterior cranial fossa with it known as the trigeminal cave or Meckel's cave. It contains the trigeminal ganglion from which three divisions of the nerve arise. The ophthalmic division goes through the supraorbital fissure, the maxillary through the foramen rotundum and the mandibular division through the foramen ovale.

There are grooves for the middle meningeal artery and vein on the inner aspect of the skull. These vessels

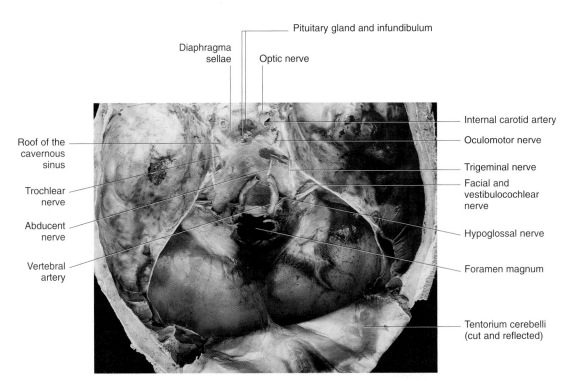

Fig. 7.10c *Middle and posterior cranial fossae and the cranial nerves.*

can rupture in head injury and produce an extradural haemorrhage. The middle meningeal artery enters the skull through the foramen spinosum.

The facial (VII) and vestibulocochlear (VIII) nerves enter the internal acoustic (auditory) meatus. The glossopharyngeal (IX), vagus (X) and accessory (XI) nerves enter the jugular foramen. The sigmoid sinus and the inferior petrosal sinus also leave the skull through this foramen. The two vertebral arteries come through the foramen magnum along with the spinal part of the accessory nerve. The hypoglossal nerve (XII) leaves the skull through the hypoglossal canal.

The meninges

The three layers of the meninges are the dura mater, the arachnoid mater and the pia mater. There are three meningeal spaces. The extradural (epidural) space is between the cranial bones and the endosteal layer of dura. This is a potential space which becomes a real space when there is an extradural haemorrhage from a torn meningeal vessel. The subdural space is also a potential space and may enlarge after head injury.

The subarachnoid space between the arachnoid and pia contains cerebrospinal fluid and the blood vessels of the brain.

The meningeal layer of dura continues into the vertebral canal as the dura mater covering the spinal cord. The two layers of dura mater are fused together except in areas where they form walls of the dural venous sinuses. The cranial cavity is divided into compartments by the three folds of dura mater. The falx cerebri lies between the two cerebral hemispheres, attached anteriorly to the crista galli and posteriorly to the tentorium cerebelli. The superior sagittal sinus lies along its superior border and the inferior sagittal sinus along its inferior free margin. The straight sinus is seen where the falx cerebri meets the tentorium cerebelli. The tentorium cerebelli is attached anteriorly to the posterior clinoid process of the sphenoid bone and its attachment runs posterolaterally along the superior border of the petrous temporal bone where the superior petrosal sinus is enclosed. Where the latter empties into the transverse sinus, the attached border turns

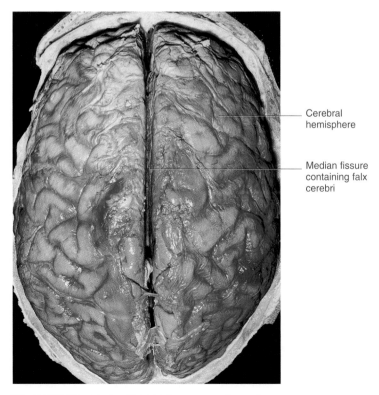

Cerebral hemisphere

Median fissure containing falx cerebri

Fig. 7.10d *The cerebral hemispheres seen from above.*

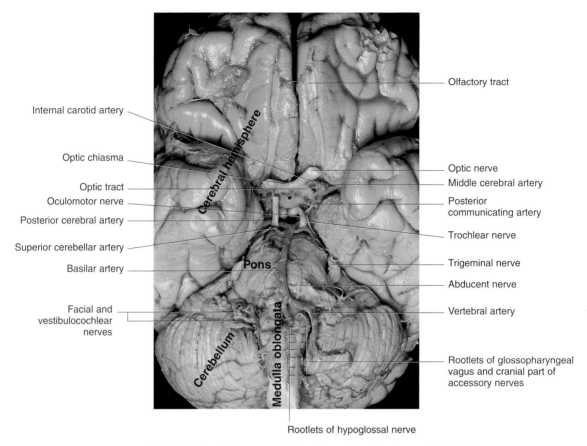

Olfactory tract

Internal carotid artery

Cerebral hemisphere

Optic chiasma

Optic nerve
Middle cerebral artery

Optic tract

Posterior communicating artery

Oculomotor nerve

Posterior cerebral artery

Trochlear nerve

Superior cerebellar artery

Basilar artery

Pons

Trigeminal nerve

Abducent nerve

Facial and vestibulocochlear nerves

Vertebral artery

Cerebellum

Medulla oblongata

Rootlets of glossopharyngeal vagus and cranial part of accessory nerves

Rootlets of hypoglossal nerve

Fig. 7.10e *Cranial nerves and blood vessels at the base of the brain.*

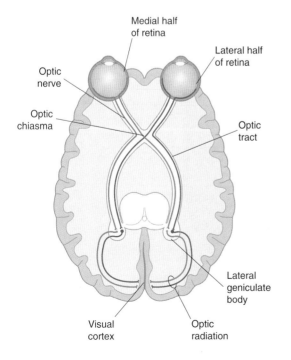

Medial half of retina

Lateral half of retina

Optic nerve

Optic chiasma

Optic tract

Lateral geniculate body

Visual cortex

Optic radiation

posteromedially along the lips of the transverse sinus to reach the internal occipital protuberance and continues round on the opposite side of the skull to the other posterior clinoid process. The free border of the tentorium cerebelli is attached to the anterior clinoid process and running posteriorly and then medially it curves round the midbrain forming the tentorial notch which surrounds the midbrain. Just behind the apex of the petrous temporal bone the inferior layer of the tentorium prolongs into the middle cranial fossa as the trigeminal cave. The falx cerebelli is a small fold of dura below the tentorium in the posterior cranial fossa. It lies between the two lateral lobes of the cerebellum.

Fig. 7.10f *The visual pathways.*

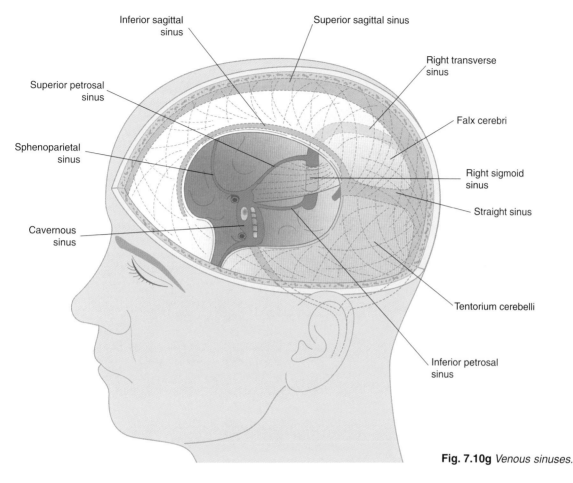

Inferior sagittal sinus

Superior sagittal sinus

Right transverse sinus

Superior petrosal sinus

Falx cerebri

Sphenoparietal sinus

Right sigmoid sinus

Straight sinus

Cavernous sinus

Tentorium cerebelli

Inferior petrosal sinus

Fig. 7.10g *Venous sinuses.*

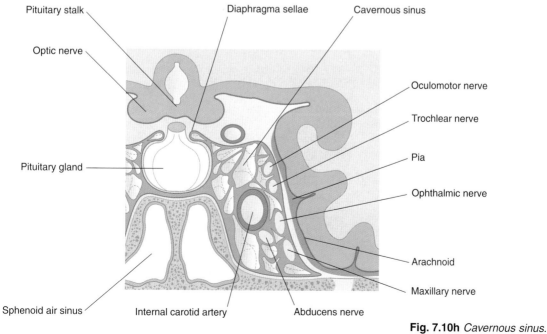

Pituitary stalk

Diaphragma sellae

Cavernous sinus

Optic nerve

Oculomotor nerve

Trochlear nerve

Pia

Pituitary gland

Ophthalmic nerve

Arachnoid

Maxillary nerve

Sphenoid air sinus

Internal carotid artery

Abducens nerve

Fig. 7.10h *Cavernous sinus.*

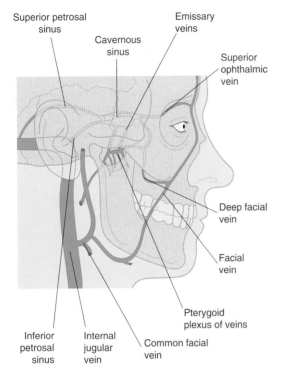

Superior petrosal sinus

Cavernous sinus

Emissary veins

Superior ophthalmic vein

Deep facial vein

Facial vein

Pterygoid plexus of veins

Inferior petrosal sinus

Internal jugular vein

Common facial vein

Fig. 7.10i *Connections of the cavernous sinus.*

The arterial supply to the brain

The brain is supplied by the two vertebral arteries and the two internal carotid arteries.

After entering the cranial cavity through the foramen magnum, the two vertebral arteries ascend on the surface of the medulla to the lower border of the pons where they unite to form the basilar artery. The posterior cerebral arteries are the terminal branches of the basilar artery. Each posterior cerebral winds round the midbrain to reach the medial surface of the cerebral hemisphere and supplies the occipital lobe, including the visual area, as well as the temporal lobe. Occlusion of the posterior cerebral artery causes blindness in the contralateral visual field.

The anterior cerebral artery, the smaller of the two terminal branches of the internal carotid artery, supplies the medial part of the inferior surface of the frontal lobe, and courses along the upper surface of the corpus callosum supplying the medial surface of the frontal and parietal lobes and the corpus callosum. It also supplies a narrow strip on the upper part of the lateral surface. The motor and sensory areas of the lower extremity are supplied by this artery, resulting in characteristic paralysis when the artery is occluded.

The middle cerebral artery is the larger of the

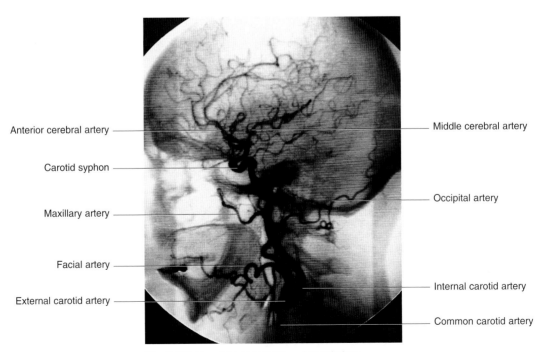

Anterior cerebral artery

Carotid syphon

Maxillary artery

Facial artery

External carotid artery

Middle cerebral artery

Occipital artery

Internal carotid artery

Common carotid artery

Fig. 7.10j *Carotid angiogram — lateral view.*

terminal branches of the internal carotid artery. It lies in the lateral sulcus and its branches supply the lateral surface of the frontal, parietal and temporal lobes, except the narrow strip in the upper part supplied by the anterior cerebral. Occlusion of the artery results in contralateral motor and sensory paralysis of the face and arm.

The two internal carotids and the two vertebral arteries form an anastomosis known as the circle of Willis on the inferior surface of the brain. Though the

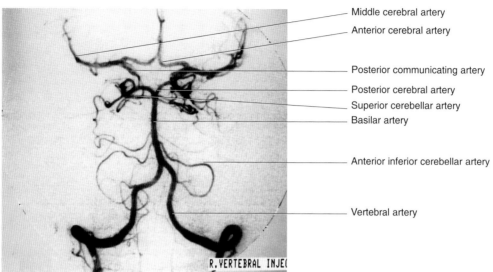

Middle cerebral artery
Anterior cerebral artery

Posterior communicating artery
Posterior cerebral artery
Superior cerebellar artery
Basilar artery

Anterior inferior cerebellar artery

Vertebral artery

R.VERTEBRAL INJE

Fig. 7.10k *Circle of Willis — arteriogram.*

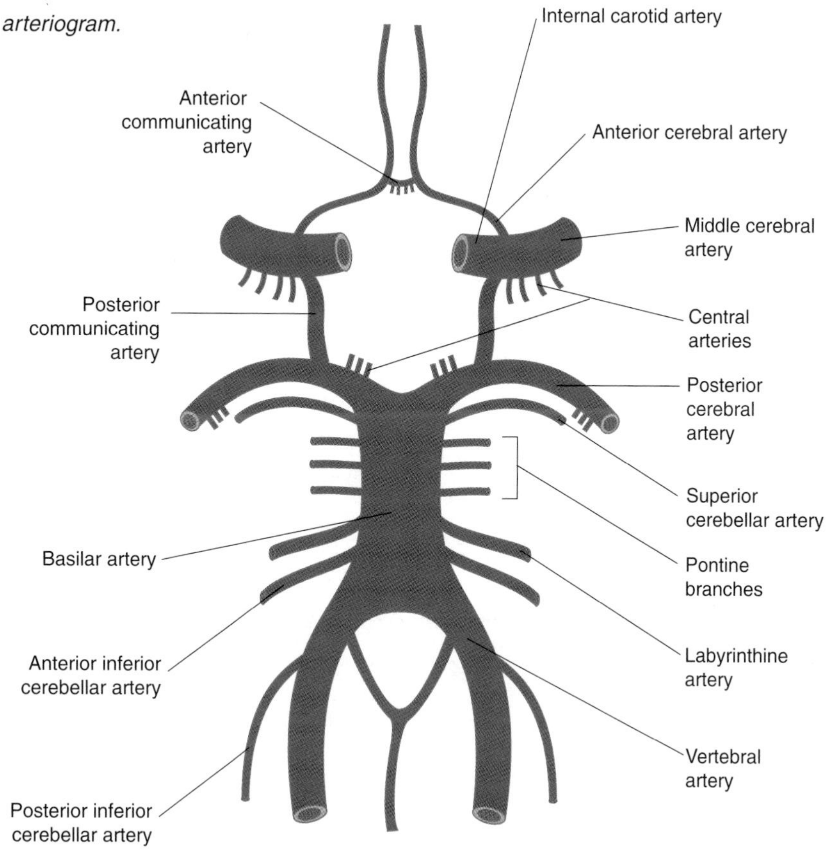

Internal carotid artery

Anterior communicating artery

Anterior cerebral artery

Middle cerebral artery

Posterior communicating artery

Central arteries

Posterior cerebral artery

Superior cerebellar artery

Basilar artery

Pontine branches

Labyrinthine artery

Anterior inferior cerebellar artery

Vertebral artery

Fig. 7.10l *Circle of Willis. The central arteries supply the corpus striatum, internal capsule, diencephalon and midbrain.*

Posterior inferior cerebellar artery

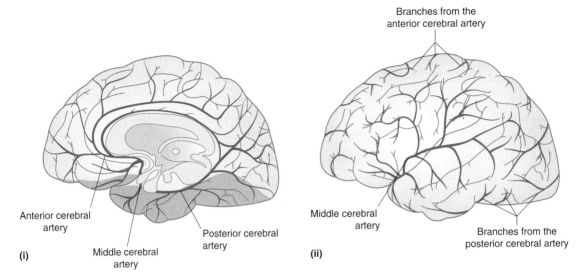

Fig. 7.10m *The cerebral arteries of the cerebral hemisphere:* **(i)** *medial view;* **(ii)** *lateral view.*

majority are thus interconnected, there is normally only minimal mixing of the blood passing through them. When one artery is blocked the arterial circle may provide collateral circulation.

The venous drainage of the brain

The veins of the brain, lying along with the arteries in the subarachnoid space, are thin-walled vessels without valves. They pierce the arachnoid and drain into the cranial dural venous sinuses which are situated within the dura mater. The dural venous sinuses are devoid of valves. They eventually drain into the internal jugular vein.

The superior sagittal sinus begins in front of the crista galli and courses backwards along the attached border of the falx cerebri and usually becomes continuous with the right transverse sinus near the internal occipital protuberance. At its commencement it may communicate with the nasal veins. A number of venous lacunae lie along its course and open into the sinus. The sinus and the lacunae are invaginated by arachnoid granulations. The superior cerebral veins drain into the superior sagittal sinus.

The inferior sagittal sinus lies along the inferior border of the falx cerebri and is much smaller than the superior sagittal sinus. It receives the cerebral veins from the medial surface of the hemisphere and joins the great cerebral vein to form the straight sinus.

The straight sinus, formed by the union of the

inferior sagittal sinus and the great cerebral vein, lies in the attachment of the falx cerebri to the tentorium cerebelli. It usually becomes continuous with the left transverse sinus near the internal occipital protuberance.

The transverse sinus lies in the groove on the inner surface of the occipital bone along the posterior attachment of the tentorium cerebelli. On reaching the petrous temporal bone, it curves downwards into the posterior cranial fossa to follow a curved course as the sigmoid sinus.

The sigmoid sinus passes through the jugular foramen and becomes continuous with the internal jugular vein.

The confluence of sinuses is formed by two transverse sinuses connected by small venous channels near the internal occipital protuberance.

The occipital sinus, a small venous sinus extending from the foramen magnum, drains into the confluence of sinuses. It lies along the falx cerebelli and connects the vertebral venous plexuses to the transverse sinus.

The cavernous sinus

The cavernous sinus, one on each side, situated on the body of the sphenoid bone, extends from the superior orbital fissure to the apex of the petrous temporal bone. Medially, the cavernous sinus is related to the pituitary gland and the sphenoid sinus. Laterally it is related to the temporal lobe of the brain. The internal carotid

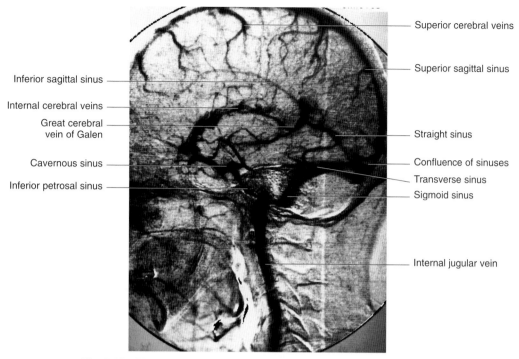

Inferior sagittal sinus

Internal cerebral veins

Great cerebral
vein of Galen

Cavernous sinus

Inferior petrosal sinus

Superior cerebral veins

Superior sagittal sinus

Straight sinus

Confluence of sinuses

Transverse sinus

Sigmoid sinus

Internal jugular vein

Fig. 7.10n *Venous phase of carotid angiogram — dural venous sinuses.*

artery and the abducens nerve pass through the cavernous sinus. On its lateral wall from above downwards lie the oculomotor, trochlear and ophthalmic nerves. The maxillary division of the trigeminal goes through the lower part of the lateral wall or just outside the sinus. The endothelial lining separates these structures from the cavity of the sinus.

Posteriorly, the sinus drains into the transverse/sigmoid sinus through superior petrosal sinus and via the inferior petrosal sinus, passing through the jugular foramen, into the internal jugular vein. The ophthalmic veins drain into the anterior part of the sinus. Emissary veins passing through the foramina in the middle cranial fossa connect the cavernous sinus to the pterygoid plexus of veins and to the facial veins. The superficial middle cerebral vein drains into the cavernous sinus from above. The two cavernous sinuses are connected to each other by anterior and posterior cavernous sinuses lying in front and behind the pituitary.

Intracranial haemorrhage

Bleeding into extradural space is classically from injury to middle meningeal artery from fracture of temporal bone. The haematoma between the dura and the skull bone compresses the brain. There is a lucid interval followed by rapid increase in intracranial tension. Transtentorial herniation of the brain may occur and may cause stem compression. In a subdural haemorrhage bleeding is usually from small bridging veins crossing the subdural space. The usual cause is trauma but it may happen in the elderly following a trivial head injury as the bridging veins are more vulnerable due to brain shrinkage. Causes of bleeding into subarachnoid space between arachnoid and pia include rupture of berry aneurysm, rupture of vascular malformation, hypertensive haemorrhage, coagulation disorders and head injury. Approximately 15% are instantly fatal and a further 45% die due to rebleed. In survivors, organisation of blood clot can obliterate subarachnoid space causing hydrocephalus.

INDEX